American Joint Committee on Cancer

MANUAL
for
STAGING
of
CANCER

This manual was prepared and published through the support of American Cancer Society Grant CCG #99BB and Grant Number CA 11606-17 awarded by the National Cancer Institute, National Institutes of Health.

Edited by

OLIVER H. BEAHRS, M.D.

Mayo Clinic and Mayo Foundation
Professor of Surgery, Emeritus
Mayo Medical School
Rochester, Minnesota

DONALD EARL HENSON, M.D.

U.S. Public Health Service
Division of Cancer Prevention and Control
National Cancer Institute
Bethesda, Maryland

ROBERT V. P. HUTTER, M.D.

Chairman, Department of Pathology
St. Barnabas Medical Center
Livingston, New Jersey

B. J. KENNEDY, M.D.

Regents' Professor of Medicine, Emeritus
Masonic Professor of Oncology, Emeritus
University of Minnesota
Minneapolis, Minnesota

MANUAL
for
STAGING
of
CANCER

Fourth Edition

American Joint Committee on Cancer
Executive Office
55 East Erie Street
Chicago, Illinois 60611

Sponsoring Organizations
American Cancer Society
National Cancer Institute
College of American Pathologists
American College of Physicians
American College of Radiology
American College of Surgeons

Fourth Printing

J. B. LIPPINCOTT COMPANY
Philadelphia

Production Supervisor: Robert D. Bartleson
Production: Tapsco, Inc.
Compositor: Tapsco, Inc.
Printer/Binder: The Murray Printing Company

FOURTH EDITION

First printing 1977
Revised and reprinted 1978
Reprinted 1980
Second edition 1983
Third edition 1988

Library of Congress Cataloging-in-Publication Data

Manual for staging of cancer / American Joint Committee on Cancer; sponsoring organization, American Cancer Society . . . [et al.]; edited by Oliver H. Beahrs . . . [et al.].—4th ed.
    p. cm.
  "Prepared and published through the support of American Cancer Society grant CCG 99BB and grant number CA 11606-17 awarded by the National Cancer Institute, National Institutes of Health."
  Includes bibliographical references.
  ISBN 0-397-51264-3 (soft cover)
  1. Tumors—Classification. 2. Cancer—Diagnosis. I. Beahrs, Oliver Howard, 1914– II. American Joint Committee on Cancer. III. American Cancer Society. IV. Title: Staging of cancer. [DNLM: 1. Neoplasm Staging. 2. Neoplasms—classification. QZ 241 M293]
RC258.M36 1992
616.99'4'0012—dc20
DNLM/DLC
for Library of Congress   92–6216
                                               CIP

The authors and publisher have exerted every effort to ensure that drug selections and dosages set forth in this text are in accordance with current recommendations and practice at the time of publication. However, in view of ongoing research, changes in government regulations, and the constant flow of information relating to drug therapy and drug reactions, the reader is urged to check the package insert for each drug for any change in indications and dosage and for added warnings and precautions. This is particularly important when the recommended agent is a new or infrequently used drug.

Fourth Edition
Dedicated to the memory of
Harvey Baker, M. D.

Doctor Baker was a quiet, unassuming, gentle man who, as Chairman of the American Joint Committee on Cancer (1982–1985), initiated the conferences with the TNM Committee of the International Union Against Cancer that has led to universal agreement on the anatomic staging of cancer. Harvey Baker graduated from the College of Physician and Surgeon School of Medicine, followed by a fellowship in Surgical Oncology at Memorial Hospital for Cancer and Allied Diseases. He practiced surgical oncology in Portland, Oregon. Among his many contributions to oncology, he served as Chairman of the Commission on Cancer of the American College of Surgeons.

Third Edition
Dedicated to the memory of
W. A. D. Anderson, M.D.
Marvin Pollard, M.D.
Paul Sherlock, M.D.

and all others who contributed greatly to the deliberations of the American Joint Committee and to the recommendations on Staging of Cancer.

Second Edition
Dedicated to the memory of
Murray M. Copeland, M.D.

The first chairman of the American Joint Committee on Cancer Staging and End-Results Reporting.

A native of McDonough, Georgia, Murray Copeland received his medical degree from Johns Hopkins University School of Medicine in 1927, followed by training in surgery and oncology at the Mayo Clinic, Memorial Hospital in New York City, and Union Memorial Hospital in Baltimore.

Among Dr. Copeland's numerous distinctions were his leadership positions as national president of the American Cancer Society in 1965 and secretary general of the 1970 UICC Cancer Congress.

He was known and loved by physicians around the world for his willingness and ability to support organizations designed to facilitate the spread of knowledge about cancer.

Murray Copeland was internationally acclaimed for his superior knowledge of and efforts against large bowel cancer and bone cancer.

Preface

The editors of this, the fourth edition of the Manual for Staging of Cancer of the American Joint Committee on Cancer, wish to recognize the contributions of 500 participants who have volunteered their time over 32 years in the evolution of the recommendations for staging cancer. Retrospective studies were carried out at some anatomic sites. In addition, reviewing available literature and information from personal experience of participants as well as reviewing staging recommendations previously brought forward by others were considered. These deliberations led to the recommendations published in the first comprehensive Manual in 1977.

Subsequently, the Committee has continued to review its definitions and fine-tune the recommendations and stage groupings for all anatomic sites with the hope that staging of cancer will be most helpful in arriving at decisions regarding appropriate treatment of malignant tumors and in determining prognosis and end results.

Unfortunately, recommendations regarding staging of cancer by individual researchers, specialties, committees, and other groups have not been uniform. This has been true in some instances in the published reports of the TNM Committee of the International Union Against Cancer (UICC) and the American Joint Committee on Cancer (AJCC). Under the leadership of Dr. Harvey Baker as Chairman of the AJCC, discussions were first undertaken with the TNM Committee to reach uniform recommendations by the two groups so that one system of staging might be used worldwide. These efforts have been actively pursued under the subsequent chairmanships of Drs. Robert Hutter and Donald Henson, with the cooperation of Dr. Leslie Sobin, Chairman of the TNM Committee, and with the aid of Professor Paul Hermanek and his associates.

Through multiple meetings with worldwide input, agreements have been reached on all definitions of T, N, and M and on stage groupings for cancers at all anatomic sites. The recommendations of the AJCC in the third edition revised Manual and the publications of the UICC, published in 1987, are identical. Thus, an international system of staging cancer is now available. Using this system will enable appropriate decisions regarding treatment and, more importantly, evaluation of end results and comparability of data.

Although recommendations for staging at most anatomic sites remain as those published in the third edition, those for the gynecologic sites have been modified to be consistent with the recommendations of the International Federation of Gynecology and Obstetrics (FIGO). Likewise, the prostate staging recommendations have been changed to be consistent with recommendations of urologists. The ICD-O codes have been revised in accordance with the recently published second edition. These changes are in agreement with the TNM Committee of the UICC, including new chapters on staging of cancer of the small intestine and mesothelioma. Also in the fourth edition, typographical errors have been corrected and some text changes made to clarify instructions and explanations.

Credit is due all members of the American Joint Committee and its Task Forces on cancer for individual anatomic sites. Special credit in preparation of the fourth edition is given to those in leadership positions and to staff support persons—in particular, Kathleen Zuber, Lisa Richards, and LeAnn Krueger. We are also grateful for the assistance provided by members of the Surveillance, Epidemiology, and End Results Program of the National Cancer Institute and the National Tumor Registrars Association. Personnel of J.B. Lippincott Company, including J. Stuart Freeman and others, have been most cooperative and helpful. The interest and help of the publisher is greatly appreciated.

Oliver H. Beahrs, M.D.
Donald Earl Henson, M.D.
Robert V.P. Hutter, M.D.
B. J. Kennedy, M.D.

Introduction

This manual brings together all currently available information on staging of cancer at various anatomic sites as developed by the American Joint Committee on Cancer (AJCC) in cooperation with the TNM Committee of the International Union Against Cancer (UICC). All of the schemes included here are uniform between the two organizations. The manual permits consistency in describing the extent of the neoplastic diseases in different anatomic parts, systems, or organs.

Proper classification and staging of cancer will allow the physician to determine treatment more appropriately, to evaluate results of management more reliably, and to compare worldwide statistics reported from various institutions on a local, regional, and national basis more confidently.

Staging of cancer is not a fixed science. As new information about etiology and various diagnostic and treatment methods becomes available, the classification and staging of cancer will change. Periodically, at reasonable intervals, this manual will be revised to reflect this changing knowledge and new technology. Currently, the anatomic extent of the disease provides the primary basis for staging; the histopathologic grade and age of the patient are also factors in some tumors. In the future, biologic, molecular, genetic, and other prognostic indicators may play a part.

It is hoped that the staging recommendations included in this manual will be used as published—or at least modified only minimally—so that consistency in data gathering will be possible. These recommendations are to be used in the cancer programs approved by the multidisciplinary Approvals Committee of the Commission on Cancer of the American College of Surgeons and is being considered as a requirement by the Joint Commission on Accreditation of Health Care Organizations in recordkeeping. Also, future reports by the Surveillance, Epidemiology, and End-Results Program (SEER) of the National Cancer Institute (NCI) will be based on the classifications recommended by the AJCC.

The AJCC was first organized on January 9, 1959, as the American Joint Committee for Cancer Staging and End-Results Reporting (AJC), for the purpose of developing a system of clinical staging for cancer acceptable to the American medical profession. The sponsoring organizations are the American College of Surgeons, the American College of Radiology, the College of American Pathologists, the American College of Physicians, the American Cancer Society, and the National Cancer Institute. Each sponsoring organization designates three representatives to the Committee. The American College of Surgeons serves as administrative sponsor. Subcommittees, called "task forces," have been established to consider malignant neoplasms of selected anatomic sites in order to develop or to review current classifications. Each task force comprises committee members and other professional appointees whose special interests and skills are appropriate to the site under consideration.

During its 33 years of activity, various special consultants have worked with the Committee, as have liaison representatives from the American Academy of Pediatrics, the American College of Obstetricians and Gynecologists, the American Urological Association, the Association of American Cancer Institutes, and the SEER program of the NCI. More than 400 individuals have contributed to the work of the various task forces. Dr. Murray Copeland served as chairman from the Committee's inception until 1969. Subsequent chairmen included Dr. W. A. D. Anderson from 1969 to 1974, Dr. Oliver H. Beahrs from 1974 to 1979, Dr. David T. Carr from 1979 to 1982, Dr. Harvey W. Baker from 1982 to 1985, and Dr. Robert V. P. Hutter from 1985 to 1990. The current chairman is Dr. Donald Earl Henson.

Pioneer work on the clinical classification of cancer was done by the League of Nations Health Organization (1929), the International Commission on Stage Grouping and Presentation of Results (ICPR) of the International Congress of Radiology (1953), and the International Union Against Cancer (Union Internationale Contre le Cancer, UICC). The latter organization became most active in the field through its Committee on Clinical Stage Classification and Applied Statistics (1954), later known as the TNM Committee.

The AJC decided to use the TNM system, when applicable, to describe the anatomic extent of the cancer at the time of diagnosis (before the application of definitive treatment), and from this to develop classification into stages to serve as a guide for treatment and prognosis and for comparing the end results of treatment. Subsequently, the system has been extended to other periods during the natural history and treatment of a cancer. Task forces to accomplish this extension were established to focus on particular sites of cancer. Retrospective studies have led to recommendations for stage classifications for cancer at various sites or systems, which have been published and distributed in separate fascicles and articles.

The AJC sponsored a National Cancer Conference on Classification and Staging in Atlanta on March 27–28, 1976. This conference delineated the accomplishments to that time and brought into focus future needs and activities.

In January 1970, a revised statement of the "Objectives, Rules and Regulations of the American Joint Committee" was adopted. This statement broadened the scope of the Committee by including in its objectives the formulation and publication of classification systems for cancer including but not limited to staging and end-results reporting.

It was recognized that for cancer of certain sites, the information made available by observation at the time of a surgical procedure, as well as information from the pathologic examination of the surgically removed cancer, could form the basis for useful classifications. From this evolved a "surgical evaluative staging" and a "postsurgical treatment-pathologic staging." Surgical evaluative staging subsequently has been dropped. Information obtained during surgical exploration may be used for clinical staging.

Further consideration of the chronology of staging has led to recognition of two main time periods. First is the clinical stage, which uses all data available to the time of first definitive treatment. Second is the pathologic stage, which can be established if a completely resected specimen of the lesion is available.

It is also evident that for certain organs (e.g., thyroid), the biologic potential of different histologic types of cancer is such that different types cannot be mixed together in a meaningful classification. Therefore, cases should be analyzed separately by histologic type. In some cancers, such as soft-tissue sarcomas, histologic grading is of such significance that it becomes a necessary component of the classification system. For certain cancers, widely used and accepted classifications, such as the Ann Arbor classification of Hodgkin's disease and the FIGO classification for carcinoma of the cervix, are considered in the recommendations. Whenever possible, established and accepted classifications are considered.

The various data published previously in individual-site fascicles, with revisions and the addition of other material, were brought together to form a Manual for Staging of Cancer, the first edition of which was published in 1977. A second printing, slightly revised, appeared in 1978. The 1983 edition of the Manual updated the earlier publications and included additional sites. It also brought the recommendations more closely in conformity with those of the TNM Committee.

The need for a staging form for use in the staging system of each site has been recognized for some years. Such a form can ensure the uniform recording of data necessary for stage classification. Recent emphasis has been given to the development of a data form for each cancer site for which there is a stage classification and to the availability of such data forms as a part of each staging recommendation.

The expanding role of the Committee in a variety of cancer classifications, including its significance and value and the promotion of indicated usage in cancer diagnosis and therapy, suggested that the original name of the Committee no longer portrayed the broader scope of its interests and activities. Thus, in 1980 the name was changed to the American Joint Committee on Cancer (AJCC). The publication of this new edition of the Manual reflects the widening interests and activities of the Committee.

The TNM Committee of the UICC and the AJCC have been working along similar lines and with similar objectives. In the past, points of view and methods have occasionally differed. Cooperation between the two groups during 1982–1991 has resulted in uniform and identical definitions and stage grouping of cancers for all anatomic sites, so that a universal system is now available.

Members of the AJCC, its task forces, and its committees, as well as the sponsoring organizations, owe a debt of gratitude to the many physicians and others who have voluntarily contributed to this effort in the hope that patients with cancer would survive and enjoy an enhanced quality of life. The contributions of the TNM Committee of the UICC and other international organizations are gratefully acknowledged.

Contents

PART I

General Information on Cancer Staging and End-Results Reporting

1 Purposes and Principles of Staging   3

    Philosophy of Classification and Staging by the
      TNM System   3
    Nomenclature in Cancer Morphology   4
    General Rules for Staging of Cancer   6
    General Rules of the TNM System   6
    Cancer Staging Data Form   9

2 Reporting of Cancer Survival and End Results   11

PART II

Staging of Cancer at Specific Anatomic Sites

HEAD AND NECK   27

3 Lip and Oral Cavity   27
4 Pharynx *(Including Base of Tongue, Soft Palate, and Uvula)*   33
5 Larynx   39
6 Maxillary Sinus   45

7   Salivary Glands *(Including Parotid,*
      Submandibular, and Sublingual)   49
8   Thyroid Gland   53

      DIGESTIVE SYSTEM   **57**

9   Esophagus   57
10 Stomach   63
11 Small Intestine   69
12 Colon and Rectum   75
13 Anal Canal   83
14 Liver *(Including Intrahepatic Bile Ducts)* 89
15 Gallbladder   93
16 Extrahepatic Bile Ducts   99
17 Ampulla of Vater   105
18 Exocrine Pancreas   109

      THORAX   **115**

19 Lung   115
20 Pleural Mesothelioma   123

      MUSCULOSKELETAL   **127**

21 Bone   127
22 Soft Tissues   131

      SKIN   **137**

23 Carcinoma of Skin *(Excluding Eyelid, Vulva,*
      and Penis)   137
24 Malignant Melanoma of the Skin
      (Excluding Eyelid)   143

      BREAST   **149**

25 Breast   149

      GYNECOLOGIC TUMORS   **155**

26 Cervix Uteri   155
27 Corpus Uteri   161
28 Ovary   167
29 Vagina   173
30 Vulva   177

GENITOURINARY CANCERS 181

31 Prostate 181
32 Testis 187
33 Penis 191
34 Urinary Bladder 195
35 Kidney 201
36 Renal Pelvis and Ureter 205
37 Urethra 209

OPHTHALMIC CANCERS 213

38 Carcinoma of the Eyelid 213
39 Malignant Melanoma of the Eyelid 217
40 Carcinoma of the Conjunctiva 221
41 Malignant Melanoma of the
Conjunctiva 225
42 Malignant Melanoma of the Uvea 229
43 Retinoblastoma 235
44 Sarcoma of the Orbit 239
45 Carcinoma of the Lacrimal Gland 243

CENTRAL NERVOUS SYSTEMS 247

46 Brain 247

LYMPHOMAS 253

47 Hodgkin's Disease 253
48 Non-Hodgkin's Lymphoma 257

PEDIATRIC CANCERS 263

49 Nephroblastoma *(Wilms' Tumor)* 263
50 Neuroblastoma 269
51 Soft-Tissue Sarcoma—Pediatric 275

PART III

**Personnel of the American
Joint Committee on Cancer**

PART I

General Information on Cancer Staging and End-Results Reporting

1

Purposes and Principles of Staging

Philosophy of Classification and Staging by the TNM System

A classification scheme for cancer must encompass all attributes of the tumor that define its life history. The American Joint Committee on Cancer (AJCC) classification is based on the premise that cancers of similar histology or site of origin share similar patterns of growth and extension.

The size of the untreated primary cancer or tumor (T) increases progressively, and at some point in time regional lymph node involvement (N) and, finally, distant metastases (M) occur. A simple classification scheme, which can be incorporated into a form for staging and universally applied, is the goal of the TNM system as proposed by the AJCC. This classification is identical with that of the Union Internationale Contre le Cancer (UICC) and is a distillate of several existing systems.

For most cancer sites, the staging recommendations in this manual are concerned only with anatomic extent of disease, but in several instances grade (e.g., soft-tissue sarcoma) and age (e.g., thyroid cancer) are factors that must be considered. In the future, biologic markers and other parameters may have to be added to those of anatomic extent in classifying cancer, but they are not necessarily components of stage.

As the primary tumor increases in size throughout its time span, at some point (probably early) local invasion occurs, followed by spread to the regional lymph nodes draining the area of the tumor. The period when this spread is manifest or discernible by available methods of clinical examination is thus another significant marker in the progression of the cancer (N). It is usually later, often in the middle or older period of the cancer life span, that distant spread or metastasis (M) becomes evident from clinical examination. Thus, metastasis (M) is the third and usually the latest time marker.

These three significant events in the life history of a cancer—tumor growth (T), spread to primary lymph nodes (N), and metastasis (M)—are used as they appear (or do not appear) on clinical examination, before definitive therapy begins, to indicate the extension of the cancer. This shorthand method of indicating the extension of disease at a particular designated time is the stage of the cancer in its progression. It may be used, however, sometimes with other features added, in a scheme of stage classification. When retrospective or prospective studies of cases show that certain groupings of TNM or other features can be identified that have valid significance for staging, a stage classification may be devised.

Events such as local spread (including spread to primary regional lymph nodes) and distant metastasis sometimes occur before they are discernible by clinical examination. Thus, examination at the time of a surgical procedure and histologic examination of the surgically removed tissues may identify the significant markers of the life history of the cancer (T, N, and M) as being different from what could be discerned clinically before therapy. Although this may be the basis of a stage classification (pathological, based on examination of a surgically resected specimen), it should be identified separately from clinical classification. Nevertheless, it may be a more accurate depiction of the period in the life history of the cancer and may be valuable for prognostic purposes.

Therapeutic procedures, even if not curative, may alter the course and life history of cancer. Although cancers that recur after therapy may be staged with the same markers as are used in pretreatment clinical staging, the significance of cancer markers may not be the same. Hence the stage classification of recurrent cancer must be considered separately for therapeutic guidance, prognosis, and end-results reporting.

The significance of the marker points in their life history differs for tumors of different sites and of different histologic types. Therefore, the marker points,

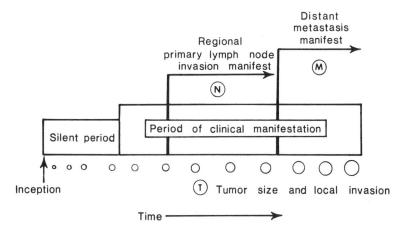

even if T, N, and M, must be defined for each type of tumor in order to be valid and to have maximum significance. In certain types of tumors, such as Hodgkin's disease and lymphomas, a different system for designating the extent of the disease and for classifying its stage is necessary to accomplish the goal of usefulness. In these cases other symbols or descriptive markers are used rather than T, N, and M.

Classification and stage-grouping is thus a method of designating the extent of a cancer and is related to the natural course of the particular type of cancer. It is intended to provide a way by which this information can be readily communicated to others, to assist in decisions regarding treatment, and to be a factor in determining prognosis. Ultimately, it provides a mechanism for comparing groups of cases, particularly in regard to the results of different therapeutic procedures.

In addition to anatomic extent, the histologic analysis and grade of the tumor may be important determinants in classification. The type of tumor and the grade are also most important variables affecting choices of treatment. For sarcomas the tumor grade may prove to be the most important index.

Nomenclature in Cancer Morphology

Cancer therapy decisions are made after an assessment of the patient and tumor, using many methods that often include sophisticated technical procedures. For most types of cancer, the extent to which the disease has spread is probably the most important factor determining prognosis and must be given prime consideration in evaluating and comparing different therapeutic regimens.

Staging classifications are based on description of the extent of disease, and their design requires a thorough knowledge of the natural history of each type of cancer. Such knowledge has been and continues to be derived primarily from morphologic studies, which also provide us with the definitions and classifications of tumor types.

An accurate histologic diagnosis, therefore, is an essential element in a meaningful evaluation of the tumor. In certain types of cancer, biochemical, molecular, genetic or immunologic measurements of normal or abnormal cellular function have become important elements in typing tumors precisely. Increasingly, definitions and classifications should include function as a component of the pathologist's anatomic diagnosis. One may also anticipate that special techniques in histochemistry, cytogenetics, and tissue culture will be used more routinely for typing and characterizing tumor behavior.

The most complete and best known compendium of tumor definitions and illustrations in English is the Atlas of Tumor Pathology, published in many volumes by the Armed Forces Institute of Pathology in Washington, D.C. These are under constant revision and are used as a basic reference by pathologists throughout the world.

RELATED CLASSIFICATIONS

Since 1958, the World Health Organization (WHO) has been involved in a program aimed at providing internationally acceptable criteria for the histologic diagnosis of tumors. This has resulted in the International Histological Classification of Tumours, which contains, in an illustrated 25-volume series, definitions of tumor types and a proposed nomenclature. This is now in a second edition.

The WHO International Classification of Diseases for Oncology (ICD-O), second edition, provides a coding system for neoplasms by topography and morphology and for indicating behavior (e.g., malignant, benign, in situ). This coded nomenclature is identical to the morphology field for neoplasms in the Systematized Nomenclature of Medicine (SNOMED) published by the College of American Pathologists.

In the interest of promoting national and international collaboration in cancer research and specifically to facilitate cooperation in clinical investigations, it is recommended to use the International Histological Classification of Tumours for classification and definition of tumor types and the ICD-O codes for storage and retrieval of data.

BIBLIOGRAPHY

1. Atlas of Tumor Pathology. Washington DC, Armed Forces Institute of Pathology, various dates
2. World Health Organization: WHO International Classification of Diseases for Oncology, 2nd ed. Geneva, WHO, 1990
3. World Health Organization: WHO International Histological Classification of Tumors, Vol 1-25. Geneva, WHO, 1967 to 1981; 2nd edition, Berlin-New York, Springer-Verlag, 1988 to 1992

General Rules for Staging of Cancer

The practice of dividing cancer cases into groups according to "stages" arose from the fact that survival rates were higher for cases in which the disease was localized than for those in which the disease had extended beyond the organ or site of origin. These groups were often referred to as "early cases" and "late cases," implying some regular progression with time. Actually, the stage of disease at the time of diagnosis may be a reflection not only of the rate of growth and extension of the neoplasm but also of the type of tumor and of the tumor-host relationship.

The staging of cancer is hallowed by tradition, and, for the purpose of analysis of groups of patients, it is often necessary to use such a method. It is preferable to reach agreement on the recording of accurate information on the extent of the disease for each site, because the precise clinical description and histopathological classification (when possible) of malignant neoplasms may serve a number of related objectives, namely:

1. To aid the clinician in planning treatment
2. To give some indication of prognosis
3. To assist in evaluating the results of treatment
4. To facilitate the exchange of information between treatment centers
5. To contribute to the continuing investigation of human cancers.

The principal purpose to be served by international agreement on the classification of cancer cases by extent of disease, however, is to provide a method of conveying clinical experience to others without ambiguity.

There are many bases or axes of classification; for example, the anatomic site and the clinical and pathologic extent of disease, the reported duration of symptoms or signs, the sex and age of the patient, and the histologic type and grade. All of these represent variables that are known to have an influence on the outcome of the disease. Classification by anatomic extent of disease, as determined clinically and histopathologically (when possible), is the classification to which the attention of the AJCC and the UICC is primarily directed.

The clinician's immediate task is to make a decision as to the most effective course of treatment and to make a judgment as to prognosis. This decision and this judgment require, among other things, an objective assessment of the anatomic extent of the disease. In accomplishing this, the trend is away from staging and toward meaningful description, with or without some form of summarization.

To meet the stated objectives, we need a system of classification:

1. With basic principles applicable to all sites regardless of treatment; and
2. Which may be supplemented later by information that becomes available from histopathology or surgery.

The TNM system meets these requirements.

General Rules of the TNM System

The TNM system for describing the anatomic extent of disease is based on the assessment of three components:

T   The extent of the primary tumor
N   The absence or presence and extent of regional lymph node metastasis
M   The absence or presence of distant metastasis.

The addition of numbers to these three components indicates the extent of the malignant disease, thus showing progressive increase in tumor size or involvement:

T0, T1, T2, T3, T4   N0, N1, N2, N3   M0, M1

In effect, the system is a shorthand notation for describing the clinical extent of a particular malignant tumor.

The general rules applicable to all sites are as follows:

1. All cases should be confirmed microscopically. Any cases not confirmed must be reported separately.
2. Four classifications are described for each site, namely:
   Clinical Classification, designated cTNM or TNM. Clinical classification is based on evidence acquired before treatment. Such evidence arises from physical examination, imaging, endoscopy, biopsy, surgical exploration, and other relevant findings. In other words, all information available prior to first definitive treatment is used.
   Pathologic Classification, designated pTNM. Pathologic classification is based on the evidence acquired before treatment, supplemented or modified by the additional evidence acquired from surgery and from pathologic examination. The pathologic assessment of the primary tumor (pT) entails a resection of the primary tumor or biopsy adequate to evaluate the highest pT category. The pathologic assessment of the regional lymph nodes (pN) entails removal of nodes adequate to validate the absence (pN0) of regional lymph node metastasis and sufficient to evaluate the highest pN category. Metastatic nodules in

the fat adjacent to colorectal, gastric, or mammary carcinomas, without evidence of residual lymph node tissue, are considered regional lymph node metastases. The pathologic assessment of distant metastasis (pM) implies microscopic examination of distant lesions.

Retreatment Classification. Retreatment classification is used after a disease-free interval and when further definitive treatment is planned. All information available at the time of retreatment should be used in determining the stage of the recurrent tumor (rTNM). Biopsy confirmation of the cancer is required.

Autopsy Classification. If classification of a cancer is done after the death of a patient and a postmortem examination has been done, all pathologic information should be used. The chronologic stage should be indicated as aTNM.

3. After assigning T, N, and M and/or pT, pN, and pM categories, these may be grouped into stages. The TNM classification and stage grouping, once established, must remain unchanged in the medical records. The clinical stage is essential to select and evaluate therapy, and the pathologic stage provides the most precise data to estimate prognosis and calculate end results.

4. If there is doubt concerning the correct T, N, or M category to which a particular case should be allotted, then the lower (less advanced) category is chosen. This will also be reflected in the stage-grouping.

5. In the case of multiple, simultaneous tumors in one organ, the tumor with the highest T category should be identified and the multiplicity, or the number of tumors, indicated in parentheses; for example, T2(m) or T2(5). In simultaneous bilateral cancers of paired organs, each tumor is classified independently. In tumors of the thyroid, liver, and ovary, as well as in nephroblastomas and neuroblastomas, multiplicity is a criterion of T classification.

6. Definitions of TNM categories and stage grouping may be telescoped or expanded for clinical or research purposes as long as basic definitions as recommended are not changed. For instance, any T, N, or M can be divided into subgroups.

THE ANATOMIC REGIONS AND SITES

The sites in this classification are listed by code number of the WHO International Classification of Diseases for Oncology, second edition. Each chapter devoted to a specific form of cancer is constructed according to the following outline:

Introduction
Anatomy

Primary site
Regional lymph nodes
Metastatic sites

Rules for Classification
   Clinical (TNM or cTNM)
   Pathologic (pTNM)

Definition of TNM
   T   Primary tumor size/extent
   N   Regional lymph node involvement
   M   Distant metastasis absent/present

Stage Grouping
Histopathologic Type
Histopathologic Grade

TNM CLINICAL CLASSIFICATION

The following general definitions are used throughout:

Primary Tumor (T)

TX	Primary tumor cannot be assessed
T0	No evidence of primary tumor
Tis	Carcinoma *in situ*
T1, T2, T3, T4	Increasing size and/or local extent of the primary tumor

Regional Lymph Nodes (N)

NX	Regional lymph nodes cannot be assessed
N0	No regional lymph node metastasis
N1, N2, N3	Increasing involvement of regional lymph nodes

Note: Direct extension of the primary tumor into lymph nodes is classified as lymph node metastasis.

Note: Metastasis in any lymph node other than regional is classified as a distant metastasis.

A *grossly* recognizable metastatic nodule in the connective tissue of a lymph drainage area without histologic evidence of residual lymph node is classified in the N category as a regional lymph node metastasis. A *microscopic* deposit, up to 2 or 3 millimeters, is classified in the T category, that is, as discontinuous extension.

Distant Metastasis (M)

MX	Presence of distant metastasis cannot be assessed
M0	No distant metastasis
M1	Distant metastasis

Note: For pathologic stage grouping, M1 may be either clinical (cM1) or pathologic (pM1).

The category M1 may be further specified according to the following notation:

Pulmonary	PUL
Osseous	OSS
Hepatic	HEP
Brain	BRA
Lymph Nodes	LYM
Bone Marrow	MAR
Pleura	PLE
Peritoneum	PER
Adrenals	ADR
Skin	SKI
Other	OTH

Subdivisions of TNM. Subdivisions of some main categories are available for those who need greater specificity (e.g., T1a, 1b or N2a, 2b).

HISTOPATHOLOGIC TYPE

The histopathologic type is a qualitative assessment whereby a tumor is categorized (typed) according to the normal tissue type or cell type it most closely resembles (e.g., lobular carcinoma, osteosarcoma, or squamous cell carcinoma).

HISTOPATHOLOGIC GRADE (G)

The histopathologic grade is a quantitative assessment of the extent to which a tumor resembles the normal tissue at that site, expressed in numerical grades of differentiation (e.g., squamous cell carcinoma, Grade 2, moderately differentiated).

GX Grade cannot be assessed
G1 Well differentiated
G2 Moderately differentiated
G3 Poorly differentiated
G4 Undifferentiated

If there are variations in the differentiation of the tumor, the least favorable variation should be recorded as the grade, using only G1 through G3. For example, a partially well differentiated, partially moderately differentiated adenocarcinoma of the colon is graded as G2. The growing edge of a tumor generally is not assessed in grading, as it may appear to be a high grade.

For some sites, grades 3 and 4 are combined into a single grade, G3-4. This combination is valid for carcinomas of the uterine corpus, ovary, prostate, urinary bladder, kidney, renal pelvis, ureter, and urethra. Only three grades are used for melanomas of the conjunctiva and uvea. Grading does not apply to carcinomas of the thyroid, melanoma of the skin and eyelids, retinoblastoma, malignant testicular tumor, nephroblastoma, and neuroblastoma.

Histologic grade G4 applies to undifferentiated carcinomas of the esophagus, stomach, pancreas, and colorectum. According to the definition of grading, an adenocarcinoma arising in these organs (or in any other site) can be classified only as G1, G2, or G3, because an adenocarcinoma by definition has glandular differentiation. Tumors containing areas of undifferentiation adjacent to areas of glandular differentiation are classified as poorly differentiated adenocarcinomas. The same rules apply to squamous cell carcinomas.

The use of G4 is reserved for those tumors that show no specific differentiation. In some sites, the WHO histologic classification includes undifferentiated carcinomas; for example, in the stomach or gallbladder. In these cases, the tumor is graded as G4.

Some histologic tumor types are by definition listed as G4. These include:

Undifferentiated carcinomas, any site
Small cell carcinomas, any site
Large cell carcinomas of the lung
Ewing's sarcomas of bone and soft tissue
Rhabdomyosarcomas of soft tissue.

ADDITIONAL DESCRIPTORS

For identification of special cases of TNM or pTNM classifications, the m, y, r, and a symbols are used. Although they do not affect the stage grouping, they indicate cases needing separate analysis.

m Symbol. The suffix m, in parenthesis, is used to indicate the presence of multiple primary tumors in a single site.

y Symbol. In those cases in which classification is performed during or following initial multimodality therapy, the TNM or pTNM categories are identified by a y prefix.

r Symbol. Recurrent tumors, when staged after a disease-free interval, are identified by the prefix r.

a Symbol. This descriptor designates that classification was first determined at autopsy.

OPTIONAL DESCRIPTORS

Lymphatic Invasion (L)

LX Lymphatic invasion cannot be assessed
L0 No lymphatic invasion
L1 Lymphatic invasion

Venous Invasion (V)

VX Venous invasion cannot be assessed
V0 No venous invasion
V1 Microscopic venous invasion
V2 Macroscopic venous invasion

Residual Tumor (R) Classification

The absence or presence of residual tumor after treatment is described by the symbol R.

COLORECTAL CARCINOMA
Observed survival (Kaplan–Meier), surgical mortality not excluded,
1978–1988

TNM and pTNM describe the anatomic extent of cancer in general without consideration of treatment. The TNM and pTNM can be supplemented by the R classification, which deals with tumor status after treatment. It reflects the effects of therapy, influences further therapeutic procedures and is a strong predictor of prognosis.

The definition of the R category is:

RX Presence of residual tumor cannot be assessed
R0 No residual tumor
R1 Microscopic residual tumor
R2 Macroscopic residual tumor

The graph above shows the different categories of R.

STAGE GROUPING

Classification by the TNM system achieves a reasonably precise description and recording of the apparent anatomic extent of disease. A tumor with four degrees of T, three degrees of N, and two degrees of M will have 24 TNM categories. For purposes of tabulation and analysis, except in very large series, it is necessary to condense these categories into a convenient number of TNM stage-groupings.

Carcinoma *in situ* is categorized Stage 0; cases with distant metastasis are categorized Stage IV. The grouping adopted is such as to ensure, as far as possible, that each group is more or less homogeneous in respect to survival, and that the survival rates of these groups for each cancer site are distinctive.

Cancer Staging Data Form

Each site staging form is to be used for recording the classification of the tumor and the stage of the cancer. The

anatomic site of the cancer should be indicated, as well as the histologic type and grade. The appropriate period of the chronology of classification must be recorded. If a cancer is staged during several time periods in the chronology, separate forms must be used for each time period; if a single form is used, it must clearly identify the stage for each period.

The T, N, and M classification can be checked opposite the appropriate definitions of the extent of the primary tumor, the regional nodes, and distant metastasis. The lesion(s) can be marked on a diagram and, finally, the stage can be checked according to the grouping of TNM. In some instances, information regarding other characteristics of the tumor (not leading to stage) might be requested. These data may be pertinent in deciding management of the cancer. On the reverse side of the staging form is information and definitions that are important in proper classification of a cancer.

The cancer staging form is not a replacement for history, treatment, or follow-up records, but should become part of the patient file. The cancer staging form may be duplicated for individual or local institutional use.

In addition, staging forms using AJCC recommendations are available from other sources. The forms for some sites have been separately published by the American Cancer Society, the American Joint Committee on Cancer, the College of American Pathologists, the International Federation of Gynecology and Obstetrics (FIGO), UICC, and the Commission on Cancer of the American College of Surgeons.

The data form presented in this manual may be duplicated for individual or institutional use without permission from the AJCC or the publisher.

2
Reporting of Cancer Survival and End Results

To evaluate the efficacy of treatment and to provide a sound base for therapeutic planning for cancer patients, it is necessary to describe in comparable form the survival and the results of treatment of different patient groups. The objective of this report is to define several widely used methods of reporting end results. Throughout this chapter, the term survival time is used, although the guidelines apply equally to reporting length of response time, time to recurrence of disease, time to development of tumor following exposure to a risk factor, or any other function of time until the event of interest.

Certain basic information must be included in every report on cancer survival and end results. Such information should include:

1. A description of the cancer patients whose survival experience is to be summarized, including basic demographic characteristics such as age, race, and sex, as well as a description of the disease in terms of basis of diagnosis, histology, anatomic site, extent of disease (or stage), treatment, and calendar year of observation
2. The size of the study group and the number of patients lost to follow-up or the percent of patients successfully followed up
3. A definition of the starting time or "zero" time for the measurement of survival
4. An explanation of the method used in calculating survival rates.

DESCRIPTION OF CASE MATERIAL

Before any meaningful interpretation of survival data can be made, the case material from which the data are derived must be described. A fact not adequately appreciated is that the description of the case material is as important as the description of the actual mechanics of handling the data and method of calculating survival rates.

In organizing the material for presentation, consideration should be given to the following:

1. Reports should account for every case diagnosed as having the particular cancer under consideration. If some cases are excluded, the characteristics and number of these cases should be stated. The report should give the dates during which the patients were studied and should state whether the results are based on the experience of an entire institution, on the experience of a single clinic or hospital service, or on the experience of a single physician or group of physicians. The general nature of the institution and the general characteristics of the patients should be indicated, because factors such as race and socioeconomic status may influence end results.
2. All diagnoses should be confirmed histologically or cytologically. Those not confirmed at any time during the course of the disease or at autopsy should be reported and tabulated separately. When indicated, the findings for histologically distinct types of cancers should be reported separately. So that the effects of morphology on survival may be appreciated, reports should be stratified by histologic type when it is indicated.
3. The clinical or pathologic extent of disease or stage at the time of diagnosis is of particular importance in evaluating treatment and in making valid comparisons of end results reported from different sources. When it is applicable, patients should be stratified by stage of disease. The TNM system provides a convenient and widely used language for categorizing the primary lesion and the extent of involvement. The TNM assignments are grouped into appropriate summary combinations to create a small number of stages, usually four, so that the force of mortality increases from one stage to the next.

Specific criteria modify this system according to the primary site. The clinical classification for cancer at certain accessible sites, such as the uterine cervix, includes all diagnostic and evaluative information (including surgical exploration) obtained up to the date that tumor-directed treatment begins or the decision for no treatment is made. Information obtained by surgical resection and histopathologic studies is used in describing extent of disease at sites inaccessible to clinical evaluation, such as carcinoma of the ovary, kidney, and stomach. Extent of disease for these cancers is usually reported in terms of the pathologic classification.

4. Data on groups of patients previously treated should be presented separately from the data on patients not previously treated. Retreated patients should be classified according to stage at retreatment.

5. The number of groups into which a patient series is subdivided will depend on the total number of patients, the purpose of the study, and the nature of the case material. For example, in reporting on cancer of the prostate, the patients might be grouped into three age groups, such as under 60, 60 to 69, and 70 and over. An entirely different age grouping would be used in reporting on patients with leukemia. For most sites it is desirable to subdivide with respect to histologic type, sex, stage, and treatment, although this is not always possible with small numbers of patients.

DEFINITION OF STARTING TIME

The starting time for determining survival of patients depends on the purpose of the study. For example, the starting time for studying the natural history of a particular cancer might be defined in reference to the appearance of the first symptom. Various reference dates are commonly used as starting times for evaluating the effects of therapy. These include (1) date of diagnosis, (2) date of first visit to physician or clinic, (3) date of hospital admission, and (4) date of treatment initiation. If the time to recurrence of a tumor after apparent complete remission is being studied, the starting time is the date of apparent complete remission. The specific reference date used should be clearly specified in every report.

The date of initiation of therapy should be used as the starting time for evaluating therapy. For untreated patients, the most comparable date is the time at which it was decided that no tumor-directed treatment would be given. For both treated and untreated patients, the above times from which survival rates are calculated will usually coincide with the date of the initial staging of cancer.

VITAL STATUS

At any given time the vital status of each patient is defined as alive, dead, or unknown (i.e., lost to follow-up). The end point of each patient's participation in the study is either (1) a specified "terminal event" such as death, (2) survival to the completion of the study, or (3) loss to follow-up. In each case, survival time is the time from the starting point to the terminal event, to the end of the study, or to the date of last observation. This survival time may be further described in terms of patient status at the end point, such as:

Alive; tumor-free; no recurrence
Alive; tumor-free; after recurrence
Alive with persistent, recurrent, or metastatic disease
Alive with primary tumor
Dead; tumor-free
Dead; with cancer (primary, recurrent, or metastatic disease)
Dead; postoperative
Unknown; lost to follow-up.

Completeness of the follow-up is crucial in any study of survival time because even a small number of patients lost to follow-up may bias the data. The maximum possible effects of bias from patients lost to follow-up may be ascertained by calculating a maximum survival rate, assuming that all lost patients lived to the end of the study. A minimum survival rate may be calculated by assuming that all patients lost to follow-up died at the time they were lost.

SURVIVAL INTERVALS

The total survival time is broken up into intervals in units of weeks, months, or years. This provides a description of the population under study with respect to the dynamics of survival over a specified time. The time interval used should be selected with regard to the natural history of the disease under consideration. In diseases with a long natural history, the duration of study could be 5 to 20 years and survival intervals of 6 to 12 months will provide a meaningful description of the survival dynamics. If the population being studied has a very poor prognosis (e.g., patients with carcinoma of the esophagus or pancreas), the total duration of study may be 2 to 3 years and the survival intervals described in terms of 1 to 3 months. In interpreting survival rates one must also take into account the number of individuals entering a survival interval. Survival rates probably should not be computed for intervals in which fewer than 10 patients enter the interval alive.

CALCULATION OF SURVIVAL RATES

A properly calculated survival rate is the best single statistical index available for measuring the efficacy of one cancer therapy compared with another, administered to a comparable group of patients who also have similar disease characteristics. The basic concept is simple: Of a given number of patients, what percentage will be alive at the end of a specified interval, such as 5 years? For example, let us begin with 1,000 patients in a defined diagnostic category such as stage I carcinoma of the uterine cervix. If we observe each member of this group until death and enumerate those alive 5 years, 10 years, and 15 years after initiation of therapy, then the ratios of these numbers to the original 1,000 patients give the respective 5-year, 10-year, and 15-year survival rates. In practice, however, we do not begin literally with a given group and follow them all continuously until death before calculating survival rates. In a body of actual data, the group considered would generally contain persons who were treated at different times, so that different persons would have been observed for different lengths of time. On the closing date of the study, some would be known to be dead, others known to be alive, and some would have been lost to follow-up, and it would not be known whether they are alive or dead.

To illustrate the approach to dealing with this type of situation, let us consider in detail a small series of patients. Table 2-1 lists 40 patients with Stage II colon cancer treated in one hospital during the 8-year period from January 1975 to December 1982. The survival experience of these patients is to be assessed on the basis of information available through March 1986. For each patient, the table provides the following basic information:

1. Sex
2. Race
3. Age at initiation of treatment
4. Primary site
5. Histologic type
6. Treatment
7. Date treatment started (month and year)
8. Date of last contact (month and year)
9. Vital status at date of last contact (alive or dead)
10. Presence of colon cancer at date of last contact (yes or no).

Patients are listed consecutively by date of first treatment.

Calculation by the Direct Method. The simplest procedure for summarizing patient survival is to calculate the percentage of patients alive at the end of a specified interval, such as 5 years, using for this purpose only patients at risk of dying for at least 5 years. This approach is known as the *direct method*.

When we closed the study in March 1986, the latest available follow-up information was from February 1986. Therefore, patients must have been treated in February 1981 or earlier in order to be at risk of dying

for 5 years. Patients 1–30 all were diagnosed at least 5 years prior; however, patients 24, 27, and 30 have not had 5 full years of follow-up (in a strict statistical sense, these were lost to follow-up because their vital status was alive and their date of last contact was prior to the close of the study, March 1986). This means that 13 of the 40 patients (patients 24, 27, and 30 through 40) must be excluded from the calculation by the direct method.

Examining the entries in the "vital status" column in Table 2-1 for the 27 patients at risk for at least 5 years, we find that 11 patients were alive at last contact and 16 had died before February 1986. However, patient 3, although known to have died in March 1981, had been alive on his fifth anniversary. Patients 10 and 21 also lived at least 5 years. Therefore, we have 14 of the 27 patients alive 5 years after their respective dates of first treatment and, thus, the 5-year survival rate is 52%.

Calculation by the Actuarial Method. The direct method may be difficult for many hospital tumor registrars to use because of the limited number of patients with a particular type of disease who have been under follow-up for a full 5 years. In addition, the direct method does not provide for use of the survival information available on the most recently treated patients. For example, we know that patient 39 lived for 2 years and 9 months after treatment was started. Such information is valuable, but could not be used under the rules for the direct method because this patient was treated after February 1981.

The *actuarial*, or *life-table*, method provides a means for using all follow-up information accumulated up to the closing date of the study. The actuarial method has the further advantage of providing information on the survival pattern, that is, the manner in which the patient group was depleted during the total period of observation. For example, do most patients die during the first year or is there a uniform death rate over 5 years?

The procedures described here are designed for the individual investigator who wants to analyze carefully the survival experience of a series of patients either manually or by using a computer.

Patient Information. Both the manual and computer approaches to survival analysis require recording on a data card, magnetic tape, or a disk, basic information on the patient, his disease, and outcome.

For purposes of clarifying the methodology and principles underlying the actuarial approach, we shall illustrate the steps in the manual approach to calculating survival rates. This might be done by employing a data card such as the one shown in Figure 2-1, with data fields providing for the following information:

Table 2-1. Stage II Colon Cancer Patients Diagnosed: 1975–1982

OBS	RACE	SEX	AGE	SITE	HISTOL	TREAT	RX DATE	FUP DATE	CANCER STATUS	VITAL STATUS	SURV
1	WHITE	F	67	C18.2	8140	S	02-75	01-77	YES	D	01Y–11M
2	WHITE	M	79	C18.5	8140	S	06-75	09-75	NO	D	00Y–03M
3	WHITE	M	63	C18.6	8140	S	10-75	03-81	YES	D	05Y–05M
4	WHITE	F	65	C18.7	8010	S	05-76	10-85	NO	A	09Y–05M
5	WHITE	M	66	C18.7	8140	S	06-76	02-77	YES	D	00Y–08M
6	WHITE	M	77	C18.0	8140	S	07-76	10-78	YES	D	02Y–03M
7	WHITE	M	55	C18.6	8140	S	08-76	10-85	NO	A	09Y–02M
8	WHITE	F	78	C18.4	8140	S C	09-76	10-84	UNK	A	08Y–01M
9	WHITE	M	83	C18.7	8140	S	09-76	05-81	NO	D	04Y–08M
10	WHITE	F	71	C18.7	8140	S	12-76	03-82	YES	D	05Y–03M
11	WHITE	M	92	C18.7	8140	S	01-77	06-84	NO	A	07Y–05M
12	WHITE	F	80	C18.2	8140	S	05-77	05-84	NO	A	07Y–00M
13	WHITE	F	85	C18.7	8140	S	01-78	12-81	YES	D	03Y–11M
14	WHITE	F	67	C18.0	8140	S	02-78	07-80	NO	D	02Y–05M
15	WHITE	F	72	C18.0	8140	S	02-78	06-79	NO	D	01Y–04M
16	WHITE	F	96	C18.3	8140	S	03-78	03-81	NO	D	03Y–00M
17	WHITE	F	56	C18.6	8140	S	05-78	12-85	NO	A	07Y–07M
18	WHITE	M	65	C18.0	8140	S C	10-78	04-85	NO	A	06Y–06M
19	WHITE	F	62	C18.7	8140	SR	01-79	06-85	NO	A	06Y–05M
20	WHITE	M	82	C18.7	8480	S	02-79	01-82	NO	D	02Y–11M
21	WHITE	M	78	C18.7	8140	S	02-79	08-84	YES	D	05Y–06M
22	WHITE	M	71	C18.7	8140	S	05-79	06-85	NO	A	06Y–01M
23	WHITE	F	64	C18.7	8140	S	06-79	09-85	NO	A	06Y–03M
24	WHITE	F	72	C18.2	8140	S	07-79	08-82	NO	A	03Y–01M
25	WHITE	M	66	C18.7	8140	SR	01-80	06-84	YES	D	04Y–05M
26	WHITE	M	68	C18.4	8140	S	05-80	07-85	NO	A	05Y–02M
27	WHITE	M	86	C18.2	8140	S	05-80	12-84	NO	A	04Y–07M
28	WHITE	F	71	C18.2	8140	S	10-80	02-85	YES	D	04Y–04M
29	WHITE	M	67	C18.0	8140	S	12-80	10-84	YES	D	03Y–10M
30	WHITE	F	66	C18.4	8140	S	12-80	04-85	NO	A	04Y–04M
31	WHITE	F	45	C18.7	8140	S	03-81	01-84	NO	A	02Y–10M
32	WHITE	F	61	C18.0	8480	S	05-81	05-85	NO	A	04Y–00M
33	WHITE	M	70	C18.0	8140	S	05-81	06-82	NO	D	01Y–01M
34	WHITE	F	79	C18.4	8140	S	07-81	10-85	YES	A	04Y–03M
35	WHITE	F	66	C18.0	8140	NONE	08-81	09-81	YES	D	00Y–01M
36	WHITE	F	66	C18.4	8140	S C	10-81	05-83	YES	D	01Y–07M
37	WHITE	F	81	C18.2	8140	S	11-81	10-84	UNK	A	02Y–11M
38	WHITE	M	66	C18.4	8480	S	03-82	01-83	YES	D	00Y–10M
39	WHITE	F	65	C18.3	8140	S	10-82	02-86	NO	A	03Y–04M
40	WHITE	M	68	C18.6	8140	S	12-82	07-85	NO	A	02Y–07M

1. Name or case number
2. Age: completed years of age at time of initiation of treatment
3. Race and sex
4. Dates of first treatment and of last contact: month and year
5. Survival time (years-months)
6. Vital status and presence of disease: reliable information on presence or absence of cancer at time of death is highly desirable
7. Diagnosis: site of the tumor, histologic type, and stage of disease
8. Treatment: brief summary.

Observed Survival Rate. The life-table method of calculating a survival rate, using all the follow-up information available on the 40 patients under study, is illustrated in Table 2-2. There are seven steps necessary in preparing such a table:

1. The number of intervals and the length of each interval for survival time are chosen. One-year intervals were chosen for this example. The first interval is defined as up to but not including 1 year (survival years = 0), the second interval as surviving 1 year up to but not including 2 years (survival years = 1), and so on.
2. The patient data are tallied for vital status and survival time (columns 3 and 4). The sum of the totals for columns 3 and 4 must equal the total number of patients alive at the beginning of the study.
3. The number of patients alive at the beginning of each year is entered in column 2 and is obtained by successive subtraction of patients dying or last seen alive during the previous year. Thus, of 40 patients alive at start of treatment—that is, at the beginning of the first year of observation—4 died during the first year and 36 were alive at the beginning of the second year.

John Doe	63	W	M		October, 1975
(Name)	(Age)	(Race)	(Sex)		(Date Treatment Started)
March, 1981		Dead			Yes
(Date of Last Contact)		(Vital Status)			(Colon Cancer Present?)
Descending Colon		Adenocarcinoma		Stage II	Surgery
(Site)		(Type)		(Stage)	(Treatment)
Survival Time		Age at Entry		Year of Entry	Expected Survival Probability
5 yrs. 5 mos.		63		1975	0.834

Fig. 2-1. Data card: Patient 3, Table 2-1

4. The "effective number exposed to risk of dying" (column 5) is based on the assumption that patients last seen alive during any year of follow-up were, on the average, observed for one-half of that year. Thus, for the third interval the "effective number" is 32 - (1/2 × 3) = 30.5; for the fourth interval, it is 26 - (1/2 × 2) = 25.0. This is equivalent to person-years at risk.

5. The proportion dying during any year (column 6) is found by dividing the entry in column 3 by the entry in column 5. Thus, for the first interval, the proportion dying is 4/40 = 0.100; for the second interval, it is 4/36 = 0.111.

6. The proportion surviving the year (column 7)—that is, the observed annual survival rate—is obtained by subtracting the proportion dying (column 6) from 1.000.

7. The proportion surviving from first treatment to the end of each year (column 8)—that is, the observed cumulative survival rate—is the product of the annual survival rates for the given year and all preceding years. For example, for the fifth interval, the proportion 0.587 is the product of all entries in column 7 from the first through the fifth years.

The 5-year survival rate calculated by the life-table method is 0.535 or 54%. In this instance, the calculation obtained by using the information available on all 40 patients agrees well with the rate (52%) based on the 27 patients eligible for inclusion in the calculation by the direct method. Such close agreement by the two methods usually will not occur when patients are excluded from the calculation of a survival rate by the direct method. In such instances, the life-table method is more reliable because it is based on more information.

The cumulative rates in column 8 may be used to plot a survival curve and therefore provide a pictorial description of the survival pattern as shown in Figure 2-2. In Figure 2-3, the survival pattern for patients with colon cancer (based on a large series) is compared with the patterns for cancer of the lung and melanoma of the skin for a 10-year period of observation.

The same set of survival rates was plotted in Figure 2-4 using a logarithmic scale, which provides a pictorial representation of changes in the rate at which patients died. A steep slope indicates a high rate; a shallow slope, a low rate. For each disease group, the death rate slowed appreciably after the third year and the slope of each curve became shallower. However, it is clear from Figure 2-4 that patients with lung cancer were dying at a greater rate from the third through the tenth years than patients with cancer of the colon or

Table 2-2. Calculation of Observed Survival Rate by the Actuarial (Life-Table) Method

INTERVAL OF LAST OBSERVATION (YEARS) (1)	NO. ALIVE AT BEGINNING OF YEAR (2) l	NO. DYING DURING YEAR (3) d	NO. LAST SEEN ALIVE DURING YEAR (4) w	EFFECTIVE NO. EXPOSED TO RISK OF DYING (5) l'	PROPORTION DYING DURING YEAR (6) q	PROPORTION SURVIVING THE YEAR (7) p	PROP. SURV. FROM 1ST RX TO END OF INTERVAL (8) CP
0 — <1	40	4	0	40.0	0.100	0.900	0.900
1 — <2	36	4	0	36.0	0.111	0.889	0.800
2 — <3	32	3	3	30.5	0.098	0.902	0.722
3 — <4	26	3	2	25.0	0.120	0.880	0.635
4 — <5	21	3	4	19.0	0.158	0.842	0.535
5 or more	14	3	11				
Total		20	20				

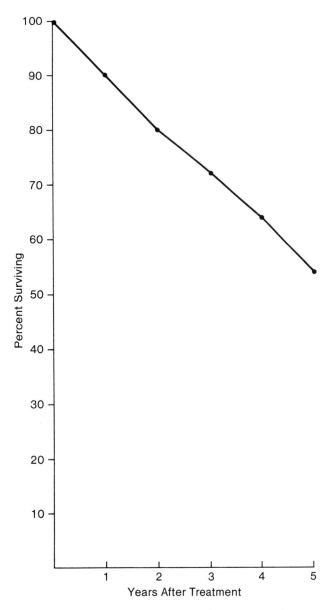

Fig. 2-2. Survival curve for 40 Stage II colon cancer patients

Fig. 2-3. Survival curves for patients with melanoma, colon cancer, and lung cancer: arithmetic scale. (Data from End-Results Group: End Results in Cancer, Report No. 4, DHEW Publication NIH 73-272. Bethesda, MD, National Cancer Institute, 1972)

not operating. Examination of Table 2-1 reveals that in seven instances colon cancer was not present at time of death (patients 2, 9, 14, 15, 16, 20, and 33). All of these deaths occurred within the first 5 years of follow-up and thus influenced the 5-year *observed* survival rate calculated in Table 2-2.

Whenever reliable information on cause of death is available, an adjustment can be made for deaths due to causes other than the disease under study. The procedure is shown in Table 2-3. Observed deaths are recorded as "with disease" (column 3a) or "without

with melanoma. In contrast, examination of Figure 2-3 might lead one to the erroneous conclusion that beyond the third year, lung cancer patients died at a lower rate. This is because Figure 2-3 portrays *absolute* changes, while Figure 2-4 provides a true picture of *relative* changes.

Adjusted Survival Rate. The observed survival rate described above accounts for all deaths, regardless of cause. Although this is a true reflection of total mortality in the patient group, we are frequently interested in describing mortality attributable to the disease under study. The *adjusted* survival rate is the proportion of the initial patient group that escaped death due to cancer if all other causes of death were

Fig. 2-4. Survival curves for patients with melanoma, colon cancer, and lung cancer: logarithmic scale. (Data from End-Results Group: End Results in Cancer, Report No. 4, DHEW Publication NIH 73-272. Bethesda, MD, National Cancer Institute, 1972)

Table 2-3. Calculation of Adjusted Survival Rate

INTERVAL OF LAST OBSERVATION (1)	NO. ALIVE AT BEGINNING OF YEAR (2)	NO. DYING DURING YEAR		NO. LAST SEEN ALIVE DURING YEAR (4)	EFFECTIVE NO. EXPOSED TO RISK OF DYING (5)	PROPORTION DYING DURING YEAR (6)	PROPORTION SURVIVING TO END OF YEAR (7)	CUMULATIVE PROPORTION SURVIVING (8)
		WITH DISEASE (3a)	WITHOUT DISEASE (3b)					
Years								
1	40	3	1	0	39.5	.076	.924	.924
2	36	2	2	0	35	.057	.943	.871
3	32	1	2	3	29.5	.034	.966	.842
4	26	2	1	2	24.5	.082	.918	.773
5	21	2	1	4	18.5	.108	.892	.689
≥6	14	3	—	11				
Total		13	7	20				

disease" (column 3b). Patients who died without disease are treated in the same manner as patients "last seen alive during year" (column 4); that is, both groups are withdrawn from the risk of dying from colon cancer. Thus, "the effective number exposed to risk of dying" (from colon cancer) in the third year of observation is 32 - (1/2 [2 + 3]) = 29.5.

The 5-year *adjusted* survival rate is 69%, compared to an observed rate of 54%. The adjusted rate indicates that 69% of patients with colon cancer escaped the risk of death from colon cancer for 5 years after treatment.

Use of the adjusted rate is particularly important in comparing patient groups that may differ with respect to factors such as sex, age, race, and socioeconomic status. Of the 40 patients listed in Table 2-1, 18 are males and 22 are females. The observed survival curves are plotted in the upper part of Figure 2-5. There is an apparent difference in survival between male and female patients. However, 4 of the 9 males who died during the first 5 years of observation had no evidence of colon cancer at time of death. Colon cancer was present at time of death in 5 of the 8 females who died. The effect of the adjustment for cause of death is shown in the lower portion of Figure 2-5. The survival curve for males is now very close to that for females. The 5-year adjusted survival rate is 66% for males and 71% for females, but the corresponding observed rates are 48% and 59%—a much larger difference.

Relative Survival Rates. Information on cause of death is sometimes unavailable or unreliable. Under such circumstances, it is not possible to compute an adjusted survival rate. However, it is possible to account for differences among patient groups in "normal mortality expectation"; that is, differences in the risk of dying from causes other than the disease under study. This can be done by means of the relative survival rate, the ratio of the observed survival rate to the expected rate for a group of people in the general population similar to the patient group with respect to race, sex, age, and calendar period of observation.

Table 2-4 provides 5-year expected survival probabilities for white males and females in the United States, based on mortality experience in calendar years 1950, 1955, 1960, 1965, 1970, 1975, and 1980. The appropriate probability, depending on the sex and age of the patient and the calendar year of entry to observation, is taken from this table and entered in the lower portion of the patient data card (Figure 2-1). Thus, for example, for patient 3 (Table 2-1), a 63-year-old man with a 1975 date of entry, the 5-year expected survival probability is 0.834. For patient 17, a 56-year-old woman who entered observation in 1978, the expected survival probability is 0.966. Thus, for the hypothetical group of patients in Table 2-1, the average expected 5-year survival probability is the sum of the individual expected probabilities (31.241) divided by the number of patients (40), and equals 0.781. The ratio of the observed (0.535) to the expected (0.781) survival rate is 0.685 or 69%. This is the relative rate and in this instance is identical with the adjusted rate.

Although in this illustration 5-year results were used to depict the relative survival rate calculation, it is conventional to calculate relative survival rates for each interval and cumulatively for successive follow-up intervals. For detailed analysis, one must consult more extensive expected rate tables and more explicit methodology (see bibliography entry 8). In publishing relative survival rates, it is important to report the method used for calculation and the source of expected rates.

In Figure 2-6, comparison is made between the survival curves based on the observed, adjusted, and relative rates on a logarithmic scale. It can be seen that the values along the adjusted and relative survival

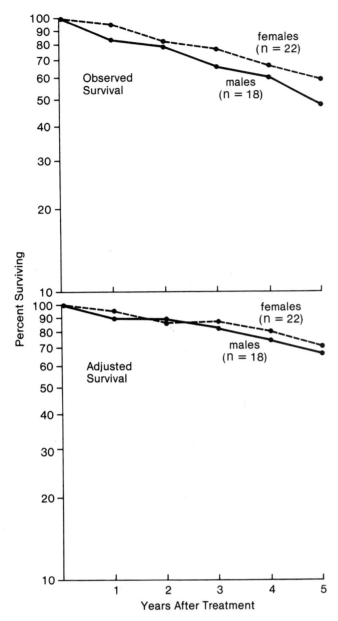

Fig. 2-5. Comparison of survival curves (logarithmic scale) for males and females with colon cancer: observed and adjusted survival rates

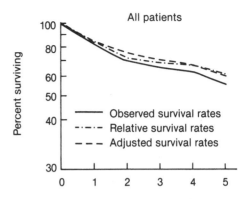

Fig. 2-6. Comparison of survival curves based on observed, adjusted, and relative rates (logarithmic scale)

cated. The different types of rates described above are all useful, but rates computed by different methods are not directly comparable with each other. Thus, in comparing the survival of different patient groups, rates must be computed by the same method.

Calculation by the Kaplan-Meier Method. Another method of survival analysis that is widely used and for which computer programs are easily available is the Kaplan-Meier method (see bibliography entry 13). It is similar to the life-table method but also provides for calculating the proportion surviving to each point in time that a death occurs. The life-table and Kaplan-Meier methods give identical results in the absence of withdrawals.

As a simple introduction to Kaplan-Meier, consider five patients who died at 1, 4, 7, 10, and 19 months, respectively. The first survival proportion is calculated at 1 month, the time of the first death. Because 4 of the 5 patients survived beyond that point, the resulting proportion surviving to that time is 4 out of 5, or 0.80. Similarly, at 4 months (the time of the second death), 3 of the 4 (0.75) who survived the first month are still alive after 4 months. Thus, the cumulative 4-month survival rate is 0.80 × 0.75 = 0.60. The third interval of interest is from 4 to 7 months, the time of the third death. For this interval, the proportion surviving is 2/3 (0.67). From 7 to 10 months, the next interval of interest, the proportion surviving is 1/2 (0.50). In the last interval, 10 to 19 months, the proportion surviving is 0/1 (0.00). This is shown in Table 2-5. The 6-month and 1-year survival rates are 60% and 20%, respectively. This is because until a death occurs, the survival proportion last calculated remains in effect. This survival pattern is shown in Figure 2-7. Note that the survival curve proceeds in steps rather than as a sloped line.

In contrast to the life-table method, if a patient had been lost or withdrawn during an interval (e.g., interval 5), that person's experience would have been

curves are not always identical. In practice, if the series is not too small and the patients are roughly representative of the population of the United States (taking race, sex, and age into account), the relative survival rate provides a useful estimate of the probability of escaping death from the specific cancer under study. However, if reliable information on cause of death is available, it is preferable to use the adjusted rate. This is particularly true if the series is small or if the patients are largely drawn from a particular socioeconomic segment of the population.

In reporting on patient survival, the specific method used in calculating the rates must be indi-

Table 2-4. Expected Probabilities for Surviving Five Years for U.S. Whites:
1950, 1955, 1960, 1965, 1970, 1975 and 1980

AGE IN YEARS (INCLUSIVE RANGE)	1950 (1948–1952)	1955 (1953–1957)	1960 (1958–1962)	1965 (1963–1967)	1970 (1968–1972)	1975 (1973–1977)	1980 (1978–1982)
Male							
<1	0.964	0.969	0.970	0.972	0.977	0.981	0.985
1 and 2	0.995	0.996	0.996	0.996	0.996	0.997	0.997
5 (3–7)	0.997	0.997	0.998	0.998	0.998	0.998	0.998
10 (8–12)	0.997	0.997	0.997	0.998	0.998	0.998	0.998
15 (13–17)	0.993	0.994	0.994	0.994	0.993	0.993	0.993
20 (18–22)	0.991	0.991	0.992	0.991	0.990	0.991	0.991
25 (23–27)	0.992	0.992	0.992	0.992	0.992	0.992	0.991
30 (28–32)	0.991	0.991	0.991	0.991	0.991	0.992	0.992
35 (33–37)	0.986	0.987	0.988	0.987	0.987	0.989	0.990
40 (38–42)	0.978	0.979	0.980	0.980	0.979	0.982	0.984
45 (43–47)	0.963	0.965	0.966	0.966	0.967	0.970	0.974
50 (48–52)	0.942	0.944	0.943	0.944	0.947	0.952	0.958
55 (53–57)	0.912	0.916	0.915	0.913	0.915	0.926	0.934
60 (58–62)	0.869	0.873	0.872	0.873	0.873	0.884	0.898
65 (63–67)	0.814	0.815	0.815	0.813	0.816	0.834	0.848
70 (68–72)	0.741	0.746	0.745	0.741	0.745	0.759	0.777
75 (73–77)	0.633	0.642	0.650	0.649	0.642	0.658	0.687
80 (78–82)	0.499	0.504	0.509	0.520	0.523	0.547	0.565
≥85 (83+)	0.350	0.349	0.349	0.350	0.379	0.421	0.426
Female							
<1	0.972	0.976	0.977	0.979	0.982	0.985	0.988
1 and 2	0.996	0.997	0.997	0.997	0.997	0.997	0.998
5 (3–7)	0.998	0.998	0.998	0.998	0.998	0.999	0.999
10 (8–12)	0.998	0.998	0.999	0.999	0.999	0.999	0.999
15 (13–17)	0.997	0.997	0.998	0.998	0.997	0.997	0.998
20 (18–22)	0.996	0.997	0.997	0.997	0.997	0.997	0.997
25 (23–27)	0.996	0.996	0.996	0.997	0.996	0.997	0.997
30 (28–32)	0.994	0.995	0.995	0.995	0.995	0.996	0.996
35 (33–37)	0.991	0.992	0.993	0.993	0.993	0.994	0.995
40 (38–42)	0.987	0.988	0.988	0.988	0.988	0.990	0.991
45 (43–47)	0.980	0.982	0.982	0.982	0.982	0.984	0.986
50 (48–52)	0.969	0.972	0.972	0.972	0.973	0.975	0.978
55 (53–57)	0.953	0.959	0.960	0.959	0.960	0.963	0.966
60 (58–62)	0.925	0.934	0.937	0.939	0.941	0.944	0.948
65 (63–67)	0.883	0.890	0.900	0.901	0.908	0.920	0.922
70 (68–72)	0.816	0.832	0.841	0.846	0.854	0.869	0.879
75 (73–77)	0.708	0.727	0.746	0.754	0.761	0.784	0.812
80 (78–82)	0.558	0.580	0.592	0.611	0.633	0.672	0.695
≥85 (83+)	0.406	0.394	0.400	0.405	0.472	0.512	0.542

(Demographic Analysis Section, National Cancer Institute, Bethesda, Maryland)

included to the end of the last completed interval (ending at 4 months) and not entered into any of the subsequent calculations.

The Kaplan-Meier method applied to the data for our series of 40 stage II colon cancer cases (Table 2-1) is shown in Table 2-6. The 5-year survival rate is 0.529, which is very similar to the rate of 0.535 found by the life-table method. Figure 2-8 shows the comparison of survival curves based on life-table and Kaplan-Meier calculations on this series of 40 colon cancer patients. An adjusted rate can be calculated by the Kaplan-Meier method by handling noncancer deaths and withdrawals in a manner similar to that illustrated above for the life-table method.

A relative survival rate can also be calculated by using the observed rate derived by the Kaplan-Meier method and dividing it by the expected rate, as was done for the life-table method.

STANDARD ERROR OF A SURVIVAL RATE

A survival rate describes the experience of the specific group of patients from which it is computed. These results are frequently used to generalize to a larger population. The existence of population values is postulated and these values are estimated from the group under study, which thus represents a sample from the larger population. If a survival rate was calculated from a second sample taken from the same population, it is unlikely that the results would be exactly the same. The difference between the two results is called the sampling variation (or chance variation or sampling error). The standard error is a measure of the extent to

Table 2-5. Example of Kaplan-Meier Survival Calculations

TIME (MONTHS)	ALIVE	DIED	WITHDRAWN	PROPORTION DYING	PROPORTION SURVIVING	SURVIVAL RATE
1	5	1	0	0.200	0.800	0.800
4	4	1	0	0.250	0.750	0.600
7	3	1	0	0.333	0.667	0.400
10	2	1	0	0.500	0.500	0.200
19	1	1	0	1.000	0.000	0.000

which sampling variation influences the computed survival rate. In repeated observations under the same conditions, the true or population survival rate will lie within the range of two standard errors on either side of the computed rate about 95 times in 100. This range is called the 95% confidence interval.

When the observed survival rate has been computed by the direct method, the standard error is computed from the formula

$$\frac{\sqrt{CP(1-CP)}}{n}$$

in which CP is the survival rate and n is the number of patients at risk of death. In the illustration of the direct method, a 5-year survival rate of 52% (or p = 0.52) was obtained based on the experience of 27 patients.

Thus, the standard error is equal to 0.096 (square root of [0.52 × 0.48 ÷ 27]). To obtain the 95% confidence interval, twice the standard error (0.19) is subtracted from and then added to the survival rate. This means that the chances are about 95 in 100 that the true 5-year rate is between 0.33 and 0.71 for our example.

Standard Error of the Actuarial Survival Rate. To calculate the standard error of the 5-year survival rate when the actuarial method is used (see bibliography entries 6, 14, and 16), two columns of figures may be added to Table 2-2, as shown in Table 2-7. The first additional column (column 9) is obtained by subtracting the values in column 3 from the values in column 5 of Table 2-2. The last column needed (column 10) is obtained by dividing the entries in column 6 by the corresponding figures in column 9. The sum of the figures in column 10 is also entered into the table and in this example equals 0.0253.

The standard error of the 5-year survival rate by the actuarial method is the calculated 5-year survival rate multiplied by the square root of the total of the entries in column 10 of Table 2-5; that is, 0.535 × $\sqrt{0.0253}$ = 0.085. The approximate 95% confidence interval for the population 5-year survival rate is found, as shown earlier for the direct method, by adding and subtracting two times the standard error to and from the 5-year survival rate that has been calculated—that is, 0.535 plus and minus (2 × 0.085)—which gives an interval from 0.36 to 0.70.

If the above computations seem to be too involved, an approximation to the standard error of the actuarial survival rate may be quickly obtained from published tables prepared by Ederer (see bibliography entry 7).

It is noteworthy that the standard error of the survival rate obtained by the actuarial method is smaller

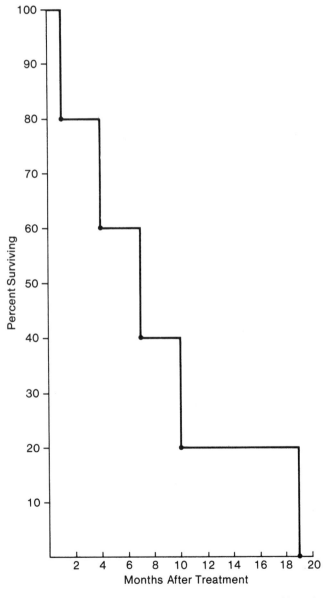

Fig. 2-7. Observed survival for five patients (data from Table 2-5), Kaplan-Meier method

Table 2-6. Calculation of Observed Survival by the Kaplan-Meier
Method: 40 Stage II Colon Cancer Patients

TIME (MONTHS)	ENTERED ALIVE	DIED	WITHDRAWN	PROPORTION DYING	PROPORTION SURVIVING	SURVIVAL RATE
1	40	1	0	0.025	0.975	0.975
3	39	1	0	0.026	0.974	0.950
8	38	1	0	0.026	0.974	0.925
10	37	1	0	0.027	0.973	0.900
13	36	1	0	0.028	0.972	0.875
16	35	1	0	0.029	0.971	0.849
19	34	1	0	0.029	0.971	0.825
23	33	1	0	0.030	0.970	0.800
27	32	1	0	0.031	0.969	0.775
29	31	1	0	0.032	0.968	0.750
31	30	0	1			
34	29	0	1			
35	28	1	1	0.036	0.964	0.723
36	26	1	0	0.038	0.962	0.696
37	25	0	1			
40	24	0	1			
46	23	1	0	0.043	0.957	0.666
47	22	1	0	0.045	0.955	0.636
48	21	0	1			
51	20	0	1			
52	19	1	1	0.053	0.947	0.602
53	17	1	0	0.059	0.941	0.567
55	16	0	1			
56	15	1	0	0.067	0.933	0.529
≥60		3	11			

than the standard error of the survival rate calculated by the direct method (0.085 versus 0.096). This difference reflects the advantage in terms of statistical precision of using all available information; that is, including information on patients under observation for less than 5 years. The issue is discussed in detail by Cutler in bibliography entry 6.

The standard error of a survival rate obtained by the Kaplan-Meier method may be calculated as shown in bibliography entry 13.

Standard Error of Relative Survival Rate. The standard error of the relative survival rate is easily obtained by dividing the standard error of the observed survival rate (obtained by either the direct or actuarial method) by the expected survival rate. To illustrate these calculations, consider results for the 40 Stage II colon cancer patients. The expected 5-year survival rate was 0.781, and the standard error of the observed survival rate was 0.085. Therefore, in this example the standard error of the 5-year relative survival rate is:

$$\frac{\text{Standard error of observed rate}}{\text{Expected survival rate}} = \frac{0.085}{0.781} = 0.109.$$

Table 2-7. Calculation of Standard Error of Survival Rate by Actuarial (Life-Table) Method

INTERVAL OF LAST OBSERVATION (YEARS) (1)	NO. ALIVE AT BEGINNING OF YEAR (2) l	NO. DYING DURING YEAR (3) d	NO. LAST SEEN ALIVE DURING YEAR (4) w	EFFECTIVE NO. EXPOSED TO RISK OF DYING (5) l'	PROPORTION DYING DURING YEAR (6) q	PROPORTION SURVIVING THE YEAR (7) p	PROP. SURV. FROM 1ST RX TO END OF INTERVAL (8) CP	ENTRY (5) MINUS ENTRY (3) (9)	ENTRY (6) DIVIDED BY ENTRY (9) (10)
0 — <1	40	4	0	40.0	0.100	0.900	0.900	36.0	.0028
1 — <2	36	4	0	36.0	0.111	0.889	0.800	32.0	.0035
2 — <3	32	3	3	30.5	0.098	0.902	0.722	27.5	.0036
3 — <4	26	3	2	25.0	0.120	0.880	0.635	22.0	.0055
4 — <5	21	3	4	19.0	0.158	0.842	0.535	16.0	.0099
5 or more	14	3	11						
Total		20	20						0.0253

Standard Error of 5-Year Survival Rate = 5 Year Survival Rate × √Total of Column (10)

= 0.535 × √0.0253 = 0.535 × 0.1591 = 0.085

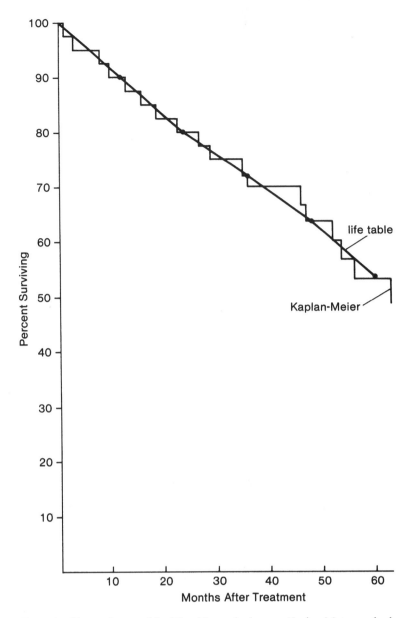

Fig. 2-8. Observed survival for life-table method versus Kaplan-Meier method calculations: 40 Stage II colon cancer patients

The 95% confidence limits of the 5-year relative survival rate therefore are:

$$0.69 \pm 2 \times (0.109) = 0.47, 0.91$$

Comparison of Survival Rates in Two Patient Groups. In comparing survival rates of two patient groups, the statistical significance of the observed difference is of interest. The essential question is: What is the probability that the observed difference may have occurred by chance? The standard error of the survival rate provides a simple means for appraising this question. If the 95% confidence intervals of two survival rates do not overlap, the observed difference would be customarily considered as statistically significant; that is, unlikely to be due to chance.

Standard statistical texts describe the z-test, which provides a numeric estimate of the probability that a difference as large as that observed would have occurred if only chance were operating. The statistic z is calculated by the formula:

$$z = \frac{|CP_1 - CP_2|}{\sqrt{(SE_1)^2 + (SE_2)^2}}$$

in which:

1. CP_1 is the survival rate for group 1
2. CP_2 is the survival rate for group 2
3. $|CP_1\text{-}CP_2|$ is the absolute value of the difference (i.e., the magnitude of the difference, whether positive or negative)
4. SE_1 is the standard error of CP_1
5. SE_2 is the standard error of CP_2.

If $z \geq 1.96$, the probability that a difference as large as that observed occurred by chance is $\leq 5\%$. If $z \geq 2.56$, the probability is $\leq 1\%$. It is conventional in most (but not all) applications to regard as statistically significant a difference that would occur by chance with a probability of 5% or less.

For example, let us apply the z-test to the difference in observed 5-year survival rates by the actuarial method for the 18 males and 22 females among the 40 colon cancer patients; that is, let us test whether there is a statistically significant difference in survival of the males with colon cancer compared with the females.

Designate the 5-year survival rate for males by CP_1 and for females by CP_2. We find $CP_1 = 0.475$ and $CP_2 = 0.591$. Employing the method shown in Table 2-5, $SE_1 = 0.122$ and $SE_2 = 0.116$. Then:

$$z = \frac{|0.475 - 0.591|}{\sqrt{0.122^2 + 0.116^2}} = \frac{0.116}{0.168} = 0.69$$

The calculated z value is smaller than 1.96 and therefore not statistically significant at the 5% level. This result indicates that for a study of this size (18 males and 22 females) the difference in CPs (0.475 versus 0.591) is not large enough for us to reject chance or sampling variation as the cause.

In a study with more patients, the same size difference in survival rates as seen here would be less likely to be due to chance and might be statistically significant; that is, z might equal or exceed 1.96. In order for this to occur, the value of the denominator in the equation for z would have to decrease in value. The denominator,

$$\sqrt{(SE_1)^2 + (SE_2)^2}$$

is called the standard error of the difference in rates and tends to become smaller as study size increases. It should also be noted that superior survival of females with colon cancer compared with males has been observed in large series of patients with resultant significant z values.

Great care must be exercised in interpreting tests of statistical significance. For example, if differences exist in the patient and disease characteristics of two treatment groups, a statistically significant difference in survival results may primarily reflect differences in the two patient series rather than differences in the efficacy of the treatment regimens. A more definitive approach to therapy evaluation requires a randomized clinical trial that helps ensure comparability of the two treatment groups and their disease.

The methods of survival analysis presented in this chapter are appropriate for a single group of patients or may be applied to subgroups derived by cross-classifying patients with respect to several variables of interest. Multivariate models, although beyond the scope of this chapter, have now been used extensively to assess the relationship to survival time of a number of variables simultaneously. One of the most commonly used is the Cox proportional hazards model (see bibliography entry 5). Bibliography entry 12 is an excellent source for additional information on multivariate survival analysis.

BIBLIOGRAPHY

1. Berkson J, Gage RP: Calculation of survival rates for cancer. Proc Staff Meet Mayo Clin 25:270–286, 1950
2. Breslow N: A generalized Kruskal-Wallis test for comparing samples subject to unequal patterns of censoring. Biometrika 57:579–594, 1970
3. Chiang CL: A stochastic study of the life table and its applications. I. Probability distributions of the biometric functions. Biometrics 16:618–635, 1960
4. Chiang CL: The Life Table and Its Applications, p. 316. Malabar, FL, Robert E. Krieger Pub., 1984
5. Cox DR: Regression models and life tables. J R Stat Soc B 34:187–220, 1972
6. Cutler SJ, Ederer F: Maximum utilization of the life table method in analyzing survival. J Chronic Dis 8:699–712, 1958
7. Ederer F: A simple method for determining standard errors of survival rates, with tables. J Chronic Dis 11:632–645, 1960
8. Ederer F, Axtell LM, Cutler SJ: The relative survival rate: A statistical methodology. Natl Cancer Inst Monogr 6:101–121, 1961
9. Gehan EA: A generalized Wilcoxon test for comparing arbitrarily single-censored samples. Biometrika 52:203–224, 1965
10. Gehan EA: Estimating survival functions from the life table. J Chronic Dis 21:629–644, 1969
11. Hankey BF, Myers MH: Evaluating differences in survival between two groups of patients. J Chronic Dis 24:523–531, 1971
12. Kalbfleisch JD, Prentice RL: The Statistical Analysis of Failure Time Data, p. 321. New York, John Wiley and Sons, 1980
13. Kaplan EL, Meier P: Nonparametric estimation from incomplete observations. J Am Stat Assn 53:457–481, 1958
14. MacDonald EJ: Method of analysis for evaluation of treatment in cancer of the oropharynx. Radiology 78:783–788, 1962
15. Mantel N: Evaluation of survival data and two new rank order statistics arising in its consideration. Cancer Chemother Rep 50:163–170, 1966
16. Merrell M, Shulman LE: Determination of prognosis in chronic disease, illustrated by systemic lupus erythematosus. J Chronic Dis 1:12–32, 1955
17. Peto R, Pike MC, Armitage P, et al: Design and analysis of randomized clinical trials requiring prolonged observation of each patient: II. Analysis and examples. Br J Cancer 35:1–35, 1977

PART II

Staging of Cancer at Specific Anatomic Sites

HEAD AND NECK

Cancers of the head and neck may arise on all lining membranes of the upper aerodigestive tract. The T classifications indicating the extent of the primary tumor are generally similar but differ in specific details for each site because of anatomic considerations. The N classification for cervical lymph node metastasis is uniform for all sites. The staging systems presented in this section are all clinical staging, based on the best possible estimate of the extent of the disease before first treatment. Although pathologic classification is possible, it is of less practical importance in the management of these tumors. However, when surgical treatment is carried out, cancer of the head and neck can be staged (pathologic stage) during this period of management using all information available from the resected specimen and from before treatment.

In reviewing these staging systems, task forces from the UICC and the AJCC made minor changes in the T classifications formerly in use, and several major changes in the previous N classifications of cervical node metastasis. Bilateral cervical node metastases previously classified as N3 by the AJCC were changed to N2 as suggested by the UICC in view of their somewhat more favorable prognosis with current therapy. The term fixed, previously applied to cervical nodes in the N3 category by the UICC, was abandoned because the degree of fixation varies and is prone to subjective interpretation by different observers. It was replaced by the AJCC definition of N3 as a node 6 cm or more in greatest diameter. This is an objective measurement, and most nodes this size formerly would have been considered fixed.

This section presents the staging classification for six major head and neck sites: the oral cavity, the pharynx (nasopharynx, oropharynx, and hypopharynx), the larynx, the maxillary sinus, the salivary glands, and the thyroid gland.

3

Lip and Oral Cavity

C00.0 External upper lip
C00.1 External lower lip
C00.2 External lip, NOS
C00.3 Mucosa of upper lip
C00.4 Mucosa of lower lip
C00.5 Mucosa of lip, NOS
C00.6 Commissure
C00.8 Overlapping lesion
C00.9 Lip, NOS

C02.0 Dorsal surface of tongue, NOS
C02.1 Border of tongue
C02.2 Ventral surface of tongue, NOS
C02.3 Anterior two-thirds of tongue, NOS
C02.4 Lingual tonsil
C02.8 Overlapping lesion
C02.9 Tongue, NOS

C03.0 Upper gum
C03.1 Lower gum
C03.9 Gum, NOS

C04.0 Anterior floor of mouth
C04.1 Lateral floor of mouth
C04.8 Overlapping lesion
C04.9 Floor of mouth, NOS

C05.0 Hard palate
C05.8 Overlapping lesion
C05.9 Palate, NOS

C06.0 Cheek mucosa
C06.1 Vestibule of mouth
C06.2 Retromolar area
C06.8 Overlapping lesion of other and unspecified parts of mouth
C06.9 Mouth, NOS

ANATOMY

Primary Site. The oral cavity extends from the skin-vermilion junction of the lips to the junction of the hard and soft palate above and to the line of circumvallate papillae below and is divided into the following specific areas:

Lip. The lip begins at the junction of the vermilion border with the skin and includes only the vermilion surface or that portion of the lip that comes into contact with the opposing lip. It is well defined into an upper and lower lip joined at the commissures of the mouth.

Buccal Mucosa. This includes all the membrane lining of the inner surface of the cheeks and lips from the line of contact of the opposing lips to the line of attachment of mucosa of the alveolar ridge (upper and lower) and pterygomandibular raphe.

Lower Alveolar Ridge. This ridge includes the alveolar process of the mandible and its covering mucosa, which extends from the line of attachment of mucosa in the buccal gutter to the line of free mucosa of the floor of the mouth. Posteriorly it extends to the ascending ramus of the mandible.

Upper Alveolar Ridge. The upper ridge is the alveolar process of the maxilla and its covering mucosa, which extends from the line of attachment of mucosa in the upper gingival buccal gutter to the junction of the hard palate. Its posterior margin is the upper end of the pterygopalatine arch.

Retromolar Gingiva (Retromolar Trigone). This is the attached mucosa overlying the ascending ramus of the mandible from the level of the posterior surface of the last molar tooth to the apex superiorly, adjacent to the tuberosity of the maxilla.

Floor of the Mouth. This is a semilunar space over the myelohyoid and hyoglossus muscles, extending from the inner surface of the lower alveolar ridge to the undersurface of the tongue. Its posterior boundary is the base of the anterior pillar of the tonsil. It is divided into two sides by the frenulum of the tongue and contains the ostia of the submaxillary and sublingual salivary glands.

Hard Palate. This is the semilunar area between the upper alveolar ridge and the mucous membrane covering the palatine process of the maxillary palatine bones. It extends from the inner surface of the superior alveolar ridge to the posterior edge of the palatine bone.

Anterior Two-Thirds of the Tongue (Oral Tongue). This is a freely mobile portion of the tongue that extends anteriorly from the line of circumvallate papillae to the undersurface of the tongue at the junction of the floor of the mouth. It is composed of four areas: the tip, the lateral borders, the dorsum, and the undersurface (nonvillous surface of the tongue). The undersurface of the tongue is considered as a separate category by the World Health Organization (WHO).

Regional Lymph Nodes. These are the cervical lymph nodes, which include:

Internal jugular
   jugulodigastric
   jugulo-omohyoid
   upper deep cervical
   lower deep cervical
Parotid
   preauricular
   infraparotid
   subparotid
   posterior auricular
Submandibular (submaxillary)
Submental
Cervical, NOS

Some primary sites drain bilaterally.

In clinical evaluation, the actual size of the nodal mass should be measured, and allowance should be made for intervening soft tissues. It is recognized that most masses over 3 cm in diameter are not single nodes but are confluent nodes or tumor in soft tissues of the neck. There are three categories of clinically positive nodes: N1, N2, and N3. The use of subgroups a, b, and c is not required but is recommended. Midline nodes are considered homolateral nodes.

Metastatic Sites. Distant spread to the lungs is common; skeletal or hepatic metastases occur less often. Mediastinal lymph node metastases are considered distant metastases.

RULES FOR CLASSIFICATION

Clinical Staging. The assessment of the primary tumor is based on inspection and palpation of the oral cavity and neck. Additional studies may include plane tomographic, or contrast roentgenograms, particularly evaluating bone invasion of the mandible or upper alveoli. Examinations for distant metastases include chest film, blood chemistries, blood count, and other routine studies as indicated. The tumor must be confirmed histologically. All clinical and pathologic data available before first definitive treatment may be used for clinical staging.

Pathologic Staging. Complete resection of the primary site, radical nodal dissections, and pathologic examination of the resected specimens allow the use of this designation. Specimens that are resected after radiation or chemotherapy need to be especially noted.

DEFINITION OF TNM

Primary Tumor (T)

TX Primary tumor cannot be assessed
T0 No evidence of primary tumor
Tis Carcinoma *in situ*
T1 Tumor 2 cm or less in greatest dimension
T2 Tumor more than 2 cm but not more than 4 cm in greatest dimension
T3 Tumor more than 4 cm in greatest dimension
T4 (lip) Tumor invades adjacent structures (e.g., through cortical bone, tongue, skin of neck)
T4 (oral cavity) Tumor invades adjacent structures (e.g., through cortical bone, into deep [extrinsic] muscle of tongue, maxillary sinus, skin)

Regional Lymph Nodes (N)

NX Regional lymph nodes cannot be assessed
N0 No regional lymph node metastasis
N1 Metastasis in a single ipsilateral lymph node, 3 cm or less in greatest dimension
N2 Metastasis in a single ipsilateral lymph node, more than 3 cm but not more than 6 cm in greatest dimension; or in multiple ipsilateral lymph nodes, none more than 6 cm in greatest dimension; or in bilateral or contralateral lymph nodes, none more than 6 cm in greatest dimension
    N2a Metastasis in single ipsilateral lymph node more than 3 cm but not more than 6 cm in greatest dimension
    N2b Metastasis in multiple ipsilateral lymph nodes, none more than 6 cm in greatest dimension
    N2c Metastasis in bilateral or contralateral lymph nodes, none more than 6 cm in greatest dimension
N3 Metastasis in a lymph node more than 6 cm in greatest dimension

Distant Metastasis (M)

MX Presence of distant metastasis cannot be assessed
M0 No distant metastasis
M1 Distant metastasis

STAGE GROUPING

Stage	T	N	M
Stage 0	Tis	N0	M0
Stage I	T1	N0	M0
Stage II	T2	N0	M0
Stage III	T3	N0	M0
	T1	N1	M0
	T2	N1	M0
	T3	N1	M0
Stage IV	T4	N0	M0
	T4	N1	M0
	Any T	N2	M0
	Any T	N3	M0
	Any T	Any N	M1

HISTOPATHOLOGIC TYPE

The predominant cancer is squamous cell carcinoma; tumors of minor salivary glands are included. Pathologic confirmation of diagnosis is required. Tumor grading is recommended using Broders' classification. Other non-epithelial tumors such as those of lymphoid tissue, soft tissue, bone and cartilage are not included. Although the grade of the tumor does not enter into staging of the tumor, it should be recorded.

HISTOPATHOLOGIC GRADE (G)

GX Grade cannot be assessed
G1 Well differentiated
G2 Moderately differentiated
G3 Poorly differentiated
G4 Undifferentiated

BIBLIOGRAPHY

1. Bloom ND, Spiro RH: Carcinoma of the cheek mucosa. Am J Surg 140:556–559, 1980
2. Evans JF, Shah VP: Epidermoid carcinoma of the palate. Am J Surg 142:451–455, 1981
3. Fayos JF, Lampe I: Treatment of squamous cell carcinoma of the tongue. Am J Surg 124:493–500, 1972
4. Feind CR, Cole RM: Cancer of the floor of the mouth and its lymphatic spread. Am J Surg 116:482–486, 1968
5. Flynn MB, Mullins FX, Moore C: Selection of treatment in squamous carcinoma of the floor of the mouth. Am J Surg 126:477–481, 1973
6. Guillamondegui OM, Oliver B, Hayden R: Cancer of the anterior floor of the mouth. Am J Surg 140:560–562, 1980
7. Harrold CC Jr: Management of cancer of the floor of the mouth. Am J Surg 122:487–493, 1971

8. Kalnins IK, Leonard AG, Sako K, et al: Correlation between prognosis and degree of lymph node involvement in carcinoma of the oral cavity. Am J Surg 134:450–454, 1977

9. Marchetta FC, Sako K: Results of radical surgery for intraoral carcinoma related to tumor size. Am J Surg 112:554–557, 1966

10. Shah JP, Cendon RA, Farr HW, et al: Carcinoma of the oral cavity: Factors affecting treatment failure at the primary site and neck. Am J Surg 132:504–507, 1976

11. Spiro RH, Alfonso AE, Farr HW, et al: Cervical node metastasis from epidermoid carcinoma of the oral cavity: A critical assessment of current staging. Am J Surg 128:562–567, 1974

12. Spiro RH, Strong EW: Epidermoid carcinoma of the mobile tongue. Am J Surg 122:707–713, 1971

13. Wahi PN, et al: Histological typing of oral tumors. WHO International Histological Classification of Tumors. Geneva, WHO, 1971.

LIP AND ORAL CAVITY

Data Form for Cancer Staging

Patient identification
Name _____
Address _____
Hospital or clinic number _____
Age _____ Sex _____ Race _____

Institution identification
Hospital or clinic _____
Address _____

Oncology Record

Anatomic site of cancer _____
Histologic type _____
Grade (G) _____
Date of classification _____

Chronology of classification
[　] Clinical (use all data prior to first treatment)
[　] Pathologic (if definitively resected specimen available)

DEFINITIONS

Clin	Path		
		Primary Tumor (T)	
[ ]	[ ]	TX	Primary tumor cannot be assessed
[ ]	[ ]	T0	No evidence of primary tumor
[ ]	[ ]	Tis	Carcinoma *in situ*
[ ]	[ ]	T1	Tumor 2 cm or less in greatest dimension
[ ]	[ ]	T2	Tumor more than 2 cm but not more than 4 cm in greatest dimension
[ ]	[ ]	T3	Tumor more than 4 cm in greatest dimension
[ ]	[ ]	T4	(lip) Tumor invades adjacent structures, *e.g.*, through cortical bone, tongue, skin of neck
[ ]	[ ]	T4	(oral cavity) Tumor invades adjacent structures, *e.g.*, through cortical bone, into deep (extrinsic) muscle of tongue, maxillary sinus, skin
		Lymph Node (N)	
[ ]	[ ]	NX	Regional lymph nodes cannot be assessed
[ ]	[ ]	N0	No regional lymph node metastasis
[ ]	[ ]	N1	Metastasis in a single ipsilateral lymph node, 3 cm or less in greatest dimension
[ ]	[ ]	N2	Metastasis in a single ipsilateral lymph node, more than 3 cm but not more than 6 cm in greatest dimension, or multiple ipsilateral lymph nodes, none more than 6 cm in greatest dimension, or bilateral or contralateral lymph nodes, none more than 6 cm in greatest dimension
[ ]	[ ]	N2a	Metastasis in a single ipsilateral lymph node more than 3 cm but not more than 6 cm in greatest dimension
[ ]	[ ]	N2b	Metastasis in multiple ipsilateral lymph nodes, none more than 6 cm in greatest dimension
[ ]	[ ]	N2c	Metastasis in bilateral or contralateral lymph nodes, none more than 6 cm in greatest dimension
[ ]	[ ]	N3	Metastasis in a lymph node more than 6 cm in greatest dimension
		Distant Metastasis (M)	
[ ]	[ ]	MX	Presence of distant metastasis cannot be assessed
[ ]	[ ]	M0	No distant metastasis
[ ]	[ ]	M1	Distant metastasis

Stage Grouping

Clin	Path				
[ ]	[ ]	0	Tis	N0	M0
[ ]	[ ]	I	T1	N0	M0
[ ]	[ ]	II	T2	N0	M0
[ ]	[ ]	III	T3	N0	M0
			T1	N1	M0
			T2	N1	M0
			T3	N1	M0
[ ]	[ ]	IV	T4	N0	M0
			T4	N1	M0
			Any T	N2	M0
			Any T	N3	M0
			Any T	Any N	M1

Staged by _____ M.D.
_____ Registrar
Date _____

(continued on next page)

American Joint Committee on Cancer—1992

Location of Tumor

[ ] Lips: Upper
       Lower
[ ] Buccal mucosa
[ ] Floor of mouth
[ ] Oral tongue
[ ] Hard palate
[ ] Gingivae: Upper
          Lower
          Retromolar trigone

Characteristics of Tumor

[ ] Exophytic
[ ] Superficial
[ ] Moderately infiltrating
[ ] Deeply infiltrating
[ ] Ulcerated
[ ] Extends to or overlies bone
[ ] Gross erosion of bone
[ ] Radiographic destruction of bone

Involvement of Neighboring Regions

[ ] Tonsillar pillar or soft palate
[ ] Nasal cavity or antrum
[ ] Nasopharynx
[ ] Pterygoid muscles
[ ] Soft tissues or skin of neck

Histopathologic Type

Predominant cancer is squamous cell carcinoma

Histopathologic Grade (G)

[ ] GX   Grade cannot be assessed
[ ] G1   Well differentiated
[ ] G2   Moderately differentiated
[ ] G3   Poorly differentiated
[ ] G4   Undifferentiated

Illustrations

Tumor size: _____cm

Indicate on diagram primary tumor and regional nodes involved.

4

Pharynx (Including Base of Tongue, Soft Palate, and Uvula)

C01.9 Base of tongue, NOS

C05.1 Soft palate, NOS
C05.2 Uvula

C09.0 Tonsillar fossa
C09.1 Tonsillar pillar
C09.8 Overlapping lesion
C09.9 Tonsil, NOS

C10.0 Vallecula
C10.2 Lateral wall of oropharynx
C10.3 Posterior wall of oropharynx
C10.4 Branchial cleft
C10.8 Overlapping lesion
C10.9 Oropharynx, NOS

C11.0 Superior wall of nasopharynx
C11.1 Posterior wall of nasopharynx
C11.2 Lateral wall of nasopharynx
C11.3 Anterior wall of nasopharynx
C11.8 Overlapping lesion
C11.9 Nasopharynx, NOS

C12.9 Pyriform sinus

C13.0 Postcricoid region
C13.1 Hypopharyngeal aspect of aryepiglottic fold
C13.2 Posterior wall of hypopharynx
C13.8 Overlapping lesion
C13.9 Hypopharynx, NOS

C14.0 Pharynx, NOS
C14.1 Laryngopharynx
C14.2 Waldeyer's ring
C14.8 Overlapping lesion of lip, oral cavity, and pharynx

ANATOMY

Primary Sites and Subsites. The pharynx (including base of tongue, soft palate, and uvula) is divided into three regions: oropharynx; nasopharynx; and hypopharynx. Each region is further subdivided into specific sites:

Oropharynx
Nasopharynx
Hypopharynx

Pharyngo-esophageal junction (postcricoid area), extends from the level of the arytenoid cartilages and connecting folds to the inferior border of the cricoid cartilage
Pyriform sinus, extends from the pharyngo-epiglottic fold to the upper end of the esophagus, bounded laterally by the thyroid cartilage and medially by the hypopharyngeal surface of the aryepiglottic fold and the arytenoid and cricoid cartilages
Posterior pharyngeal wall, extends from the level of the floor of the vallecula to the level of the crico-arytenoid joints

Regional Lymph Nodes. These are the cervical lymph nodes, which include:

Internal jugular
  jugulodigastric
  jugulo-omohyoid
  upper deep cervical
  lower deep cervical
Submandibular (submaxillary)
Submental
Retropharyngeal
Cervical, NOS

Some primary sites drain bilaterally.

In clinical evaluation the actual size of the nodal mass should be measured, and allowance should be made for intervening soft tissues. It is recognized that most masses over 3 cm in diameter are not single nodes but are confluent nodes or tumor in soft tissues of the neck. There are three stages of clinically positive nodes: N1, N2, and N3. The use of subgroups a, b, and c is not required but is recommended. Midline nodes are considered homolateral nodes.

Metastatic Sites. Distant spread to the lungs is common; skeletal or hepatic metastases occur less often. Mediastinal lymph node metastases are considered distant metastases.

RULES FOR CLASSIFICATION

Clinical Staging. Clinical staging is generally employed for squamous cell carcinomas of the pharynx because many of these tumors are treated by nonsurgical methods. Assessment is based primarily on inspection by indirect mirror examination and by direct endoscopy. Palpation of sites (when feasible) and neck nodes is essential. Neurologic evaluation of all cranial nerves is required. A variety of imaging procedures, including tomograms, CT scans, and bone scans, are extremely useful in evaluating the extent of disease, particularly for locally advanced tumors. The tumor must be confirmed histologically, and any other data obtained by biopsies may be included.

Pathologic Staging. Pathologic staging requires the use of all information obtained in clinical staging in addition to histologic study of the surgically resected specimen. The surgeon's evaluation of gross unresected residual tumor must also be included.

DEFINITION OF TNM

Primary Tumor (T)

TX   Primary tumor cannot be assessed
T0   No evidence of primary tumor
Tis   Carcinoma *in situ*

Oropharynx

T1   Tumor 2 cm or less in greatest dimension
T2   Tumor more than 2 cm but not more than 4 cm in greatest dimension
T3   Tumor more than 4 cm in greatest dimension
T4   Tumor invades adjacent structures (e.g., through cortical bone, soft tissues of neck, deep [extrinsic] muscle of tongue)

Nasopharynx

T1   Tumor limited to one subsite of nasopharynx (refer to text page 33)
T2   Tumor invades more than one subsite of nasopharynx
T3   Tumor invades nasal cavity and/or oropharynx
T4   Tumor invades skull and/or cranial nerve(s)

Hypopharynx

T1   Tumor limited to one subsite of hypopharynx (refer to text page 33)
T2   Tumor invades more than one subsite of hypopharynx or an adjacent site, without fixation of hemilarynx
T3   Tumor invades more than one subsite of hypopharynx or an adjacent site, with fixation of hemilarynx
T4   Tumor invades adjacent structures (e.g., cartilage or soft tissues of neck)

Regional Lymph Nodes (N)

NX   Regional lymph nodes cannot be assessed
N0   No regional lymph node metastasis
N1   Metastasis in a single ipsilateral lymph node, 3 cm or less in greatest dimension
N2   Metastasis in a single ipsilateral lymph node, more than 3 cm but not more than 6 cm in greatest dimension; or in multiple ipsilateral lymph nodes, none more than 6 cm in greatest dimension; or in bilateral or contralateral lymph nodes, none more than 6 cm in greatest dimension

    N2a   Metastasis in a single ipsilateral lymph node more than 3 cm but not more than 6 cm in greatest dimension
    N2b   Metastasis in multiple ipsilateral lymph nodes, none more than 6 cm in greatest dimension
    N2c   Metastasis in bilateral or contralateral lymph nodes, none more than 6 cm in greatest dimension

N3   Metastasis in a lymph node more than 6 cm in greatest dimension

Distant Metastasis (M)

MX   Presence of distant metastasis cannot be assessed
M0   No distant metastasis
M1   Distant metastasis

STAGE GROUPING

Stage 0	Tis	N0	M0
Stage I	T1	N0	M0
Stage II	T2	N0	M0
Stage III	T3	N0	M0
	T1	N1	M0
	T2	N1	M0
	T3	N1	M0
Stage IV	T4	N0	M0
	T4	N1	M0
	Any T	N2	M0
	Any T	N3	M0
	Any T	Any N	M1

HISTOPATHOLOGIC TYPE

The predominant cancer is squamous cell carcinoma. Pathologic diagnosis is required to use this classification. Other nonepithelial tumors such as those of lymphoid tissue, soft tissue, bone, and cartilage are not included.

HISTOPATHOLOGIC GRADE (G)

GX   Grade cannot be assessed
G1   Well differentiated
G2   Moderately differentiated
G3   Poorly differentiated
G4   Undifferentiated

BIBLIOGRAPHY

1. Barkley HT Jr, Fletcher GT, Jesse RH, et al: Management of cervical lymph node metastases in squamous carcinoma of the tonsillar fossa, base of tongue, supraglottic larynx and hypopharynx. Am J Surg 124:462–467, 1972
2. Futrell JW, Bennett SH, Hoye RC, et al: Predicting survival in cancer of the larynx or hypopharynx. Am J Surg 122:451–457, 1971
3. Garrett PG, Beale FA, Cummings BJ, et al: Cancer of the tonsil: Results of radical radiation therapy with surgery in reserve. Am J Surg 146:432–435, 1983
4. Jesse RH, Sugarbaker EV: Squamous cell carcinoma of the oral pharynx: Why we fail. Am J Surg 132:435–439, 1976
5. Ring AH, Sako K, Razack MS, et al: Nasopharyngeal carcinomas: Results of treatment over a 27 year period. Am J Surg 146:429–431, 1983
6. Shanmugaratnan K: Histological typing of tumors of the upper respiratory tract. WHO International Histological Classification of Tumors, 2nd ed. Berlin-New York, Springer-Verlag, 1991
7. Silver AJ, Mawad ME, Hilal SK, et al: Computed tomography of the nasopharynx and related spaces. Radiology 147:733–738, 1983
8. Wahi PN, et al: Histological typing of oral tumors. WHO International Histological Classification of Tumors. Geneva, WHO, 1971

Data Form for Cancer Staging

Patient identification
Name _____
Address _____
Hospital or clinic number _____
Age _____ Sex _____ Race _____

Institution identification
Hospital or clinic _____
Address _____

Oncology Record

Anatomic site of cancer _____
Histologic type _____
Grade (G) _____
Date of classification _____

Chronology of classification
[ ] Clinical (use all data prior to first treatment)
[ ] Pathologic (if definitively resected specimen available)

DEFINITIONS

Clin	Path		

Primary Tumor (T)

Clin	Path		
[ ]	[ ]	TX	Primary tumor cannot be assessed
[ ]	[ ]	T0	No evidence of primary tumor
[ ]	[ ]	Tis	Carcinoma *in situ*

Oropharynx

Clin	Path		
[ ]	[ ]	T1	Tumor 2 cm or less in greatest dimension
[ ]	[ ]	T2	Tumor more than 2 cm but not more than 4 cm in greatest dimension
[ ]	[ ]	T3	Tumor more than 4 cm in greatest dimension
[ ]	[ ]	T4	Tumor invades adjacent structures, *e.g.*, through cortical bone, soft tissues of neck, deep (extrinsic) muscle of tongue

Nasopharynx

Clin	Path		
[ ]	[ ]	T1	Tumor limited to one subsite of nasopharynx
[ ]	[ ]	T2	Tumor invades more than one subsite of nasopharynx
[ ]	[ ]	T3	Tumor invades nasal cavity and/or oropharynx
[ ]	[ ]	T4	Tumor invades skull and/or cranial nerve(s)

Hypopharynx

Clin	Path		
[ ]	[ ]	T1	Tumor limited to one subsite of hypopharynx
[ ]	[ ]	T2	Tumor invades more than one subsite of hypopharynx or an adjacent site, without fixation of hemilarynx
[ ]	[ ]	T3	Tumor invades more than one subsite of hypopharynx or an adjacent site, with fixation of hemilarynx
[ ]	[ ]	T4	Tumor invades adjacent structures, *e.g.*, cartilage or soft tissues of neck

Lymph Node (N)

Clin	Path		
[ ]	[ ]	NX	Regional lymph nodes cannot be assessed
[ ]	[ ]	N0	No regional lymph node metastasis
[ ]	[ ]	N1	Metastasis in a single ipsilateral lymph node, 3 cm or less in greatest dimension
[ ]	[ ]	N2	Metastasis in a single ipsilateral lymph node, more than 3 cm but not more than 6 cm in greatest dimension, or multiple ipsilateral lymph nodes, none more than 6 cm in greatest dimension, or bilateral or contralateral lymph nodes, none more than 6 cm in greatest dimension
[ ]	[ ]	N2a	Metastasis in a single ipsilateral lymph node more than 3 cm but not more than 6 cm in greatest dimension
[ ]	[ ]	N2b	Metastasis in multiple ipsilateral lymph nodes, none more than 6 cm in greatest dimension
[ ]	[ ]	N2c	Metastasis in bilateral or contralateral lymph nodes, none more than 6 cm in greatest dimension
[ ]	[ ]	N3	Metastasis in a lymph node more than 6 cm in greatest dimension

Distant Metastasis (M)

Clin	Path		
[ ]	[ ]	MX	Presence of distant metastasis cannot be assessed
[ ]	[ ]	M0	No distant metastasis
[ ]	[ ]	M1	Distant metastasis

(continued on next page)

Clin	Path	Stage Grouping			
[ ]	[ ]	0	Tis	N0	M0
[ ]	[ ]	I	T1	N0	M0
[ ]	[ ]	II	T2	N0	M0
[ ]	[ ]	III	T3	N0	M0
			T1	N1	M0
			T2	N1	M0
			T3	N1	M0
[ ]	[ ]	IV	T4	N0	M0
			T4	N1	M0
			Any T	N2	M0
			Any T	N3	M0
			Any T	Any N	M1

Staged by _____ M.D.
_____ Registrar

Date _____

Histopathologic Grade (G)

[ ] GX   Grade cannot be assessed
[ ] G1   Well differentiated
[ ] G2   Moderately differentiated
[ ] G3   Poorly differentiated
[ ] G4   Undifferentiated

Location of Tumor

Oropharynx
[ ]   Faucial arch
[ ]   Tonsillar fossa, tonsil
[ ]   Base of tongue
[ ]   Pharyngeal wall

Nasopharynx
[ ]   Posterosuperior wall
[ ]   Lateral wall

Hypopharynx
[ ]   Piriform fossa
[ ]   Postcricoid area
[ ]   Posterior wall

Characteristics of Tumor

[ ]   Superficial
[ ]   Exophytic
[ ]   Moderate infiltration
[ ]   Deep infiltration

Histopathologic Type

Predominant cancer is squamous cell carcinoma.

Postsurgical Resection—Pathologic Residual Tumor (R)

Does not enter into staging but may be a factor in deciding further treatment
[ ] R0   No residual tumor
[ ] R1   Microscopic residual tumor
[ ] R2   Macroscopic residual tumor
      Specify _____

Illustrations

Size of primary tumor: _____ cm

Regional lymph nodes; illustrate if metastatic.

American Joint Committee on Cancer—1992

5

Larynx

C10.1 Anterior surface of
         epiglottis

C32.0 Glottis
C32.1 Supraglottis
C32.2 Subglottis
C32.3 Laryngeal cartilage
C32.8 Overlapping lesion
C32.9 Larynx, NOS

ANATOMY

Primary Site. The following anatomic definition of larynx allows classification of carcinomas arising in the encompassed mucous membranes but excludes cancers arising on the lateral or posterior pharyngeal wall, pyriform fossa, postcricoid area, and base of the tongue.

The anterior limit of the larynx comprises the anterior or lingual surface of the suprahyoid epiglottis, the thyrohyoid membrane, the anterior commissure, and the anterior wall of the subglottic region, which includes the thyroid cartilage, the cricothyroid membrane, and the anterior arch of the cricoid cartilage.

The posterior and lateral limits include the laryngeal aspect of the arytenoepiglottic folds, the arytenoid region, the interarytenoid space, and the posterior surface of the subglottic space, represented by the mucous membrane covering the cricoid cartilage.

The superolateral limits comprise the tip and the lateral borders of the epiglottis. The inferior limits are made up of the plane passing through the inferior edge of the cricoid cartilage.

For purposes of this clinical-stage classification, the larynx is divided into three regions: supraglottis, glottis, and subglottis. The supraglottis comprises the epiglottis (both its lingual and laryngeal aspects), arytenoepiglottic folds (laryngeal aspect), arytenoids, and ventricular bands (false cords). The inferior boundary of the supraglottis is a horizontal plane passing through the apex of the ventricle. The glottis comprises the true vocal cords, including the anterior and posterior commissures. The lower boundary is the horizontal plane, 1 cm below the apex of the ventricle. The subglottis is the region extending from the lower boundary of the glottis to the lower margin of the cricoid cartilage.

The division of the larynx is summarized in the following table:

Site	Subsite
Supraglottis	Ventricular bands (false cords)
	Arytenoids
	Suprahyoid epiglottis (both lingual and laryngeal aspects)
	Infrahyoid epiglottis
	Arytenoepiglottic folds (laryngeal aspect)
Glottis	True vocal cords including anterior and posterior commissures
Subglottis	Subglottis

Regional Lymph Nodes. These are cervical lymph nodes, which include:

Internal jugular
  jugulodigastric
  jugulo-omohyoid
  upper deep cervical
  lower deep cervical
Anterior cervical
  Prelaryngeal
  Pretracheal
  Paratracheal
  Lateral tracheal (recurrent larengeal)

Submandibular (submaxillary)
Submental
Cervical, NOS

Some primary sites drain bilaterally.

In clinical evaluation, the actual size of the nodal mass should be measured and allowance made for intervening soft tissues. It is recognized that most masses over 3 cm in diameter are not single nodes but rather are confluent nodes or tumor in soft tissues of the neck. There are three stages of clinically positive nodes: N1, N2, and N3. The use of subgroups a, b, and c is not required but is recommended. Midline nodes are considered homolateral nodes.

Metastatic Sites. Distant spread to the lungs is common; skeletal or hepatic metastases occur less often. Mediastinal lymph node metastases are considered distant metastases.

RULES FOR CLASSIFICATION

Clinical Staging. The assessment of the larynx is accomplished primarily by inspection, using both indirect mirror examination and direct laryngoscopy. A variety of imaging procedures are valuable in evaluating the extent of disease, particularly for advanced tumors. These include laryngeal tomograms, CT scans, and MRI scans. Diagnostic ultrasound may help detect destruction of laryngeal cartilages. Palpation of neck nodes to evaluate laryngeal fremitus is essential. The tumor must be confirmed histologically, and any other data obtained by biopsies may be included.

Pathologic Staging. All information used in clinical staging and in histologic studies of the surgically resected specimen is used for pathologic staging. The surgeon's evaluation of gross unresected residual tumor must also be included.

DEFINITION OF TNM

Primary Tumor (T)

TX   Primary tumor cannot be assessed
T0   No evidence of primary tumor
Tis   Carcinoma *in situ*

Supraglottis

T1   Tumor limited to one subsite of the supraglottis with normal vocal cord mobility (refer to text page 39)
T2   Tumor invades more than one subsite of the supraglottis or glottis, with normal vocal cord mobility
T3   Tumor limited to the larynx with vocal cord fixation and/or invades the postcricoid area, medial wall of the pyriform sinus, or pre-epiglottic tissues
T4   Tumor invades through the thyroid cartilage and/or extends to other tissues beyond the larynx (e.g., to the oropharynx or soft tissues of the neck)

Glottis

T1   Tumor limited to the vocal cord(s) (may involve anterior or posterior commissures) with normal mobility
   T1a   Tumor limited to one vocal cord
   T1b   Tumor involves both vocal cords
T2   Tumor extends to the supraglottis and/or subglottis, and/or with impaired vocal cord mobility
T3   Tumor limited to the larynx with vocal cord fixation
T4   Tumor invades through the thyroid cartilage and/or extends to other tissues beyond the larynx (e.g., to the oropharynx or soft tissues of the neck)

Subglottis

T1   Tumor limited to the subglottis
T2   Tumor extends to the vocal cord(s) with normal or impaired mobility
T3   Tumor limited to the larynx with vocal cord fixation
T4   Tumor invades through the cricoid or thyroid cartilage and/or extends to other tissues beyond the larynx (e.g., to the oropharynx or soft tissues of the neck)

Regional Lymph Nodes (N)

NX   Regional lymph nodes cannot be assessed
N0   No regional lymph node metastasis
N1   Metastasis in a single ipsilateral lymph node, 3 cm or less in greatest dimension
N2   Metastasis in a single ipsilateral lymph node, more than 3 cm but not more than 6 cm in greatest dimension; or in multiple ipsilateral lymph nodes, none more than 6 cm in greatest dimension; or in bilateral or contralateral lymph nodes, none more than 6 cm in greatest dimension
   N2a   Metastasis in a single ipsilateral lymph node more than 3 cm but not more than 6 cm in greatest dimension
   N2b   Metastasis in multiple ipsilateral lymph nodes, none more than 6 cm in greatest dimension
   N2c   Metastasis in bilateral or contralateral lymph nodes, none more than 6 cm in greatest dimension
N3   Metastasis in a lymph node more than 6 cm in greatest dimension

Distant Metastasis (M)

MX Presence of distant metastasis cannot be assessed
M0 No distant metastasis
M1 Distant metastasis

STAGE GROUPING

Stage 0	Tis	N0	M0
Stage I	T1	N0	M0
Stage II	T2	N0	M0
Stage III	T3	N0	M0
	T1	N1	M0
	T2	N1	M0
	T3	N1	M0
Stage IV	T4	N0	M0
	T4	N1	M0
	Any T	N2	M0
	Any T	N3	M0
	Any T	Any N	M1

HISTOPATHOLOGIC TYPE

The predominant cancer is squamous cell carcinoma. Pathologic diagnosis is required to use this classification. Tumor grading is recommended, using Broders' classification. Other nonepithelial tumors—such as those of lymphoid tissue, soft tissue, bone, and cartilage—are not included.

HISTOPATHOLOGIC GRADE (G)

GX Grade cannot be assessed
G1 Well differentiated
G2 Moderately differentiated
G3 Poorly differentiated
G4 Undifferentiated

BIBLIOGRAPHY

1. Flynn MB, Jesse RH, Lindberg RT: Surgery and irradiation in the treatment of squamous cell cancer of the supraglottic larynx. Am J Surg 124:477–481, 1972
2. Futrell JW, Bennett SH, Hoye RC, et al: Predicting survival in cancer of the larynx or hypopharynx. Am J Surg 122:451–457, 1971
3. Harris HS, Watson FR, Spratt JS Jr: Carcinoma of the larynx. Am J Surg 118:676–684, 1969
4. Powell RW, Redd BL, Wilkins SA: An evaluation of treatment of cancer of the larynx. Am J Surg 10:635–643, 1965
5. Shah JP, Tollefson HR: Epidermoid carcinoma of the supraglottic larynx: Role of neck dissection in initial surgical treatment. Am J Surg 128:494–499, 1974
6. Shaha AR and Shah JP: Carcinoma of the supraglottic larynx. Am J Surg 144:456–458, 1982
7. Shanmugaratnam K: Histological typing of tumors of the upper respiratory tract. WHO International Histological Classification of Tumors, 2nd ed. Berlin-New York, Springer-Verlag, 1991
8. Wahi PN, et al: Histological typing of oral tumors. WHO International Histological Classification of Tumors. Geneva, WHO, 1971
9. Wang CC, Schultz MD, Miller D: Combined radiation therapy and surgery for carcinoma of the supraglottis and pyriform sinus. Am J Surg 124:551–554, 1972

Data Form for Cancer Staging

Patient identification
Name _____
Address _____
Hospital or clinic number _____
Age _____ Sex _____ Race _____

Institution identification
Hospital or clinic _____
Address _____

Oncology Record

Anatomic site of cancer _____
Histologic type _____
Grade (G) _____
Date of classification _____

Chronology of classification
[　]　Clinical (use all data prior to first treatment)
[　]　Pathologic (if definitively resected specimen available)

Clin	Path		
		DEFINITIONS	
		Primary Tumor (T)	
[ ]	[ ]	TX	Primary tumor cannot be assessed
[ ]	[ ]	T0	No evidence of primary tumor
[ ]	[ ]	Tis	Carcinoma *in situ*
		Supraglottis	
[ ]	[ ]	T1	Tumor limited to one subsite of supraglottis with normal vocal cord mobility
[ ]	[ ]	T2	Tumor invades more than one subsite of supraglottis or glottis, with normal vocal cord mobility
[ ]	[ ]	T3	Tumor limited to larynx with vocal cord fixation and/or invades postcricoid area, medial wall of piriform sinus, or pre-epiglottic tissues
[ ]	[ ]	T4	Tumor invades through thyroid cartilage, and/or extends to other tissues beyond the larynx, *e.g.*, to oropharynx, soft tissues of neck
		Glottis	
[ ]	[ ]	T1	Tumor limited to vocal cord(s) (may involve anterior or posterior commissures) with normal mobility
[ ]	[ ]	T1a	Tumor limited to one vocal cord
[ ]	[ ]	T1b	Tumor involves both vocal cords
[ ]	[ ]	T2	Tumor extends to supraglottis and/or subglottis, and/or with impaired vocal cord mobility
[ ]	[ ]	T3	Tumor limited to the larynx with vocal cord fixation
[ ]	[ ]	T4	Tumor invades through thyroid cartilage and/or extends to other tissues beyond the larynx, *e.g.*, oropharynx, soft tissues of neck
		Subglottis	
[ ]	[ ]	T1	Tumor limited to the subglottis
[ ]	[ ]	T2	Tumor extends to vocal cord(s) with normal or impaired mobility
[ ]	[ ]	T3	Tumor limited to larynx with vocal cord fixation
[ ]	[ ]	T4	Tumor invades through cricoid or thyroid cartilage and/or extends to other tissues beyond the larynx, *e.g.*, oropharynx, soft tissues of neck
		Lymph Node (N)	
[ ]	[ ]	NX	Regional lymph nodes cannot be assessed
[ ]	[ ]	N0	No regional lymph node metastasis
[ ]	[ ]	N1	Metastasis in a single ipsilateral lymph node, 3 cm or less in greatest dimension
[ ]	[ ]	N2	Metastasis in a single ipsilateral lymph node, more than 3 cm but not more than 6 cm in greatest dimension, or multiple ipsilateral lymph nodes, none more than 6 cm in greatest dimension, or bilateral or contralateral lymph nodes, none more than 6 cm in greatest dimension
[ ]	[ ]	N2a	Metastasis in a single ipsilateral lymph node more than 3 cm but not more than 6 cm in greatest dimension
[ ]	[ ]	N2b	Metastasis in multiple ipsilateral lymph nodes, none more than 6 cm in greatest dimension
[ ]	[ ]	N2c	Metastasis in bilateral or contralateral lymph nodes, none more than 6 cm in greatest dimension
[ ]	[ ]	N3	Metastasis in a lymph node more than 6 cm in greatest dimension
		Distant Metastasis (M)	
[ ]	[ ]	MX	Presence of distant metastasis cannot be assessed
[ ]	[ ]	M0	No distant metastasis
[ ]	[ ]	M1	Distant metastasis

(continued on next page)

Clin	Path	Stage Grouping			
[ ]	[ ]	0	Tis	N0	M0
[ ]	[ ]	I	T1	N0	M0
[ ]	[ ]	II	T2	N0	M0
[ ]	[ ]	III	T3	N0	M0
			T1	N1	M0
			T2	N1	M0
			T3	N1	M0
[ ]	[ ]	IV	T4	N0	M0
			T4	N1	M0
			Any T	N2	M0
			Any T	N3	M0
			Any T	Any N	M1

Staged by _____ M.D.

_____ Registrar

Date _____

Histopathologic Type

The predominant cancer is squamous cell carcinoma.

Histopathologic Grade (G)

[ ] GX   Grade cannot be assessed
[ ] G1   Well differentiated
[ ] G2   Moderately differentiated
[ ] G3   Poorly differentiated
[ ] G4   Undifferentiated

Illustrations

Indicate on diagram primary tumor and regional nodes involved.

Indicate size and location of primary tumor.

American Joint Committee on Cancer—1992

6

Maxillary Sinus

C31.0 Maxillary sinus

ANATOMY

Primary Site. Cancer of the maxillary sinus is the most common of the paranasal sinus cancers; it is the only site to which the following classification applies. The ethmoid sinuses and nasal cavity may ultimately be defined similarly with further study. Tumors of the sphenoid and frontal sinuses are so rare as to not warrant staging.

Ohngren's line, a theoretic plane joining the medical canthus of the eye with the angle of the mandible, may be used to divide the maxillary antrum into the anteroinferior portion (the infrastructure) and the superoposterior portion (the suprastructure).

Regional Lymph Nodes. These are the cervical lymph nodes, which include:

Internal jugular
    Jugulodigastric
    Jugulo-omohyoid
    Upper deep cervical
    Lower deep cervical
Submandibular (submaxillary)
Submental
Retropharyngeal
Cervical, NOS

Some primary sites drain bilaterally.

In clinical evaluation, the actual size of the nodal mass should be measured and allowance made for intervening soft tissues. It is recognized that most masses over 3 cm in diameter are not single nodes but are confluent nodes or tumor in soft tissues of the neck. There are three stages of clinically positive nodes: N1, N2, and N3. The use of subgroups a, b, and c is not required but is recommended. Midline nodes are considered homolateral nodes.

Metastatic Sites. Distant spread to lungs is most common; occasionally there is spread to bone and remote lymph nodes.

RULES FOR CLASSIFICATION

Clinical Staging. The assessment of primary maxillary antrum tumors is based on inspection and palpation of the orbit, nasal and oral cavities, and nasopharynx and on neurologic evaluation of the cranial nerves. Radiographic studies include plane films and tomograms for evaluation of bone destruction. Neck nodes are assessed by palpation. Examination for distant metastases includes chest film, blood chemistries, blood count, and other routine studies as indicated.

Pathologic Staging. Complete resection of primary sites and major nodal dissections allow the use of this designation. Specimens resected after radiation or chemotherapy need to be noted especially.

DEFINITION OF TNM

Primary Tumor (T)

TX   Primary tumor cannot be assessed

T0   No evidence of primary tumor

Tis   Carcinoma *in situ*

T1   Tumor limited to the antral mucosa with no erosion or destruction of bone

T2   Tumor with erosion or destruction of the infrastructure (see anatomic division, above), including the hard palate and/or the middle nasal meatus

T3   Tumor invades any of the following: skin of cheek, posterior wall of maxillary sinus, floor or medial wall of orbit, anterior ethmoid sinus

T4   Tumor invades orbital contents and/or any of the following: cribriform plate, posterior ethmoid or sphenoid sinuses, nasopharynx, soft palate, pterygomaxillary or temporal fossae, or base of skull

Regional Lymph Nodes (N)

NX   Regional lymph nodes cannot be assessed
N0   No regional lymph node metastasis
N1   Metastasis in a single ipsilateral lymph node, 3 cm or less in greatest dimension
N2   Metastasis in a single ipsilateral lymph node, more than 3 cm but not more than 6 cm in greatest dimension; or in multiple ipsilateral lymph nodes, none more than 6 cm in greatest dimension; or in bilateral or contralateral lymph nodes, none more than 6 cm in greatest dimension

    N2a   Metastasis in a single ipsilateral lymph node more than 3 cm but not more than 6 cm in greatest dimension

    N2b   Metastasis in multiple ipsilateral lymph nodes, none more than 6 cm in greatest dimension

    N2c   Metastasis in bilateral or contralateral lymph nodes, none more than 6 cm in greatest dimension

N3   Metastasis in a lymph node more than 6 cm in greatest dimension

Distant Metastasis (M)

MX   Presence of distant metastases cannot be assessed
M0   No distant metastasis
M1   Distant metastasis

STAGE GROUPING

Stage 0	Tis	N0	M0
Stage I	T1	N0	M0
Stage II	T2	N0	M0
Stage III	T3	N0	M0
	T1	N1	M0
	T2	N1	M0
	T3	N1	M0
Stage IV	T4	N0	M0
	T4	N1	M0
	Any T	N2	M0
	Any T	N3	M0
	Any T	Any N	M1

HISTOPATHOLOGIC TYPE

The predominant cancer is squamous cell carcinoma. Pathologic diagnosis is required to use this classification. Tumor grading is recommended, using Broders' classification. Other nonepithelial tumors—such as those of lymphoid tissue, soft tissue, bone, and cartilage—are not included.

HISTOPATHOLOGIC GRADE (G)

GX   Grade cannot be assessed
G1   Well differentiated
G2   Moderately differentiated
G3   Poorly differentiated
G4   Undifferentiated

BIBLIOGRAPHY

1. Goepfert H, Jesse RH, Lindberg RD: Arterial infusion and radiation therapy in the treatment of advanced cancer of the nasal cavity and perinasal sinuses. Am J Surg 126:464–468, 1973
2. Jesse RH: Preoperative versus postoperative radiation in the treatment of squamous carcinoma of the perinasal sinuses. Am J Surg 110:552–556, 1965
3. Shanmugaratnam K: Histological typing of tumors of the upper respiratory tract. WHO International Histological Classification of Tumors, 2nd ed. Berlin-New York, Springer-Verlag, 1991
4. Sisson GA, Johnson NE, Ammiri CS: Cancer of the maxillary sinus: Clinical classification and management. Ann Otol Rhinol Laryngol 72:1050–1059, 1963
5. Wahi PN, et al: Histological typing of oral tumors. WHO International Histological Classification of Tumors. Geneva, WHO, 1971

Data Form for Cancer Staging

Patient identification
Name _____
Address _____
Hospital or clinic number _____
Age _____ Sex _____ Race _____

Institution identification
Hospital or clinic _____
Address _____

Oncology Record

Anatomic site of cancer _____
Histologic type _____
Grade (G) _____
Date of classification _____

Chronology of classification
[   ]   Clinical (use all data prior to first treatment)
[   ]   Pathologic (if definitively resected specimen available)

DEFINITIONS

Primary Tumor (T)

Clin	Path		
[ ]	[ ]	TX	Primary tumor cannot be assessed
[ ]	[ ]	T0	No evidence of primary tumor
[ ]	[ ]	Tis	Carcinoma *in situ*
[ ]	[ ]	T1	Tumor limited to the antral mucosa with no erosion or destruction of bone
[ ]	[ ]	T2	Tumor with erosion or destruction of the infrastructure including the hard palate and/or the middle nasal meatus
[ ]	[ ]	T3	Tumor invades any of the following: skin of cheek, posterior wall of the maxillary sinus, floor or medial wall of orbit, anterior ethmoid sinus
[ ]	[ ]	T4	Tumor invades orbital contents and/or any of the following: cribriform plate, posterior ethmoid or sphenoid sinuses, nasopharynx, soft palate, pterygomaxillary or temporal fossae or base of skull

Lymph Node (N)

Clin	Path		
[ ]	[ ]	NX	Regional lymph nodes cannot be assessed
[ ]	[ ]	N0	No regional lymph node metastasis
[ ]	[ ]	N1	Metastasis in a single ipsilateral lymph node, 3 cm or less in greatest dimension
[ ]	[ ]	N2	Metastasis in a single ipsilateral lymph node, more than 3 cm but not more than 6 cm in greatest dimension, or multiple ipsilateral lymph nodes, none more than 6 cm in greatest dimension, or bilateral or contralateral lymph nodes, none more than 6 cm in greatest dimension
[ ]	[ ]	N2a	Metastasis in a single ipsilateral lymph node more than 3 cm but not more than 6 cm in greatest dimension
[ ]	[ ]	N2b	Metastasis in multiple ipsilateral lymph nodes, none more than 6 cm in greatest dimension
[ ]	[ ]	N2c	Metastasis in bilateral or contralateral lymph nodes, none more than 6 cm in greatest dimension
[ ]	[ ]	N3	Metastasis in a lymph node more than 6 cm in greatest dimension

Distant Metastasis (M)

Clin	Path		
[ ]	[ ]	MX	Presence of distant metastasis cannot be assessed
[ ]	[ ]	M0	No distant metastasis
[ ]	[ ]	M1	Distant metastasis

Stage Grouping

Clin	Path				
[ ]	[ ]	0	Tis	N0	M0
[ ]	[ ]	I	T1	N0	M0
[ ]	[ ]	II	T2	N0	M0
[ ]	[ ]	III	T3	N0	M0
			T1	N1	M0
			T2	N1	M0
			T3	N1	M0
[ ]	[ ]	IV	T4	N0	M0
			T4	N1	M0
			Any T	N2	M0
			Any T	N3	M0
			Any T	Any N	M1

Staged by _____ M.D.
_____ Registrar
Date _____

(continued on next page)

American Joint Committee on Cancer—1992

Location of Tumor

[　] Antrum
  [　] Infrastructure
  [　] Suprastructure
  [　] Both
[　] Nasal Cavity
  [　] Septum
  [　] Root
  [　] Lateral wall
  [　] Floor
[　] Ethmoid
  [　] Anterior
  [　] Posterior
[　] Sphenoid
[　] Frontal

Histopathologic Type

Predominant cancer is squamous cell or undifferentiated carcinoma. Adenocarcinoma and other cellular types also occur.

Histopathologic Grade (G)

[　] GX   Grade cannot be assessed
[　] G1   Well differentiated
[　] G2   Moderately differentiated
[　] G3   Poorly differentiated
[　] G4   Undifferentiated

Illustrations

Indicate on diagram primary tumor and regional nodes involved.

7

Salivary Glands—Parotid, Submandibular, and Sublingual

C07.9 Parotid gland

C08.0 Submandibular gland
     (submaxillary)
C08.1 Sublingual gland
C08.8 Overlapping lesion
C08.9 Major salivary gland, NOS

This staging system is based on an extensive retrospective study of malignant tumors of the major salivary glands collected from 11 participating United States and Canadian institutions. Statistical analysis of the data revealed that numerous factors affected patient survival, including the histologic diagnosis; cellular differentiation of the tumor; tumor site, size, degree of fixation, or local extension; and nerve involvement. The status of regional lymph nodes and of distant metastases were also of major significance. The classification proposed herein involves only four clinical variables: tumor size, local extension of the tumor, the palpability and suspicion of nodes, and the presence or absence of distant metastasis. It offers a simple but effective and accurate method of evaluating the stage of salivary gland cancer.

ANATOMY

Primary Site. The major salivary glands include the parotid, submandibular (submaxillary), and sublingual glands. Tumors arising in minor salivary glands (mucus-secreting glands in the lining membrane of the upper aerodigestive tract) are included at the anatomic site of origin (e.g., lip).

Regional Lymph Nodes. These are the cervical nodes, which include:

Parotid
Submandibular (submaxillary)
Submental

Deep cervical
Cervical, NOS

Other lymph node metastases are distant metastases.

Metastatic Sites. Distant spread is most frequently to the lungs.

RULES FOR CLASSIFICATION

Clinical Staging. The assessment of primary tumor includes inspection and palpation and neurologic evaluation of the seventh cranial or other nerves. Radiologic studies may include films of the mandible and possibly sialograms.

Pathologic Staging. The surgical pathology report and all other available data should be used to assign a pathologic classification to those patients who have a resection of the cancer.

DEFINITION OF TNM

Primary Tumor (T)

TX   Primary tumor cannot be assessed
T0   No evidence of primary tumor
T1   Tumor 2 cm or less in greatest dimension
T2   Tumor more than 2 cm but not more than 4 cm in greatest dimension
T3   Tumor more than 4 cm but not more than 6 cm in greatest dimension
T4   Tumor more than 6 cm in greatest dimension

Note: All categories are subdivided: (a) no local extension; (b) local extension. Local extension is clinical or macroscopic evidence of invasion of skin, soft tissues, bone, or nerve. Microscopic evidence alone is not local extension for classification purposes.

Regional Lymph Nodes (N)

NX   Regional lymph nodes cannot be assessed
N0   No regional lymph node metastasis
N1   Metastasis in a single ipsilateral lymph node, 3 cm or less in greatest dimension
N2   Metastasis in a single ipsilateral lymph node, more than 3 cm but not more than 6 cm in greatest dimension; or in multiple ipsilateral lymph nodes, none more than 6 cm in greatest dimension; or in bilateral or contralateral lymph nodes, none more than 6 cm in greatest dimension

    N2a   Metastasis in a single ipsilateral lymph node more than 3 cm but not more than 6 cm in greatest dimension
    N2b   Metastasis in multiple ipsilateral lymph nodes, none more than 6 cm in greatest dimension
    N2c   Metastasis in bilateral or contralateral lymph nodes, none more than 6 cm in greatest dimension

N3   Metastasis in a lymph node more than 6 cm in greatest dimension

Distant Metastasis (M)

MX   Presence of distant metastasis cannot be assessed
M0   No distant metastases
M1   Distant metastasis

STAGE GROUPING

Stage	T	N	M
Stage I	T1a	N0	M0
	T2a	N0	M0
Stage II	T1b	N0	M0
	T2b	N0	M0
	T3a	N0	M0
Stage III	T3b	N0	M0
	T4a	N0	M0
	Any T	N1	M0 (except T4b)
Stage IV	T4b	Any N	M0
	Any T	N2	M0
	Any T	N3	M0
	Any T	Any N	M1

HISTOPATHOLOGIC TYPE

The histologic types are:

Acinic (acinar) cell carcinoma
Adenoid cystic carcinoma (cylindroma)
Adenocarcinoma
Squamous cell carcinoma
Carcinoma in pleomorphic adenoma (malignant mixed tumor)
Mucoepidermoid carcinoma
    Well differentiated (low grade)
    Poorly differentiated (high grade)
Other

HISTOPATHOLOGIC GRADE (G)

GX   Grade cannot be assessed
G1   Well differentiated
G2   Moderately differentiated
G3   Poorly differentiated
G4   Undifferentiated

BIBLIOGRAPHY

1. Seifert G, et al: Histological typing of salivary gland tumors. WHO International Histological Classification of Tumors, 2nd ed. Berlin-New York, Springer-Verlag, 1991

SALIVARY GLANDS

Data Form for Cancer Staging

Patient identification
Name _____
Address _____
Hospital or clinic number _____
Age _____ Sex _____ Race _____

Institution identification
Hospital or clinic _____
Address _____

Oncology Record

Anatomic site of cancer _____
Histologic type _____
Grade (G) _____
Date of classification _____

Chronology of classification
[ ] Clinical (use all data prior to first treatment)
[ ] Pathologic (if definitively resected specimen available)

DEFINITIONS

Primary Tumor (T)

Clin	Path		
[ ]	[ ]	TX	Primary tumor cannot be assessed
[ ]	[ ]	T0	No evidence of primary tumor
[ ]	[ ]	T1	Tumor 2 cm or less in greatest dimension
[ ]	[ ]	T2	Tumor more than 2 cm but not more than 4 cm in greatest dimension
[ ]	[ ]	T3	Tumor more than 4 cm but not more than 6 cm in greatest dimension
[ ]	[ ]	T4	Tumor more than 6 cm in greatest dimension

Lymph Node (N)

Clin	Path		
[ ]	[ ]	NX	Regional lymph nodes cannot be assessed
[ ]	[ ]	N0	No regional lymph node metastasis
[ ]	[ ]	N1	Metastasis in a single ipsilateral lymph node, 3 cm or less in greatest dimension
[ ]	[ ]	N2	Metastasis in a single ipsilateral lymph node, more than 3 cm but not more than 6 cm in greatest dimension, or in multiple ipsilateral lymph nodes, none more than 6 cm in greatest dimension or in bilateral or in contralateral lymph nodes, none more than 6 cm in greatest dimension
[ ]	[ ]	N2a	Metastasis in a single ipsilateral lymph node more than 3 cm but not more than 6 cm in greatest dimension
[ ]	[ ]	N2b	Metastasis in multiple ipsilateral lymph nodes, none more than 6 cm in greatest dimension
[ ]	[ ]	N2c	Metastasis in bilateral or contralateral lymph nodes, none more than 6 cm in greatest dimension
[ ]	[ ]	N3	Metastasis in a lymph node more than 6 cm in greatest dimension

Distant Metastasis (M)

Clin	Path		
[ ]	[ ]	MX	Presence of distant metastasis cannot be assessed
[ ]	[ ]	M0	No distant metastasis
[ ]	[ ]	M1	Distant metastasis

Stage Grouping

Clin	Path				
[ ]	[ ]	I	T1a	N0	M0
[ ]	[ ]		T2a	N0	M0
[ ]	[ ]	II	T1b	N0	M0
[ ]	[ ]		T2b	N0	M0
[ ]	[ ]		T3a	N0	M0
[ ]	[ ]	III	T3b	N0	M0
			T4a	N0	M0
			Any T (except T4b)	N1	M0
[ ]	[ ]	IV	T4b	Any N	M0
			Any T	N2	M0
			Any T	N3	M0
			Any T	Any N	M1

Staged by _____ M.D.
_____ Registrar
Date _____

(continued on next page)

American Joint Committee on Cancer—1992

Histopathologic Grade (G)

[ ] GX   Grade cannot be assessed
[ ] G1   Well differentiated
[ ] G2   Moderately differentiated
[ ] G3   Poorly differentiated
[ ] G4   Undifferentiated

Histopathologic Type

The histologic classification recommended is a modification of the WHO classification of salivary gland tumors. The major malignant varieties include the following:

Acinic cell carcinoma
Adenoid cystic carcinoma (cylindroma)
Adenocarcinoma
Squamous cell carcinoma
Carcinoma in pleomorphic adenoma (malignant mixed tumor)
Mucoepidermoid carcinoma
    Well differentiated (low grade)
    Poorly differentiated (high grade)
Other

Other data that might be pertinent to the biologic behavior of the tumor.

_____
_____
_____
_____

Illustration

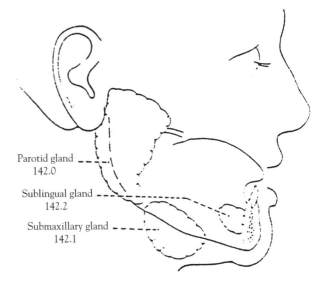

Parotid gland 142.0
Sublingual gland 142.2
Submaxillary gland 142.1

8

Thyroid Gland

C73.9 Thyroid gland

The following staging system for cancer of the thyroid gland was developed after an analysis of more than 1,000 case protocols. Although staging for cancers in other head and neck sites is based entirely on the anatomic extent of disease, it is not possible to follow this pattern for the unique group of malignant tumors that arise in the thyroid. Both the histologic diagnosis and the age of the patient are of such importance in the behavior and prognosis of thyroid cancer that these factors are included in this staging system.

ANATOMY

Primary Site. The thyroid gland ordinarily comprises a right and a left lobe lying adjacent and lateral to the upper trachea and esophagus. An isthmus connects the two lobes, and in some cases a pyramidal lobe is present, extending upward anterior to the thyroid cartilage.

Regional Lymph Nodes. Regional lymph nodes include:

Jugular (upper, middle, lower)
Pretracheal (delphian)
Lateral tracheal
Tracheoesophageal (posterior mediastinal)
Cervical, NOS
Retropharyngeal
Upper anterior mediastinal

Metastatic Sites. Distant spread occurs by contiguous lymphatic or hematogenous routes (e.g., to lungs and bones), but many other sites may be involved.

RULES FOR CLASSIFICATION

Clinical Staging. The assessment of a thyroid tumor depends on inspection and palpation of the thyroid gland and regional lymph nodes in the neck. Indirect laryngoscopy to evaluate vocal cord motion is important. Various imaging procedures can provide additional useful information. These include radioisotope thyroid scans, CT scans, MRI scans, and ultrasound examinations. The diagnosis of thyroid cancer must be confirmed by needle biopsy or open biopsy of the tumor. Further information for clinical staging may be obtained by biopsy of lymph nodes or other areas of suspected local or distant spread. All information available before first treatment should be used.

Pathologic Staging. All available clinical data are combined with pathologic study of the surgically resected specimen for pathologic staging. The surgeon's evaluation of gross unresected residual tumor must be included.

DEFINITION OF TNM

Primary Tumor (T)

Note: All categories may be subdivided: (a) solitary tumor, (b) multifocal tumor (the largest determines the classification).

TX Primary tumor cannot be assessed
T0 No evidence of primary tumor
T1 Tumor 1 cm or less in greatest dimension limited to the thyroid
T2 Tumor more than 1 cm but not more than 4 cm in greatest dimension limited to the thyroid
T3 Tumor more than 4 cm in greatest dimension limited to the thyroid
T4 Tumor of any size extending beyond the thyroid capsule

Regional Lymph Nodes (N)

Regional lymph nodes are the cervical and upper mediastinal lymph nodes.

NX Regional lymph nodes cannot be assessed
N0 No regional lymph node metastasis
N1 Regional lymph node metastasis
    N1a Metastasis in ipsilateral cervical lymph node(s)
    N1b Metastasis in bilateral, midline, or contralateral cervical or mediastinal lymph node(s)

Distant Metastasis (M)

MX   Presence of distant metastasis cannot be assessed
M0   No distant metastasis
M1   Distant metastasis

STAGE GROUPING

Separate stage groupings are recommended for papillary and follicular, medullary, and undifferentiated.

Papillary or Follicular

	UNDER 45 YEARS	45 YEARS AND OLDER
Stage I	Any T, Any N, M0	T1, N0, M0
Stage II	Any T, Any N, M1	T2, N0, M0
		T3, N0, M0
Stage III		T4, N0, M0
		Any T, N1, M0
Stage IV		Any T, Any N, M1

Medullary

Stage I	T1	N0	M0
Stage II	T2	N0	M0
	T3	N0	M0
	T4	N0	M0
Stage III	Any T	N1	M0
Stage IV	Any T	Any N	M1

Undifferentiated

All cases are stage IV.

Stage IV	Any T	Any N	Any M

HISTOPATHOLOGIC TYPE

Histopathologic types include four major areas:

Papillary carcinoma (including those with follicular foci)
Follicular carcinoma
Medullary carcinoma
Undifferentiated (anaplastic) carcinoma

BIBLIOGRAPHY

1. Bengtsson A, Malmaeus J, Grimelius L, et al: Measurement of nuclear DNA content in thyroid diagnosis. World J Surg 8:481–486, 1984
2. Cady B, Sedgwick CE, Meissner WA, et al: Changing clinical pathologic, therapeutic and survival patterns in differentiated thyroid carcinoma. Ann Surg 184:541–553, 1976
3. Cohn K, Blackdahl M, Forsslund G, et al: Prognostic value of nuclear DNA content in papillary thyroid carcinoma. World J Surg 8:474–480, 1984
4. Franssila KO: Prognosis in thyroid carcinoma. Cancer 36:1138–1146, 1975
5. Halnan KE: Influence of age and sex on incidence and prognosis of thyroid cancer: Three hundred forty-four cases followed for ten years. Cancer 19:1534–1536, 1966
6. Hedinger C, et al: Histological typing of thyroid tumors. WHO International Histological Classification of Tumors, 2nd ed. Berlin-New York, Springer-Verlag, 1988
7. Heitz P, Moser H, Staub JJ: Thyroid cancer: A study of 573 thyroid tumors and 161 autopsy cases observed over a thirty-year period. Cancer 37:2329–2337, 1976
8. Mazzaferri E, Young R: Papillary thyroid carcinoma. A ten year report of the impact of therapy in five hundred and seventy-six patients. Am J Med 70:511–517, 1981
9. Russell MA, Gilbert EF, Jaeschke WF: Prognostic features of thyroid cancer: A long-term followup of 68 cases. Cancer 36:553–559, 1975
10. Woolner LB, Beahrs OH, Black BM, et al: Thyroid carcinoma: General considerations and follow-up data on 1181 cases. In Thyroid Neoplasia, Proceedings of the 2nd Imperial Cancer Research Fund Symposium, pp 51–79. London, Academic Press, 1968

Data Form for Cancer Staging

Patient identification
Name _____
Address _____
Hospital or clinic number _____
Age _____ Sex _____ Race _____

Institution identification
Hospital or clinic _____
Address _____

Oncology Record

Anatomic site of cancer _____
Histologic type _____
Grade (G) _____
Date of classification _____

Chronology of classification
[ ] Clinical (use all data prior to first treatment)
[ ] Pathologic (if definitively resected specimen available)

DEFINITIONS

Primary Tumor (T)

All categories may be subdivided: (a) solitary; (b) multifocal—measure the largest for classification

Clin	Path		
[ ]	[ ]	TX	Primary tumor cannot be assessed
[ ]	[ ]	T0	No evidence of primary tumor
[ ]	[ ]	T1	Tumor 1 cm or less in greatest dimension limited to the thyroid
[ ]	[ ]	T2	Tumor more than 1 cm but not more than 4 cm
[ ]	[ ]	T3	Tumor more than 4 cm in greatest dimension limited to the thyroid
[ ]	[ ]	T4	Tumor of any size extending beyond the thyroid capsule

Lymph Node (N)

Regional nodes are the cervical and upper mediastinal lymph nodes

Clin	Path		
[ ]	[ ]	NX	Regional lymph nodes cannot be assessed
[ ]	[ ]	N0	No regional lymph node metastasis
[ ]	[ ]	N1	Regional lymph node metastasis
[ ]	[ ]	N1a	Metastasis in ipsilateral cervical lymph nodes
[ ]	[ ]	N1b	Metastasis in bilateral, midline, or contralateral cervical or mediastinal lymph nodes

Distant Metastasis (M)

Clin	Path		
[ ]	[ ]	MX	Presence of distant metastasis cannot be assessed
[ ]	[ ]	M0	No distant metastasis
[ ]	[ ]	M1	Distant metastasis

Stage Grouping

Separate stage groupings are recommended for papillary and follicular, medullary, and undifferentiated

Papillary or Follicular

Under 45 Years

Clin	Path		
[ ]	[ ]	Stage I	Any T, Any N, M0
[ ]	[ ]	Stage II	Any T, Any N, M1

45 Years and Over

Clin	Path		
[ ]	[ ]	Stage I	T1, N0, M0
[ ]	[ ]	Stage II	T2, N0, M0
			T3, N0, M0
[ ]	[ ]	Stage III	T4, N0, M0
			Any T, N1, M0
[ ]	[ ]	Stage IV	Any T, Any N, M1

Medullary

Clin	Path				
[ ]	[ ]	Stage I	T1	N0	M0
[ ]	[ ]	Stage II	T2	N0	M0
			T3	N0	M0
			T4	N0	M0
[ ]	[ ]	Stage III	Any T	N1	M0
[ ]	[ ]	Stage IV	Any T	Any N	M1

Undifferentiated

All cases are Stage IV

Clin	Path				
[ ]	[ ]	Stage IV	Any T	Any N	Any M

Staged by _____ M.D.
_____ Registrar
Date _____

(continued on next page)
American Joint Committee on Cancer—1992

Nodal Involvement

Cervical unilateral _____
Cervical bilateral _____
Delphian _____
Mediastinal _____

Indicate on diagram primary tumor and regional nodes involved.

Histopathologic Type

The World Health Organization (WHO) classification of thyroid cancer should be used, including at least the four major types:

Papillary carcinoma (with or without follicular foci)
Follicular carcinoma (extent of invasion of tumor capsule should be noted)
Medullary carcinoma
Undifferentiated (anaplastic) carcinoma
Unclassified malignant tumor

Illustrations

Tumor size ___ cm (greatest diameter). Indicate node(s) considered metastatic.

DIGESTIVE SYSTEM

9

Esophagus

C15.0 Cervical
C15.1 Thoracic
C15.2 Abdominal
C15.3 Upper third
C15.4 Middle third
C15.5 Lower third
C15.8 Overlapping lesion
C15.9 Esophagus, NOS

Occurring more often in males, cancers of the esophagus account for only 4% of all malignant tumors in the United States. Predisposing factors include high alcohol intake and heavy use of tobacco. The disease may be difficult to diagnose in its early stages. Most cancers arise in the middle or lower third of the esophagus. Squamous cell carcinomas account for more than 90% of all esophageal cancers. These tumors may extend over wide areas of the mucosal surface. Only the depth of penetration, however, is considered in staging. Adenocarcinomas, which account for less than 10% of all esophageal cancers, are usually found in the distal esophagus. Dysphagia is the most common clinical symptom.

ANATOMY

Primary Site. Beginning at the hypopharynx, the esophagus lies posterior to the trachea and the heart, passing through the posterior mediastinum and entering the stomach through an opening in the diaphragm called the hiatus.

Histologically, the esophagus has four layers: mucosa, submucosa, muscle coat or muscularis propria, and adventitia. There is no serosa.

For classification, staging, and reporting of cancer, the esophagus is divided into four regions. Because the behavior of esophageal cancer and its treatment vary with the anatomic divisions, these regions should be recorded and reported separately. The location of the esophageal cancer is often measured from the incisors (front teeth).

Cervical esophagus: The cervical esophagus begins at the lower border of the cricoid cartilage and ends at the thoracic inlet (the suprasternal notch), approximately 18 cm from the upper incisor teeth.

Intrathoracic esophagus:

Upper thoracic portion: This portion extends from the thoracic inlet to the level of the tracheal bifurcation, approximately 24 cm from the upper incisor teeth.

Midthoracic portion: This is the proximal half of the esophagus between the tracheal bifurcation and the esophagogastric junction. The lower level is approximately 32 cm from the upper incisor teeth.

Lower thoracic portion: Approximately 8 cm long, the lower thoracic portion (which includes the abdominal esophagus) is the distal half of the esophagus between the tracheal bifurcation and the esophagogastric junction. It is approximately 40 cm from the upper incisor teeth.

Regional Lymph Nodes

Specific regional lymph nodes are listed as follows:

Cervical esophagus:
Scalene
Internal jugular
Upper cervical
Periesophageal
Supraclavicular
Cervical, NOS

Intrathoracic esophagus—upper, middle, and lower:
Internal jugular
Tracheobronchial
Superior mediastinal

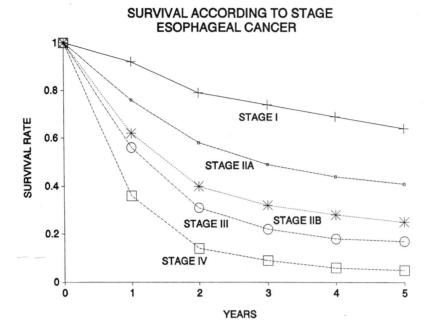

Figure 9-1. Survival according to the stage of disease. Data taken from Iizuka, et al. Chart represents 5,071 patients

Nodes (cont.)
    Peritracheal
    Perigastric (excluding celiac)
    Carinal
    Hilar (pulmonary roots)
    Periesophageal
    Left gastric
    Cardiac
    Nodes of lesser curvature of stomach
    Mediastinal, NOS

Involvement of more distant nodes is considered distant metastasis.

The listing of specific lymph nodes for each region includes those lying within the defined boundaries for that region. For example, the supraclavicular, and periesophageal nodes superior to the thoracic inlet would be considered regional for tumors located in the cervical esophagus, but distant metastasis for tumors arising in the thoracic esophagus.

Metastatic Sites

The liver, lungs, pleura, and kidneys are the most common sites of distant metastases. Occasionally, the tumor may extend directly into the mediastinum before distant spread is evident.

RULES FOR CLASSIFICATION

Clinical Staging

Clinical staging depends on the anatomic extent of the primary tumor that can be ascertained by examination before treatment. Such an examination may include physical examination, medical history, biopsy, routine laboratory studies, endoscopic examinations, and imaging. Endoscopic ultrasound and computed tomography are useful for identifying tumor location, depth of invasion, and lymph node metastasis. The location of the primary tumor should be recorded, because prognosis will vary depending on its site of origin.

Pathologic Staging. Pathologic staging is based on surgical exploration and on examination of the surgically resected esophagus and associated lymph nodes. Extension of the tumor to adjacent structures and the presence of distant metastases should be documented carefully. A single classification serves all regions of the esophagus. It serves both clinical and pathologic staging. Involvement of the adjacent structures depends on the location of the primary tumor. These structures should be specified when involved with tumor.

DEFINITION OF TNM

Primary Tumor (T)

TX   Primary tumor cannot be assessed
T0   No evidence of primary tumor
Tis   Carcinoma *in situ*
T1   Tumor invades lamina propria or submucosa
T2   Tumor invades muscularis propria
T3   Tumor invades adventitia
T4   Tumor invades adjacent structures

Regional Lymph Nodes (N)

NX   Regional lymph nodes cannot be assessed
N0   No regional lymph node metastasis
N1   Regional lymph node metastasis

Distant Metastasis (M)

MX   Presence of distant metastasis cannot be assessed
M0   No distant metastasis
M1   Distant metastasis

STAGE GROUPING

Stage	T	N	M
Stage 0	Tis	N0	M0
Stage I	T1	N0	M0
Stage IIA	T2	N0	M0
	T3	N0	M0
Stage IIB	T1	N1	M0
	T2	N1	M0
Stage III	T3	N1	M0
	T4	Any N	M0
Stage IV	Any T	Any N	M1

HISTOPATHOLOGIC TYPE

The staging classification applies to all carcinomas. Squamous cell carcinomas are most common. Adenocarcinomas that arise in Barrett's esophagus are also included in the classification.

HISTOPATHOLOGIC GRADE (G)

GX   Grade cannot be assessed
G1   Well differentiated
G2   Moderately differentiated
G3   Poorly differentiated
G4   Undifferentiated

BIBLIOGRAPHY

1. Bergman F: Cancer of the esophagus: A histological study of development and local spread of 10 cases of squamous cell carcinoma in the lower third of oesophagus. Acta Chir Scand 117:356–365, 1959

2. Bottger T, Storkel S, Stockle M, et al: DNA image cytometry. A prognostic tool in squamous cell carcinoma of the esophagus? Cancer 67:2290–2294, 1991

3. Ellis FH, Jr: Treatment of carcinoma of the esophagus or cardia. Mayo Clin Proc 64:945–955, 1989

4. Fu-Sheng L, Ling L, and Song-Liang Q: Clinical and pathological characteristics of early oesophageal cancer. Clinics in Oncology 1, No. 2:539–557, 1982

5. Gion M, Tremolada C, Mione R, et al: Tumor markers in serum of patients with primary squamous cell carcinoma of the esophagus. Tumori 75:489–493, 1989

6. Hermanek P, Husemann B, Hohenberger W: The new TNM classification and stage grouping of intrathoracic oesophageal carcinoma. Dis Esoph. In press.

7. Iizuka T, Isono K, Kakegawa T, et al: Parameters linked to ten-year survival in Japan of resected esophageal carcinoma. Chest 96:1005–1011, 1989

8. Petrovich Z, Lam K, Langholz B, et al: Surgical therapy and radiotherapy for carcinoma of the esophagus. Treatment results in 195 patients. J Thorac Cardiovasc Surg 98:614–617, 1989

9. Rice TW, Boyce GA, Sivak MV: Esophageal ultrasound and the preoperative staging of carcinoma of the esophagus. J Thorac Cardiovasc Surg 101:536–543, 1991

10. Siewert JR, Holscher AH, Dittler HJ: Preoperative staging and risk analysis in esophageal carcinoma. Hepatogastroenterology 37:382–387, 1990

11. Skinner DB, Ferguson MK, Little AG: Selection of operation for esophageal cancer based on staging. Ann Surg 204:391–400, 1986

12. Stephens JK, Bibbo M, Dytch H, et al: Correlation between automated karyometric measurements of squamous cell carcinoma of the esophagus and histopathologic and clinical features. Cancer 64:83–87, 1989

13. Tio TL, Coene PP, Hartog Jager FC, et al: Preoperative TNM classification of esophageal carcinoma by endosonography. Hepatogastroenterology 37:376–381, 1990

14. Turnbull ADM, Goodner JT: Primary adenocarcinoma of the esophagus. Cancer 22:915–918, 1968

15. Vilgrain V, Mompoint D, Palazzo L, et al: Staging of esophageal carcinoma: Comparison of results with endoscopic sonography and CT. Am J Roentgenol 155:277–281, 1990

16. Watanabe H, Jass JR, Sobin LH: Histological typing of esophageal and gastric tumors. WHO International Histological Classification of Tumors, 2nd ed. Berlin-New York, Springer-Verlag, 1990

Data Form for Cancer Staging

Patient identification
Name _____
Address _____
Hospital or clinic number _____
Age _____ Sex _____ Race _____

Institution identification
Hospital or clinic _____
Address _____

Oncology Record

Anatomic site of cancer _____
Histologic type _____
Grade (G) _____
Date of classification _____

Chronology of classification
[ ] Clinical (use all data prior to first treatment)
[ ] Pathologic (if definitively resected specimen available)

DEFINITIONS

Clin	Path		
		Primary Tumor (T)	
[ ]	[ ]	TX	Primary tumor cannot be assessed
[ ]	[ ]	T0	No evidence of primary tumor
[ ]	[ ]	Tis	Carcinoma *in situ*
[ ]	[ ]	T1	Tumor invades lamina propria or submucosa
[ ]	[ ]	T2	Tumor invades muscularis propria
[ ]	[ ]	T3	Tumor invades adventitia
[ ]	[ ]	T4	Tumor invades adjacent structures
		Lymph Node (N)	
[ ]	[ ]	NX	Regional lymph nodes cannot be assessed
[ ]	[ ]	N0	No regional lymph node metastasis
[ ]	[ ]	N1	Regional lymph node metastasis
		Distant Metastasis (M)	
[ ]	[ ]	MX	Presence of distant metastasis cannot be assessed
[ ]	[ ]	M0	No distant metastasis
[ ]	[ ]	M1	Distant metastasis

Stage Grouping

Clin	Path				
[ ]	[ ]	0	Tis	N0	M0
[ ]	[ ]	I	T1	N0	M0
[ ]	[ ]	IIA	T2	N0	M0
			T3	N0	M0
[ ]	[ ]	IIB	T1	N1	M0
			T2	N1	M0
[ ]	[ ]	III	T3	N1	M0
			T4	Any N	M0
[ ]	[ ]	IV	Any T	Any N	M1

Histopathologic Grade (G)

[ ] GX Grade cannot be assessed
[ ] G1 Well differentiated
[ ] G2 Moderately differentiated
[ ] G3 Poorly differentiated
[ ] G4 Undifferentiated

Histopathologic Type

The staging system classification applies to all squamous cell carcinomas, which are most common, and to the adenocarcinomas. Other histologic types are reported separately.

Illustration

Length of tumor: _____cm

Indicate on diagram primary tumor and regional nodes involved.

Staged by _____ M.D.
_____Registrar
Date _____

10

Stomach

C16.0 Cardia, NOS
C16.1 Fundus
C16.2 Body
C16.3 Antrum
C16.4 Pylorus
C16.5 Lesser curvature
C16.6 Greater curvature
C16.8 Overlapping lesion
C16.9 Stomach, NOS

As in most hollow organs, the prognosis of carcinomas of the stomach depends on the extent of penetration of the wall by the tumor and involvement of adjacent organs. Size, location, and the histologic type of cancer have not been found useful for estimating prognosis. The overall prognosis for carcinomas of the stomach is poor. For reasons unknown, the incidence of stomach cancer has been declining since 1930 in most developed countries. Chronic atrophic gastritis is a predisposing factor. Nearly all carcinomas arise from the mucus-secreting cells of the gastric crypts.

ANATOMY

Primary Site. The stomach is the first division of the abdominal alimentary tract. Its first part is the esophagogastric junction, which lies immediately below the diaphragm and is often called the cardia. The upper part of the stomach is the fundus; the lower part, the antrum. The pylorus is continuous with the duodenum. The shorter right border is the lesser curvature and the longer border on the left is the greater curvature. The stomach wall has five layers: mucosal, submucosal, muscular, subserosal, and serosal.

Regional Lymph Nodes

Inferior (right) gastric:
   Greater curvature
   Greater omental
   Gastroduodenal

Gastrocolic
Gastroepiploic, right, or NOS
Gastrohepatic
Pyloric, including subpyloric and infrapyloric
Pancreaticoduodenal (anteriorly along first part of
   the duodenum)

Splenic:
   Gastroepiploic, left
   Pancreaticolienal
   Peripancreatic
   Splenic hilar

Superior (left) gastric:
   Lesser curvature
   Lesser omental
   Gastropancreatic, left
   Gastric, left
   Paracardial; cardial
   Cardioesophageal
   Perigastric, NOS
   Celiac
   Hepatic (excluding gastrohepatic)

All other lymph nodes are considered distant. They include:

   Retropancreatic
   Hepatoduodenal
   Aortic
   Portal
   Retroperitoneal
   Mesenteric

Metastatic Sites. Distant spread to the liver, lungs, and supraclavicular lymph nodes is common, although widespread visceral involvement can also occur. Frequently there is direct extension to the liver, the transverse colon, the pancreas, or the diaphragm.

RULES FOR CLASSIFICATION

Clinical Staging. Designated as cTNM, clinical staging is based on evidence acquired before definitive treatment is instituted. It includes physical examination, imaging, endoscopy, biopsy, and other findings. All cases must be confirmed histologically.

Pathologic Staging. Pathologic staging depends on data acquired clinically along with results of surgical exploration and examination of the resected specimen or biopsy. Pathologic assessment of the regional lymph nodes entails removal of nodes adequate to validate the absence of metastasis and to evaluate the highest pN category. Metastatic nodules in the fat adjacent to the gastric carcinoma, without evidence of residual lymph node tissue, are considered regional lymph node metastases. If there is doubt concerning the correct T, N, or M assignment, the lower (less advanced) category should be selected. This guideline also applies to the stage grouping.

DEFINITION OF TNM

Primary Tumor (T)

TX   Primary tumor cannot be assessed
T0   No evidence of primary tumor
Tis   Carcinoma *in situ:* intraepithelial tumor without invasion of the lamina propria

T1   Tumor invades lamina propria or submucosa
T2   Tumor invades the muscularis propria or the subserosa*
T3   Tumor penetrates the serosa (visceral peritoneum) without invasion of adjacent structures**,***
T4   Tumor invades adjacent structures**,***

*Note: A tumor may penetrate the muscularis propria with extension into the gastrocolic or gastrohepatic ligaments or into the greater or lesser omentum without perforation of the visceral peritoneum covering these structures. In this case, the tumor is classified T2. If there is perforation of the visceral peritoneum covering the gastric ligaments or omenta, the tumor should be classified T3.

**Note: The adjacent structures of the stomach are the spleen, transverse colon, liver, diaphragm, pancreas, abdominal wall, adrenal gland, kidney, small intestine, and retroperitoneum.

***Note: Intramural extension to the duodenum or esophagus is classified by the depth of greatest invasion in any of these sites, including the stomach.

Regional Lymph Nodes (N) (Please see diagram below)

The regional lymph nodes are the perigastric nodes along the lesser (1, 3, 5) and greater (2, 4a, 4b, 6) curvatures and the nodes located along the left gastric (7) and common hepatic (8), splenic (10, 11), and celiac arteries (9). Involvement of other intraabdominal lymph nodes, such as hepatoduodenal (12), retropancreatic, mesenteric, and paraaortic, is classified as distant metastasis.

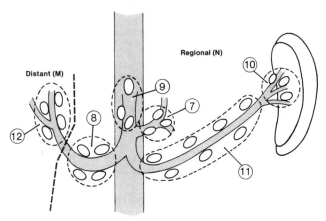

Note: The numerical order corresponds to the proposals of the Japanese Research Society for Gastric Cancer Study in Surgery and Pathology, the Japanese Journal of Surgery, Tokyo 11:127-145, 1982.

NX Regional lymph node(s) cannot be assessed
N0 No regional lymph node metastasis
N1 Metastasis in perigastric lymph node(s) within 3 cm of the edge of the primary tumor
N2 Metastasis in perigastric lymph node(s) more than 3 cm from the edge of the primary tumor, or in lymph nodes along the left gastric, common hepatic, splenic, or celiac arteries

Distant Metastasis (M)

MX Presence of distant metastasis cannot be assessed
M0 No distant metastasis
M1 Distant metastasis

STAGE GROUPING

Stage 0	Tis	N0	M0
Stage IA	T1	N0	M0
Stage IB	T1	N1	M0
	T2	N0	M0
Stage II	T1	N2	M0
	T2	N1	M0
	T3	N0	M0
Stage IIIA	T2	N2	M0
	T3	N1	M0
	T4	N0	M0
Stage IIIB	T3	N2	M0
	T4	N1	M0
Stage IV	T4	N2	M0
	Any T	Any N	M1

HISTOPATHOLOGIC TYPE

The staging recommendations apply only to carcinomas and not to other histologic types such as lymphomas, sarcomas, or carcinoid tumors. Adenocarcinomas may be divided into the subtypes intestinal, diffuse, and mixed.

The histopathologic types are:

Adenocarcinoma
Papillary adenocarcinoma
Tubular adenocarcinoma
Mucinous adenocarcinoma
Signet ring cell carcinoma
Adenosquamous carcinoma
Squamous cell carcinoma
Small cell carcinoma
Undifferentiated carcinoma

Survival for Patients with Stomach Cancer by Pathologic Stages Diagnosed in 1982

Stage IA (n=437)
Stage 0 (n=84)
Stage IB (n=672)
Stage II (n=1100)
Stage IIIA (n=1411)
Stage IIIB (n=914)
Stage IV (n=1991)

Disease specific survival data taken from the Commission on Cancer Patient Care Evaluation Study. (H. Wanebo: with permission)

HISTOPATHOLOGIC GRADE (G)

GX Grade cannot be assessed
G1 Well differentiated
G2 Moderately differentiated
G3 Poorly differentiated
G4 Undifferentiated

BIBLIOGRAPHY

1. Coller FA, Kay EB, MacIntyre RS: Regional lymphatic metastases of carcinoma of the stomach. Arch Surg 43:748–761, 1941
2. Cook AO, Levine BA, Sirinek KR, et al: Evaluation of gastric adenocarcinoma: Abdominal computed tomography does not replace celiotomy. Arch Surg 121:603–606, 1986
3. Dulchavshy S, Dahn MS, and Wilson RF: The preoperative staging of malignant tumors of the stomach by computed tomography and liver function tests. Current Surgery 46:26–28, 1989
4. Dupont JB Jr, Lee JR, Burton GR, et al: Adenocarcinoma of the stomach: Review of 1,497 cases. Cancer 41:941–947, 1978
5. Kennedy BJ: TNM classification of stomach cancer. Cancer 26:971–983, 1970
6. Kennedy BJ: The unified international gastric cancer staging classification system. Scandinavian Journal of Gastroenterology 22 (Suppl 133): 11–13, 1987

7. Lauren P: The two histological main types of gastric carcinoma. Acta Pathol Microbiol Scand 64:31–49, 1965

8. Ming SC: Tumors of the esophagus and stomach. Atlas of Tumor Pathology, Second Series, Fascicle 7. Washington DC, Armed Forces Institute of Pathology, 1973

9. Rhode H, Gebbensleben P, Bauer P, et al: Has there been any improvement in the staging of gastric cancer? Findings from the German Gastric Cancer TNM Study Group. Cancer 64:2465–2481, 1989

10. Saario I, Schroder T, Talppanen EM, et al: Factors influencing 5-year survival in gastric malignancies after total gastrectomy. Annales Chirurgiae et Gynaccologiae (Helsinki) 75:23–27, 1986

11. Serlin O, Keehn RJ, Higgins GA, et al: Factors related to survival following resection for gastric carcinoma: Analysis of 903 cases. Cancer 40:1318–1329, 1977

12. Shiu MH, Perrotti M, and Brennan MF: Adenocarcinoma of the stomach: A multivariate analysis of clinical, pathologic, and treatment factors. Hepatogastroenterology 36:7–12, 1989

13. Sunderland DA, McNeer G, Ortega LS, et al: The lymphatic spread of gastric cancer. Cancer 6:987–996, 1953

14. Wanebo HJ, Kennedy BJ, Chmiel JS, Steele GD, Winchester DP: Cancer of the Stomach—A Patient Care Study by the American College of Surgeons (in preparation)

15. Watanabe H, Jass JR, Sobin LH: Histological typing of esophageal and gastric tumors. WHO International Histological Classification of Tumors, 2nd ed. Berlin-New York, Springer-Verlag, 1991

16. Zinninger MM, Colling WT: Extension of carcinomas of the stomach into the duodenum and esophagus. Ann Surg 130:557–566, 1949

Data Form for Cancer Staging

Patient identification
Name _____

Address _____

Hospital or clinic number _____

Age _____ Sex _____ Race _____

Institution identification
Hospital or clinic _____

Address _____

Oncology Record

Anatomic site of cancer _____

Histologic type _____

Grade (G) _____

Date of classification _____

Chronology of classification
[ ]   Clinical (use all data prior to first treatment)
[ ]   Pathologic (if definitively resected specimen available)

DEFINITIONS

Primary Tumor (T)

Clin	Path		
[ ]	[ ]	TX	Primary tumor cannot be assessed
[ ]	[ ]	T0	No evidence of primary tumor
[ ]	[ ]	Tis	Carcinoma *in situ*: intraepithelial tumor without invasion of lamina propria
[ ]	[ ]	T1	Tumor invades lamina propria or submucosa
[ ]	[ ]	T2	Tumor invades muscularis propria or subserosa
[ ]	[ ]	T3	Tumor penetrates serosa (visceral peritoneum) without invasion of adjacent structures
[ ]	[ ]	T4	Tumor invades adjacent structures

Lymph Node (N)

Clin	Path		
[ ]	[ ]	NX	Regional lymph node(s) cannot be assessed
[ ]	[ ]	N0	No regional lymph node metastasis
[ ]	[ ]	N1	Metastasis in perigastric lymph node(s) within 3 cm of edge of primary tumor
[ ]	[ ]	N2	Metastasis in perigastric lymph node(s) more than 3 cm from edge of primary tumor, or in lymph nodes along left gastric, common hepatic, splenic, or celiac arteries

Distant Metastasis (M)

Clin	Path		
[ ]	[ ]	MX	Presence of distant metastasis cannot be assessed
[ ]	[ ]	M0	No distant metastasis
[ ]	[ ]	M1	Distant metastasis

Stage Grouping

Clin	Path				
[ ]	[ ]	0	Tis	N0	M0
[ ]	[ ]	IA	T1	N0	M0
[ ]	[ ]	IB	T1	N1	M0
			T2	N0	M0
[ ]	[ ]	II	T1	N2	M0
			T2	N1	M0
			T3	N0	M0
[ ]	[ ]	IIIA	T2	N2	M0
			T3	N1	M0
			T4	N0	M0
[ ]	[ ]	IIIB	T3	N2	M0
			T4	N1	M0
[ ]	[ ]	IV	T4	N2	M0
			Any T	Any N	M1

Histopathologic Grade (G)

[ ] GX   Grade cannot be assessed
[ ] G1   Well differentiated
[ ] G2   Moderately differentiated
[ ] G3   Poorly differentiated
[ ] G4   Undifferentiated

Histopathologic Type

The staging recommendations apply only to carcinomas and not to other histologic types such as lymphomas or sarcomas. Adenocarcinomas should be divided into the following subtypes and recorded.

a. Intestinal
b. Diffuse
c. Mixed

The prognosis is worse for the diffuse type.

Illustration

Mucosa
Muscularis mucosae
Muscularis propria
Serosa

Indicate on diagram primary tumor and regional nodes involved.

Staged by _____ M.D.

_____ Registrar

Date _____

11

Small Intestine

C17.0 Duodenum
C17.1 Jejunum
C17.2 Ileum
C17.8 Overlapping lesion
C17.9 Small intestine, NOS

Carcinomas of the small intestine represent less than 2% of all malignant tumors of the intestinal tract. Most occur in the first or second part of the duodenum. Adenocarcinomas comprise less than 50% of all primary malignant tumors of the small intestine. Considered together, sarcomas, lymphomas, and malignant carcinoid tumors are more common than adenocarcinomas. Because primary carcinomas of the small bowel are rare, a staging system has not been previously published by the International Union Against Cancer or by the American Joint Committee on Cancer. Because carcinomas of the small bowel are not common, information on their method of spread and biologic behavior is not complete. However, there is no reason to believe that these tumors behave differently than carcinomas arising in other parts of the gastrointestinal tract. Patients with Crohn's disease or certain familial polyposis syndromes are at a higher risk for developing carcinomas of the small intestine. *In situ* lesions occur in adenomas. This classification is used for both clinical and pathological staging.

ANATOMY

Primary Site. This classification applies to carcinomas arising in the duodenum, jejunum, and ileum. It does not apply to carcinomas arising in the ileocecal valve or to carcinomas that may arise in Meckel's diverticulum. Carcinomas arising in the ampulla of Vater are staged according to the system described on page 106. Carcinomas arising in the vermiform appendix are staged according to the classification listed for the colon; see page 77.

Duodenum. About 25 cm in length, the duodenum extends from the pyloric sphincter to the jejunum. It is usually divided into four parts, with the pancreatic duct opening into the second part.

Jejunum and Ileum. The jejunum and ileum extend from the duodenum to the ileocecal valve. The division between the jejunum and ileum is arbitrary. As a rule, the jejunum occupies about 40% of the small intestine exclusive of the duodenum; the ileum, 60%.

The small intestine is supported by a fold of the peritoneum, the mesentery. The shortest segment, the duodenum, has no mesentery and is only partially covered by peritoneum. The wall of the small intestine has five layers: mucosal, submucosal, muscular, subserosal, and serosal. A thin layer of smooth muscle cells, the muscularis mucosae, separates the mucosa from the submucosa. The small intestine is ensheathed by peritoneum except for a narrow strip that is attached to the mesentery and the part of the duodenum that is located retroperitoneally.

Regional Lymph Nodes. They are:

Duodenum:
  Duodenal
  Hepatic
  Pancreaticoduodenal
  Infrapyloric
  Gastroduodenal
  Ampulla of Vater
  Pyloric
  Cystic
  Superior mesenteric
  Hilar
  Pericholedochal
  Regional lymph nodes, NOS

Ileum and Jejunum:
    Posterior cecal (terminal ileum only)
    Ileocolic (terminal ileum only)
    Superior mesenteric
    Mesenteric, NOS
    Regional lymph nodes, NOS

Metastatic Sites. Cancers of the small intestine can metastasize to most organs. Involvement of regional lymph nodes and adjacent structures is most common.

RULES FOR CLASSIFICATION

The primary tumor is staged according to its depth of penetration and involvement of adjacent structures or distant sites. Lateral spread from the duodenum into the jejunum or jejunum into the ileum is not considered in the classification, only the depth of tumor penetration.

Differences between this staging system and that of the colon should be noted. Unlike the large intestine, there is no subdivision of the N category based on the number of lymph nodes involved with the tumor. Also, in the colon, Tis applies to intraepithelial (*in situ*) lesions as well as to intramucosal spread. In the small intestine, intramucosal spread is listed as T1. In this regard, the T1 definition for the small bowel is the same as the T1 category defined for the stomach. Invasion through the wall is staged as for the colon. Discontinuous metastasis or seeding is coded as M1.

DEFINITION OF TNM

Primary Tumor (T)

TX   Primary tumor cannot be assessed
T0   No evidence of primary tumor
Tis   Carcinoma *in situ*
T1   Tumor invades lamina propria or submucosa
T2   Tumor invades muscularis propria
T3   Tumor invades through the muscularis propria into the subserosa or into the nonperitonealized perimuscular tissue (mesentery or retroperitoneum) with extension 2 cm or less.*
T4   Tumor perforates the visceral peritoneum or directly invades other organs or structures (includes other loops of the small intestine, mesentery, or retroperitoneum more than 2 cm, and the abdominal wall by way of the serosa; for the duodenum only, includes invasion of the pancreas).

*Note: The nonperitonealized perimuscular tissue is, for the jejunum and ileum, part of the mesentery and, for the duodenum in areas where serosa is lacking, part of the retroperitoneum.

Regional Lymph Nodes (N)

NX   Regional lymph nodes cannot be assessed
N0   No regional lymph node metastasis
N1   Regional lymph node metastasis

Distant Metastasis (M)

MX   Presence of distant metastasis cannot be assessed
M0   No distant metastasis
M1   Distant metastasis

STAGE GROUPING

Stage	T	N	M
Stage 0	Tis	N0	M0
Stage I	T1	N0	M0
	T2	N0	M0
Stage II	T3	N0	M0
	T4	N0	M0
Stage III	Any T	N1	M0
Stage IV	Any T	Any N	M1

CARCINOMA OF THE SMALL INTESTINE
SURVIVAL ACCORDING TO AJCC STAGE

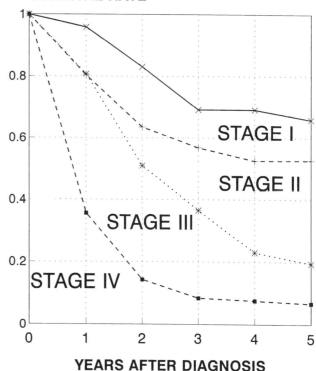

Fig. 11-1. Relative survival rates according to stage of disease. Data based on 250 cases recorded in the Surveillance, Epidemiology, and End Results Program of the National Cancer Institute. Stage I includes 13 cases; Stage II, 77; Stage III, 56; and Stage IV, 104.

HISTOPATHOLOGIC TYPE

The classification applies to all carcinomas arising in the small intestine. Lymphomas, carcinoid tumors, and sarcomas are not included.

HISTOPATHOLOGIC GRADE (G)

GX Grade cannot be assessed
G1 Well differentiated
G2 Moderately differentiated
G3 Poorly differentiated
G4 Undifferentiated

BIBLIOGRAPHY

1. Brookes VS, Waterhouse JAH, Powell DJ: Malignant lesions of the small intestine: A ten-year survey. Brit J Surg 55:405–410,1968
2. Dudiak KM, Johnson CD, Stephens DH: Primary tumors of the small intestine: CT evaluation. AJR Am J Roentgenol 152:995–998, 1989
3. Hancock RJ: An 11-year review of primary tumours of the small bowel including the duodenum. Can Med Assoc J:103:1177–1179,1970
4. Jass JR, Sobin LH: Histological typing of intestinal tumors. WHO International Histological Classification of Tumors, 2nd ed. Berlin-New York, Springer-Verlag, 1989.
5. Lien GS, Mori M, Enjoji M: Primary carcinoma of the small intestine. A clinicopathologic and immunohistochemical study. Cancer 61:316–322, 1988
6. Maglinte DD, O'Connor K, Bessette J, et al: The role of the physician in the late diagnosis of primary malignant tumors of the small intestine. Am J Gastroenterol 86:304–308, 1991
7. Mittal VK, Bodzin JH: Primary malignant tumors of the small bowel. Am J Surg 140:396–399,1980
8. Sindelar WF: Cancer of the small intestine. In DeVita VT, Hellman S, Rosenberg SA (Eds.), Cancer, Principles and Practice of Oncology, 2nd ed. Philadelphia, Lippincott, 1985

Data Form for Cancer Staging

Patient identification
Name _____
Address _____
Hospital or clinic number _____
Age _____ Sex _____ Race _____

Institution identification
Hospital or clinic _____
Address _____

Oncology Record

Anatomic site of cancer _____
Histologic type _____
Grade (G) _____
Date of classification _____

Chronology of classification
[   ] Clinical (use all data prior to first treatment)
[   ] Pathologic (if definitively resected specimen available)

DEFINITIONS

Primary Tumor (T)

Clin	Path		
[ ]	[ ]	TX	Primary tumor cannot be assessed
[ ]	[ ]	T0	No evidence of primary tumor
[ ]	[ ]	Tis	Carcinoma *in situ*
[ ]	[ ]	T1	Tumor invades lamina propria or submucosa
[ ]	[ ]	T2	Tumor invades muscularis propria
[ ]	[ ]	T3	Tumor invades through the muscularis propria into the subserosa or into the non-peritonealized perimuscular tissue (mesentery or retroperitoneum) with extension 2 cm or less
[ ]	[ ]	T4	Tumor perforates the visceral peritoneum, or directly invades other organs and structures, (includes other loops of small intestine, mesentery, or retroperitoneum more than 2 cm, and the abdominal wall by way of the serosa; for the duodenum only includes invasion of the pancreas)

Regional Lymph Nodes (N)

Clin	Path		
[ ]	[ ]	NX	Regional lymph nodes cannot be assessed
[ ]	[ ]	N0	No regional lymph node metastasis
[ ]	[ ]	N1	Regional lymph node metastasis

Distant Metastasis (M)

Clin	Path		
[ ]	[ ]	MX	Presence of distant metastasis cannot be assessed
[ ]	[ ]	M0	No distant metastasis
[ ]	[ ]	M1	Distant metastasis

Histopathologic Type

The classification applies to all carcinomas arising in the small intestine. Lymphomas, carcinoid tumors, and sarcomas are not included.

Histopathologic Grade (G)

[   ] GX Grade cannot be assessed
[   ] G1 Well differentiated
[   ] G2 Moderately differentiated
[   ] G3 Poorly differentiated
[   ] G4 Undifferentiated

Stage Grouping

Clin	Path				
[ ]	[ ]	0	Tis	N0	M0
[ ]	[ ]	I	T1	N0	M0
[ ]	[ ]		T2	N0	M0
[ ]	[ ]	II	T3	N0	M0
[ ]	[ ]		T4	N0	M0
[ ]	[ ]	III	Any T	N1	M0
[ ]	[ ]	IV	Any T	Any N	M1

Staged by _____ M.D.
_____ Registrar
Date _____

12

Colon and Rectum

C18.0 Cecum
C18.1 Appendix
C18.2 Ascending
C18.3 Hepatic flexure
C18.4 Transverse
C18.5 Splenic flexure
C18.6 Descending

C18.7 Sigmoid
C18.8 Overlapping lesion
C18.9 Colon, NOS

C19.9 Rectosigmoid junction

C20.9 Rectum

The TNM classification for carcinomas of the colon and rectum provides more detail than other staging systems. Compatible with Dukes, the TNM is based on the depth of tumor penetration into the wall of the intestine, the number and site of regional lymph nodes involved with tumor, and the presence or absence of distant metastasis. Other prognostic variables that should be considered in patient management, but do not enter into TNM, include histologic type, histologic differentiation, ploidy, invasion of blood or lymphatic vessels, and complications such as fistula formation.

The classification applies to both clinical and pathologic staging. Most cancers of the colorectum, however, are staged after pathologic examination of the resected specimen. This staging system applies to all carcinomas arising in the colon, rectum, or vermiform appendix.

ANATOMY

Anatomic Divisions of the Colon and Rectum:

Cecum
Ascending colon
Hepatic flexure
Transverse colon
Splenic flexure
Descending colon
Sigmoid colon
Rectosigmoid colon
Rectum

Cancers that originate in the anal canal are staged according to the classification used for the anus; refer to page 83.

Primary Site. The large intestine (colorectum) extends from the terminal ileum to the anal canal. Excluding the rectum and the vermiform appendix, the colon is divided into four parts: the right or ascending colon, the middle or transverse colon, the left or descending colon, and the sigmoid colon. The sigmoid is continuous with the rectum, which terminates at the anal canal. The entire colon and proximal rectum are covered, at least in part, with peritoneum (serosa).

The cecum is a large pouch that forms the proximal segment of the right colon. It usually measures 6 cm by 9 cm and is covered with peritoneum. The ascending colon is 15 to 20 cm long, located retroperitoneally. Connecting the ascending colon to the transverse colon is the hepatic flexure, which lies under the right lobe of the liver near the duodenum.

The transverse colon lies more anteriorly than the other divisions of the colon. As a result, tumors that arise in this division are more readily palpated through the anterior abdominal wall. The transverse colon is supported by the transverse mesocolon, which is attached to the pancreas. Anteriorly, its serosa is continuous with the gastrocolic ligament. The transverse colon is connected to the descending colon by the splenic flexure, located near the spleen and tail of the pancreas. The descending colon, measuring 10 to 15 cm long, is also located retroperitoneally. The descending colon becomes the sigmoid at the origin of the mesosigmoid. The sigmoid loop extends from the medial border of the left posterior major psoas muscle to the rectum, which begins at the termination of the mesosigmoid.

Normally 12 cm in length, the rectum extends from a point opposite the third sacral vertebra to the apex of the prostate gland in the male and to the apex of the perineal body in the female; that is, to a point 4 cm anterior to the tip of the coccyx. It is often defined as the distal 10 cm of the large intestine as measured from the anal verge with a sigmoidoscope. The rectosigmoid segment is usually 10 to 15 cm from the anal mucocutaneous junction. The rectum is covered by peritoneum in front and on both sides in its upper third and on the anterior wall only in its middle third. The peritoneum is reflected laterally from the rectum to form the perirectal fossa and anteriorly to form the uterine or rectovesical fold. There is no peritoneal covering in the lower third, which is often known as the rectal ampulla. The anal canal, measuring 4 to 5 cm long, courses downward and backward from the apex of the prostate gland or from the perineal body to the anal verge. This definition is similar to the international definition.

Regional Lymph Nodes. Regional nodes are those along the course of the major vessels supplying the colon and rectum, those following the vascular arcades of the marginal artery, and those adjacent to the colon; that is, located along the mesocolic border of the colon. Specifically, the regional lymph nodes are the pericolic and perirectal nodes and those located along the ileocolic, right colic, middle colic, left colic, inferior mesenteric, superior rectal (hemorrhoidal), and internal iliac arteries.

The regional lymph nodes for each segment of the colon are:

SEGMENT	REGIONAL LYMPH NODES
Cecum and appendix	Anterior cecal, posterior cecal, ileocolic, right colic
Ascending colon	Ileocolic, right colic, middle colic
Hepatic flexure	Middle colic, right colic
Transverse colon	Middle colic
Splenic flexure	Middle colic, left colic, inferior mesenteric
Descending colon	Left colic, inferior mesenteric, sigmoid
Sigmoid colon	Inferior mesenteric, superior rectal (hemorrhoidal), sigmoidal, sigmoid mesenteric
Rectosigmoid	Perirectal, left colic, sigmoid mesenteric, sigmoidal, inferior mesenteric, superior rectal (hemorrhoidal), middle rectal (hemorrhoidal)
Rectum	Perirectal, sigmoid mesenteric, inferior mesenteric, lateral sacral, presacral, internal iliac, sacral promontory (Gerota's) superior rectal (hemorrhoidal), middle rectal (hemorrhoidal), inferior rectal (hemorrhoidal)

COLORECTAL CANCER
SURVIVAL ACCORDING TO STAGE

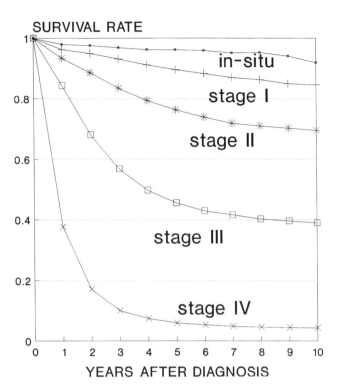

Fig. 12-1. Relative survival rates of patients with colon cancer according to the stage of disease. Rates based on 111,110 patients. Data taken from the Surveillance, Epidemiology, and End Results Program of the National Cancer Institute for the years 1973 to 1987. Patients were staged according to the current TNM. Stage 0 (*in situ*) includes 4,841 patients; Stage I, 19,623; Stage II, 33,798; Stage III, 29,615; and Stage IV, 23,233.

Metastatic Sites. Carcinomas of the colon and rectum can metastasize to almost any organ, with liver and lungs the most common sites. Seeding of other segments of the colon may also occur.

RULES FOR CLASSIFICATION

Clinical Staging. Clinical assessment is based on medical history, physical examination, routine and special roentgenograms, including barium enema, sigmoidoscopy, colonoscopy with biopsy, and special examinations used to demonstrate the presence of extracolonic metastasis, for example, chest films, liver function tests, and liver scans.

Pathologic Staging. Colorectal cancers are usually staged after pathologic examination of the resected specimen and surgical exploration of the abdomen. The definition of *in situ* carcinoma—Tis—includes cancer cells confined within the glandular basement membrane (intraepithelial) or lamina propria (intramucosal) with no extension through the muscularis mucosae into the submucosa. This definition for Tis is different from that used in other divisions of the gastrointestinal tract. Neither intraepithelial nor intramucosal carcinomas of the large intestine have a significant potential for metastasis.

Tumor that invades the stalk of a polyp is classified according to the T definitions adopted for colorectal cancers. For instance, tumor that has invaded the lamina propria only is listed as Tis, whereas tumor that has penetrated the muscularis mucosae and entered the submucosa of the stalk is listed as T1.

The number of lymph nodes should be recorded. It is desirable to obtain at least 12 lymph nodes in radical colon resections; however, in cases in which tumor is resected for palliation, only a few lymph nodes may be present.

Patients with free tumor located on the serosal surface as a result of direct extension through the colon are listed as T4. Seeding of abdominal organs—for instance, the distal ileum from a carcinoma of the transverse colon—is considered discontinuous metastasis and should be recorded as M1. Metastatic nodules or foci found in the pericolic or perirectal fat or in adjacent mesentery (mesocolic fat) without evidence of residual lymph node tissue are equivalent to regional lymph node metastasis. Multiple metastatic foci seen microscopically only in the pericolic fat should be considered as metastasis in a single lymph node for classification.

Lymph node involvement—pN—is stratified according to the number of positive nodes. Patients with 1 to 3 positive nodes have a 66% 5-year survival rate, while patients with 4 or more nodes have a 37% 5-year survival rate. (6)

Metastasis in the external iliac or common iliac nodes is classified as M1.

DEFINITION OF TNM

The same classification is used for both clinical and pathologic staging.

Primary Tumor (T)

TX   Primary tumor cannot be assessed
T0   No evidence of primary tumor
Tis   Carcinoma *in situ*: intraepithelial or invasion of the lamina propria*
T1   Tumor invades the submucosa
T2   Tumor invades the muscularis propria
T3   Tumor invades through the muscularis propria into the subserosa or into nonperitonealized pericolic or perirectal tissues
T4   Tumor directly invades other organs or structures and/or perforates the visceral peritoneum **

* Note: Tis includes cancer cells confined within the glandular basement membrane (intraepithelial) or lamina propria (intramucosal) with no extension through the muscularis mucosae into the submucosa.

** Note: Direct invasion of other organs or structures includes invasion of other segments of colorectum by way of serosa; for example, invasion of the sigmoid colon by a carcinoma of the cecum.

Regional Lymph Nodes (N)

NX   Regional lymph nodes cannot be assessed
N0   No regional lymph node metastasis
N1   Metastasis in one to three pericolic or perirectal lymph nodes
N2   Metastasis in four or more pericolic or perirectal lymph nodes
N3   Metastasis in any lymph node along the course of a named vascular trunk and/or metastasis to apical node(s) (when marked by the surgeon)

Distant Metastasis (M)

MX   Presence of distant metastasis cannot be assessed
M0   No distant metastasis
M1   Distant metastasis

STAGE GROUPING

AJCC/UICC				DUKES
Stage 0	Tis	N0	M0	—
Stage I	T1	N0	M0	A
	T2	N0	M0	
Stage II	T3	N0	M0	B
	T4	N0	M0	
Stage III	Any T	N1	M0	C
	Any T	N2	M0	
	Any T	N3	M0	
Stage IV	Any T	Any N	M1	—

Note: Dukes B is a composite of better (T3, N0, M0) and worse (T4, N0, M0) prognostic groups, as is Dukes C (Any T, N1, M0 and Any T, N2, N3, M0).

HISTOPATHOLOGIC TYPE

This staging classification applies to carcinomas that arise in the colon, rectum, or appendix. It does not apply to sarcomas, lymphomas, or carcinoid tumors. The histologic types include:

Adenocarcinoma *in situ*
Adenocarcinoma
Mucinous adenocarcinoma (colloid type; greater than 50% mucinous carcinoma)
Signet ring cell carcinoma (greater than 50% signet ring cell)

Squamous cell (epidermoid) carcinoma
Adenosquamous carcinoma
Small cell (oat cell) carcinoma
Undifferentiated carcinoma
Carcinoma, NOS

HISTOPATHOLOGIC GRADE (G)

GX   Grade cannot be assessed
G1   Well differentiated
G2   Moderately differentiated
G3   Poorly differentiated
G4   Undifferentiated

BIBLIOGRAPHY

1. Astler VB, Coller FA: The prognostic significance of direct extension of carcinoma of the colon and rectum. Ann Surg 139:846–852, 1954
2. Beart RW Jr, van Heerden JA, Beahrs OH: Evolution in the pathologic staging of carcinoma of the colon. Surg Gynecol Obstet 146:257–259, 1978
3. Blenkinsopp WK, Stewart-Brown S, Blesovsky L, et al: Histopathology reporting in large bowel cancer. J Clin Pathol 34:509–513,1981
4. Butch RJ, Stark DD, Wittenberg J, et al: Staging rectal cancer by MR and CT. Am J Roentgenol 146:1155–1160, 1986
5. Chapuis PH, Fisher R, Dent DF, et al: The relationship between different staging methods and survival in colorectal carcinoma. Dis Colon Rectum 28:158–161, 1985
6. Cohen AM, Tremiterra S, Candela F, et al: Prognosis of node-positive colon cancer. Cancer 67:1859–1861, 1991
7. Dukes CE: The classification of cancer of the rectum. J Pathol Bacteriol 35:322–332, 1932
8. Dukes CE: Cancer of the rectum: An analysis of 1000 cases. J Pathol Bacteriol 50:527–539, 1940
9. Dukes CE, Bussey HJR: The spread of rectal cancer and its effect on prognosis. Br J Cancer 12:309–320, 1958
10. Fenoglio-Preiser CM, Hutter, RVP: Colorectal polyps: Pathologic diagnosis and clinical significance. Cancer J Clin 35:322–344, 1985
11. Fielding LP: Clinicopathological staging for colorectal cancer: An International Documentation System (IDS) and an International Comprehensive Anatomical Terminology (ICAT). J Gastroenterology Hepatology, 1991
12. Fielding LP, Ballantyne GH: Classification systems for staging colorectal cancer. Problems Gen Surg 4:39–53, 1987
13. Fielding LP, Phillips RK, Frey JS, et al: The prediction of outcome after curative resection for large bowel cancer. Lancet 2:904–907, 1986
14. Fielding LP, Phillips RK, Hittinger R: Factors influencing mortality after curative resection for large bowel cancer in elderly patients. Lancet 1:595–597, 1989
15. Gabriel WB, Dukes CE, Bussey HJR: Lymphatic spread in cancer of the rectum. Br J Surg 23:395–399; 412–413, 1935
16. Griffin MR, Bergstralh EJ, Coffey RJ, et al: Predictors of survival after curative resection of carcinoma of the colon and rectum. Cancer 60:2318–2324, 1987
17. Grinnell RS: The grading and prognosis of carcinoma of the colon and rectum. Ann Surg 109:500–533, 1939
18. Hermanek P: Colorectal carcinoma: Histopathological diagnosis and staging. Baillieres Clin Gastroenterol 3:511–529,1989
19. Hermanek P, Gall FP: Early (microinvasive) colorectal carcinoma: Pathology, diagnosis, surgical treatment. Int J Colorectal Dis 1:79–84, 1986
20. Hermanek P, Giedl J, Dworak O: Two programs for examination of regional lymph nodes in colorectal carcinoma with regard to the new pN classification. Pathol Res Pract 185:867–873, 1989
21. Hermanek P, Guggenmoos-Holzmann I, Gall FP: Prognostic factors in rectal carcinoma: A contribution to the further development of tumor classification. Dis Colon Rectum 32:593–599, 1989
22. Herrera-Ornelas L, Justiniano J, Castillo, N, et al: Metastases in small lymph nodes from colon cancer. Arch Surg 122:1253–1256, 1987
23. Jass JR, Atkin WS, Cuzick J, et al: The grading of rectal cancer: Historical perspectives and a multivariate analysis of 447 cases. Histopathology 10:437–459, 1986
24. Jass JR, Love SB, Northover JMA: A new prognostic classification of rectal cancer. Lancet i:1303–1306, 1987
25. Jass JR, Mukawa K, Goh HS, et al: Clinical importance of DNA content in rectal cancer measured by flow cytometry. J Clin Pathol 42:254–259, 1989
26. Jass JR, Sobin LH: Histological typing of intestinal tumors. WHO International Histological Classification of Tumors, 2nd ed. Berlin-New York, Springer-Verlag, 1989
27. Kokal W, Sheibani K, Terz J, et al: Tumor DNA content in the prognosis of colorectal carcinoma. JAMA 255:3123–3127, 1986
28. Minsky BD, Mies C, Rich TA, et al: Lymphatic vessel invasion is an independent prognostic factor for survival in colorectal cancer. Int J Radiat Oncol 17:311–318, 1989
29. Newland RC, Chapuis PH, Pheils MT, et al: The relationship of survival to staging and grading of colorectal carcinoma: A prospective study of 503 cases. Cancer 47:1424–1429, 1981
30. Ondero H, Maetani S, Nishikawa T, et al: The reappraisal of prognostic classifications for colorectal cancer. Dis Colon Rectum 32:609–614, 1989
31. Phillips RKS, Hittinger R, Blesovsky L, et al: Large bowel cancer: Surgical pathology and its relationship to survival. Br J Surg 71:604–610, 1984
32. Qizilbash AH: Pathologic studies in colorectal cancer: A guide to the surgical pathology examination of colorectal specimens and review of features of prognostic significance. Pathol Annu 17 (part 1): 1–46, 1982

33. Scott KWM, Grace RH: Detection of lymph node metastases in colorectal carcinoma before and after fat clearance. Brit J Surg 76:1165–1167, 1989

34. Scott NA, Rainwater LM, Wieland HS, et al: The relative prognostic value of flow cytometric DNA analysis and conventional clinicopathologic criteria in patients with operative rectal carcinoma. Dis Colon Rectum 30:513–520,1987

35. Shepherd NA, Saraga EP, Love SB, et al: Prognostic factors in colonic cancer. Histopathology 14:613–620, 1989

36. Steinberg SM, Barkin JS, Kaplan RS, et al: Prognostic indicators of colon tumors: The gastrointestinal tumor study group experience. Cancer 57:1866–1870, 1986

37. Williams NS, Durdey P, Qwihe P, et al: Pre-operative staging of rectal neoplasm and its impact on clinical management. Br J Surg 72:868–874, 1985

38. Wolmark N, Fisher ER, Wieand HS, et al: The relationship of depth of penetration and tumor size to the number of positive nodes in Dukes' C colorectal cancer. Cancer 53:2707–2712, 1984

39. Wolmark N, Fisher B, Wieand HS: The prognostic value of the modifications of the Dukes' C class of colorectal cancer: An analysis of the NSABP clinical trials. Ann Surg 203:115–122, 1986

40. Wood DA, Robbins GF, Zippin C, et al: Staging of cancer of the colon and rectum. Cancer 43:961–968, 1979

Data Form for Cancer Staging

Patient identification
Name _____
Address _____
Hospital or clinic number _____
Age _____ Sex _____ Race _____

Institution identification
Hospital or clinic _____
Address _____

Oncology Record

Anatomic site of cancer _____
Histologic type _____
Grade (G) _____
Date of classification _____

Chronology of classification
[ ] Clinical (use all data prior to first treatment)
[ ] Pathologic (if definitively resected specimen available)

Clin	Path		

DEFINITIONS

Primary Tumor (T)

Clin	Path		
[ ]	[ ]	TX	Primary tumor cannot be assessed
[ ]	[ ]	T0	No evidence of primary tumor
[ ]	[ ]	Tis	Carcinoma *in situ*: intraepithelial or invasion of lamina propria
[ ]	[ ]	T1	Tumor invades submucosa
[ ]	[ ]	T2	Tumor invades muscularis propria
[ ]	[ ]	T3	Tumor invades through muscularis propria into subserosa, or into nonperitonealized pericolic or perirectal tissues
[ ]	[ ]	T4	Tumor directly invades other organs or structures, and/or perforates visceral peritoneum

Lymph Node (N)

Clin	Path		
[ ]	[ ]	NX	Regional lymph nodes cannot be assessed
[ ]	[ ]	N0	No regional lymph node metastasis
[ ]	[ ]	N1	Metastasis in 1 to 3 pericolic or perirectal lymph nodes
[ ]	[ ]	N2	Metastasis in 4 or more pericolic or perirectal lymph nodes
[ ]	[ ]	N3	Metastasis in any lymph node along course of a named vascular trunk, and/or metastasis to apical node(s) (when marked by the surgeon)

Distant Metastasis (M)

Clin	Path		
[ ]	[ ]	MX	Presence of distant metastasis cannot be assessed
[ ]	[ ]	M0	No distant metastasis
[ ]	[ ]	M1	Distant metastasis

Stage Grouping

Clin	Path	Stage				Dukes
[ ]	[ ]	0	Tis	N0	M0	
[ ]	[ ]	I	T1	N0	M0	A
			T2	N0	M0	
[ ]	[ ]	II	T3	N0	M0	B
			T4	N0	M0	
[ ]	[ ]	III	Any T	N1	M0	C
			Any T	N2	M0	
			Any T	N3	M0	
[ ]	[ ]	IV	Any T	Any N	M1	

Histopathologic Type

This staging classification applies to all carcinomas that arise in the colon and rectum or appendix.

Adenocarcinoma *in situ*
Adenocarcinoma
Mucinous adenocarcinoma
Signet cell carcinoma
Squamous cell carcinoma
Adenosquamous carcinoma
Small cell carcinoma
Undifferentiated carcinoma
Carcinoma, NOS

Staged by _____ M.D.
_____ Registrar
Date _____

Histopathologic Grade (G)

[ ] GX   Grade cannot be assessed
[ ] G1   Well differentiated
[ ] G2   Moderately differentiated
[ ] G3   Poorly differentiated
[ ] G4   Undifferentiated

(continued on next page)

American Joint Committee on Cancer—1992

Illustrations

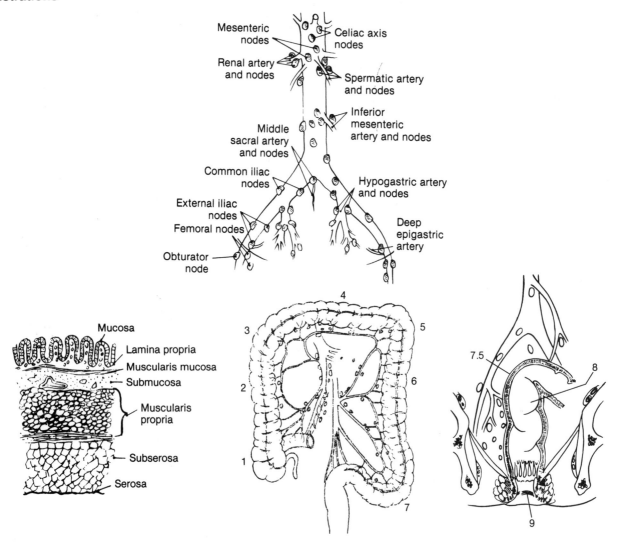

For anatomic areas corresponding to numbers, see list below.
Indicate on diagram primary and regional nodes involved.

Anatomic Areas of Colon and Rectum

1. Cecum
2. Ascending colon
3. Hepatic flexure
4. Transverse colon
5. Splenic flexure
6. Descending colon
7. Sigmoid
7.5 Rectosigmoid
8. Rectum
9. Anal canal

13
Anal Canal

C21.0 Anus, NOS
C21.1 Anal canal
C21.2 Cloacogenic zone
C21.8 Overlapping lesion of
        rectum, anus and anal
        canal

There are two staging systems for carcinomas of the anus: one for the anal canal and the other for the anal margin. The separation is important because it affects prognosis and treatment.

Cancers of the anal canal are staged clinically according to the size and extent of the primary tumor. Thus, patients with cancer of the canal can be classified at time of presentation by inspection of the lesion and palpation of adjacent structures, including the regional lymph nodes. Although additional information concerning depth of penetration is often provided by the pathologist after resection, in many cases—especially those treated with radiation and chemotherapy—the true depth of invasion cannot always be assessed. Radiation and chemotherapy not only destroy tumor cells but also cause inflammatory changes and edema, which makes it difficult for the pathologist to assess the true depth of invasion.

Cancers that arise at the anal margin—that is, the junction of the hair-bearing skin and the mucous membrane of the anal canal—or more distal are staged according to the system used for skin cancers (see page 135).

ANATOMY

Primary Site. For staging purposes, the anatomic limits of the anal canal are defined as follows. The anal canal extends from the rectum to the perianal skin and is lined by the mucous membrane overlying the internal sphincter, including the transitional epithelium and dentate line, to the junction with the hair-bearing skin.

Regional Lymph Nodes

Perirectal:
  Anorectal
  Perirectal
  Lateral sacral

Internal iliac (hypogastric)

Inguinal:
  Superficial
  Deep femoral

All other nodal groups represent sites of distant metastasis. The sites of regional node involvement are explained by the lymphatic drainage, above to the rectal ampulla and below to the perineum. Tumors that arise in the anal canal usually spread initially to the anorectal and perirectal nodes, and those that arise at the anal margin spread to the superficial inguinal nodes.

Metastatic Sites. Cancers of the anus can metastasize to most organs, especially the liver and lungs. Involvement of the abdominal cavity is not unusual.

RULES FOR CLASSIFICATION

The staging system does not preclude the surgeon from recording the depth of penetration or extension of tumor based on information provided by the pathologist or radiologist. This information, however, is not included in the staging classification.

The primary tumor is staged according to its size and local extension, as determined by clinical or pathologic examination. For most histologic types, the diameter of the tumor correlates with the depth of penetration. Extension to the anorectal, perirectal, superficial inguinal, or femoral nodes, as well as to adjacent structures, usually can be assessed by palpation. Tumor can extend to the rectal mucosa or submucosa, subcutaneous perianal tissue, perianal skin, ischiorectal fat, or local skeletal muscles, such as the external anal sphincter, levator ani, and coccygeus muscles. Tumor can also invade the perineum, vulva, prostate gland, urinary bladder, urethra, vagina, cervix uteri, corpus uteri, pelvic peritoneum, and broad ligaments. The organs invaded by tumor should be specified.

Spread to other nodal groups, such as inferior mesenteric, can often be suspected by computed tomography or magnetic nuclear imaging.

Clinical Staging. Anal cancers are staged primarily by inspection and palpation. Imaging may help to define the extent of tumor. In rare cases of rectal excision, tumors of the anal canal may be staged pathologically. Direct invasion of the rectal wall, perirectal skin, or subcutaneous tissue is not considered T4. The tumor is classified by size.

DEFINITION OF TNM

Anal Canal

The following is the TNM classification for the staging of cancers that arise in the anal canal only. Cancers that arise at the anal margin are staged according to the classification for cancers of the skin.

Primary Tumor (T)

TX Primary tumor cannot be assessed
T0 No evidence of primary tumor
Tis Carcinoma *in situ*
T1 Tumor 2 cm or less in greatest dimension
T2 Tumor more than 2 cm but not more than 5 cm in greatest dimension
T3 Tumor more than 5 cm in greatest dimension
T4 Tumor of any size invades adjacent organ(s), e.g., vagina, urethra, bladder (involvement of sphincter muscle(s) alone is not classified as T4)

Regional Lymph Nodes (N)

NX Regional lymph nodes cannot be assessed
N0 No regional lymph node metastasis
N1 Metastasis in perirectal lymph node(s)
N2 Metastasis in unilateral internal iliac and/or inguinal lymph node(s)
N3 Metastasis in perirectal and inguinal lymph nodes and/or bilateral internal iliac and/or inguinal lymph nodes

Distant Metastasis (M)

MX Presence of distant metastasis cannot be assessed
M0 No distant metastasis
M1 Distant metastasis

STAGE GROUPING

Stage 0	Tis	N0	M0
Stage I	T1	N0	M0
Stage II	T2	N0	M0
	T3	N0	M0
Stage IIIA	T1	N1	M0
	T2	N1	M0
	T3	N1	M0
	T4	N0	M0
Stage IIIB	T4	N1	M0
	Any T	N2	M0
	Any T	N3	M0
Stage IV	Any T	Any N	M1

HISTOPATHOLOGIC TYPE

The staging system applies to all carcinomas arising in the anal canal, including carcinomas that arise within anorectal fistulas. The classification also includes cloacogenic carcinomas. Melanomas are excluded.

HISTOPATHOLOGIC GRADE (G)

GX Grade cannot be assessed
G1 Well differentiated
G2 Moderately differentiated
G3 Poorly differentiated
G4 Undifferentiated

BIBLIOGRAPHY

1. Boman BM, Moertel CG, O'Connell MJ, et al: Carcinoma of the anal canal: A clinical and pathologic study of 188 cases. Cancer 54:114–125, 1984
2. Flam MS, John M, Lovalvo LJ, et al: Definitive nonsurgical therapy of epithelial malignancies of the anal canal. Cancer 51:1378–1387, 1983
3. Gabriel WB: Squamous cell carcinoma of the anus and anal canal. J Royal Soc Med 34 (Part 1):139–157, 1941
4. Greenall MJ, Quan SHQ, Stearns MW, et al: Epidermoid cancer of the anal margin. Am J Surg 149:95–101, 1985
5. Morson BC: The pathology and results of treatment of squamous cell carcinoma of the anal canal and anal margin. J Royal Soc Med 53:416–420, 1960

6. Nigro ND: An evaluation of combined therapy for squamous cell cancer of the anal canal. Dis Colon Rectum 27:763–766, 1984

7. Nigro ND: Treatment of squamous cell cancer of the anus. Cancer Treat Res 18:221–242, 1984

8. Nigro ND, Vaitkeviceus VK, Herskovic AM: Preservation of function in the treatment of cancer of the anus. Important Adv Oncol pp 161–177, 1989

9. Paradis P, Douglass HO Jr, Holyoke ED: The clinical implications of a staging system for carcinoma of the anus. Surg Gynecol Obstet 141:411–416, 1975

10. Pintor MP, Northover JM, Nicholls RJ: Squamous cell carcinoma of the anus at one hospital from 1948. Br J Surg 76:806–810, 1989

11. Salmon RJ, Fenton J, Asselain B, et al: Treatment of epidermoid anal canal cancer. Am J Surg 147:43–47, 1984

12. Salmon RJ, Zafrani B, Labib A, et al: Prognosis of cloacogenic and squamous cancers of the anal canal. Dis Colon Rectum 29:336–340, 1986

13. Schraut WH, Wang CH, Dawson PJ, et al: Depth of invasion, location, and size of cancer of the anus dictate operative treatment. Cancer 51:1291–1296, 1983

14. Scott NA, Beart RW Jr, Weiland LH, et al: Carcinoma of the anal canal and flow cytometric DNA analysis. Br J Cancer 60:56–58, 1989

15. Shank B: Treatment of anal canal carcinoma. Cancer (Suppl) 55:2156–2162, 1985

16. Spratt JS (Ed.): Neoplasms of the Colon, Rectum, and Anus. Philadelphia, WB Saunders, 1984

Data Form for Cancer Staging

Patient identification
Name _____
Address _____
Hospital or clinic number _____
Age _____ Sex _____ Race _____

Institution identification
Hospital or clinic _____
Address _____

Oncology Record

Anatomic site of cancer _____
Histologic type _____
Grade (G) _____
Date of classification _____

Chronology of classification
[ ] Clinical (use all data prior to first treatment)
[ ] Pathologic (if definitively resected specimen available)

DEFINITIONS
Primary Tumor (T)

Clin	Path		
[ ]	[ ]	TX	Primary tumor cannot be assessed
[ ]	[ ]	T0	No evidence of primary tumor
[ ]	[ ]	Tis	Carcinoma *in situ*
[ ]	[ ]	T1	Tumor 2 cm or less in greatest dimension
[ ]	[ ]	T2	Tumor more than 2 cm but not more than 5 cm in greatest dimension
[ ]	[ ]	T3	Tumor more than 5 cm in greatest dimension
[ ]	[ ]	T4	Tumor of any size invades adjacent organ(s): *e.g.*, vagina, urethra, bladder (involvement of sphincter muscle(s) *alone* is not classified as T4)

Lymph Node (N)

Clin	Path		
[ ]	[ ]	NX	Regional lymph nodes cannot be assessed
[ ]	[ ]	N0	No regional lymph node metastasis
[ ]	[ ]	N1	Metastasis in perirectal lymph node(s)
[ ]	[ ]	N2	Metastasis in unilateral internal iliac and/or inguinal lymph node(s)
[ ]	[ ]	N3	Metastasis in perirectal and inguinal lymph nodes and/or bilateral internal iliac and/or inguinal lymph nodes

Distant Metastasis (M)

Clin	Path		
[ ]	[ ]	MX	Presence of distant metastasis cannot be assessed
[ ]	[ ]	M0	No distant metastasis
[ ]	[ ]	M1	Distant metastasis

Stage Grouping

Clin	Path				
[ ]	[ ]	0	Tis	N0	M0
[ ]	[ ]	I	T1	N0	M0
[ ]	[ ]	II	T2	N0	M0
			T3	N0	M0
[ ]	[ ]	IIIA	T1	N1	M0
			T2	N1	M0
			T3	N1	M0
			T4	N0	M0
[ ]	[ ]	IIIB	T4	N1	M0
			Any T	N2	M0
			Any T	N3	M0
[ ]	[ ]	IV	Any T	Any N	M1

Histopathologic Type

The staging system applies to all carcinomas arising in the anal canal, including carcinomas that arise within an anorectal fistula. Melanomas are excluded.

Histopathologic Grade (G)

[ ] GX Grade cannot be assessed
[ ] G1 Well differentiated
[ ] G2 Moderately differentiated
[ ] G3 Poorly differentiated
[ ] G4 Undifferentiated

Illustration

Indicate on diagram primary tumor and regional nodes involved.

Staged by _____ M.D.
_____ Registrar
Date _____

14

Liver (Including Intrahepatic Bile Ducts)

C22.0 Liver
C22.1 Intrahepatic bile duct

The largest parenchymatous organ in the body, the liver is often the site of metastatic cancer, especially from carcinomas originating in abdominal viscera. Primary cancers of the liver are uncommon in the United States, but common in many other countries. Several distinctive malignant tumors are found in the liver. These include hepatocellular carcinomas originating from hepatocytes, cholangiocarcinomas or intrahepatic bile duct carcinomas arising from bile ducts, and sarcomas arising from mesenchymal elements. Hepatocellular carcinomas are often associated with pre-existing liver disease, usually cirrhosis, which may dominate the clinical picture. Cholangiocarcinomas are not associated with chronic liver disease. The liver has a dual blood supply: the hepatic artery, which branches from the celiac artery, and the portal vein, which drains the intestine. Blood from the liver passes through the hepatic vein and enters the inferior vena cava. Hepatocellular carcinomas have a proclivity to invade blood vessels, a fact that is considered in the staging classification. Invasion of adjacent structures such as the diaphragm, adrenal gland, vena cava, or hilar vessels often makes resection of the tumor difficult or impossible.

ANATOMY

Histologically, the liver is divided into lobules. Between the lobules are the portal areas that contain the intrahepatic bile ducts.

Primary Site. The liver is located in the right upper abdominal cavity below the right leaf of the diaphragm. It extends from the fifth rib and midclavicular line on the left side to the inferior costal margin and midaxillary line on the right side. Covered by a smooth, reddish-brown capsule, the organ is divided into right and left lobes, the former being much larger. The smaller lobes, the quadrate and the caudate, are subdivisions of the undersurface of the liver, located on the left side of the plane projecting between the bed of the gallbladder and the inferior vena cava. For classification, the quadrate lobe is considered part of the left lobe. The quadrate lobe is inferior and the caudate lobe superior to the porta hepatis, through which passes the hepatic artery. The caudate lobe receives its blood supply from both the right and left lobes and secretes bile into both the right and left hepatic ducts, so anatomically and functionally it is part of both the right and left lobes.

Regional Lymph Nodes. The regional lymph nodes are the hilar (i.e., those in the hepatoduodenal ligament, hepatic and periportal nodes). Regional nodes also include those along the inferior vena cava, hepatic artery, and portal vein. Any lymph node involvement beyond these nodes is considered distant metastasis and should be coded as M1.

Metastatic Sites. Hepatocellular carcinomas can spread to most organs in the body. The most common sites are the lungs and bone. Direct extension often occurs to the diaphragm.

RULES FOR CLASSIFICATION

T categories are based on the number of tumor nodules, the size of the largest nodule (2 cm is the discriminating limit), and the presence of vascular invasion. The staging system does not consider etiologic mechanisms such as whether multiple nodules represent multiple, independent primary tumors or intrahepatic metastasis from a single primary hepatic carcinoma.

Because of the tendency for vascular invasion, imaging of the liver is important for staging primary hepatocellular carcinomas, unless distant metastasis is present at the time of diagnosis.

Clinical Staging. Staging depends on some type of imaging procedure to demonstrate the size of the primary tumor and vascular invasion. Surgical exploration is usually not carried out, because the possibility for complete resection is minimal, especially for larger tumors.

Pathologic Staging. If surgical exploration is carried out and there is resection then Pathologic Staging can be recorded.

Note: For classification, the plane projecting between the bed of the gallbladder and the inferior vena cava divides the liver into two lobes.

DEFINITION OF TNM
Primary Tumor (T)

TX   Primary tumor cannot be assessed
T0   No evidence of primary tumor
T1   Solitary tumor 2 cm or less in greatest dimension without vascular invasion
T2   Solitary tumor 2 cm or less in greatest dimension with vascular invasion; or multiple tumors limited to one lobe, none more than 2 cm in greatest dimension without vascular invasion; or a solitary tumor more than 2 cm in greatest dimension without vascular invasion
T3   Solitary tumor more than 2 cm in greatest dimension with vascular invasion; or multiple tumors limited to one lobe, none more than 2 cm in greatest dimension, with vascular invasion; or multiple tumors limited to one lobe, any more than 2 cm in greatest dimension, with or without vascular invasion
T4   Multiple tumors in more than one lobe, or tumor(s) involving a major branch of the portal or hepatic vein(s)

Regional Lymph Nodes (N)

NX   Regional lymph nodes cannot be assessed
N0   No regional lymph node metastasis
N1   Regional lymph node metastasis

Distant Metastasis (M)

MX   Presence of distant metastasis cannot be assessed
M0   No distant metastasis
M1   Distant metastasis

STAGE GROUPING

Stage	T	N	M
Stage I	T1	N0	M0
Stage II	T2	N0	M0
Stage III	T1	N1	M0
	T2	N1	M0
	T3	N0	M0
	T3	N1	M0
Stage IVA	T4	Any N	M0
Stage IVB	Any T	Any N	M1

HISTOPATHOLOGIC TYPE

The staging system applies to all primary carcinomas of the liver. These include hepatomas or hepatocellular carcinomas, intrahepatic bile duct carcinomas or cholangiocarcinomas, and mixed types. (Hepatomas are by far the most common.) The classification does not apply to sarcomas. The histologic type should be recorded.

HISTOPATHOLOGIC GRADE (G)

GX   Grade cannot be assessed
G1   Well differentiated
G2   Moderately differentiated
G3   Poorly differentiated
G4   Undifferentiated

BIBLIOGRAPHY

1. Adson MA, Beart RW: Elective hepatic resections. Surg Clin North Am 57:339–360, 1977
2. Bartok I, Remenar E, Toth J, et al: Clinico-pathological studies of liver cirrhosis and hepatocellular carcinoma in a general hospital. Hum Pathol 12:794–803, 1981
3. Chuong JJ, Livstone EM, Barwick KW: The histopathologic and clinical indicators of prognosis in hepatoma. J Clin Gastroenterol 4:547–552, 1982
4. Craig JR, Peters RL, Edmondson HA: Tumors of liver and intrahepatic bile ducts. Atlas of Tumor Pathology, Fascicle 26, Second Series. Washington DC, Armed Forces Institute of Pathology, 1989
5. Liver Cancer Study Group of Japan, Primary liver cancer in Japan: Clinicopathologic features and results of surgical treatment. Ann Surg 211:277–287, 1990
6. Okuda K, Peters RL (Eds.): Hepatocellular Carcinoma. New York, Wiley Publications, 1976
7. Schaff Z, Lapis K, Henson DE: Liver. In Henson DE, Albores-Saavedra J (Eds.), The Pathology of Incipient Neoplasia. Philadelphia, WB Saunders, 1986
8. Warvi WN: Primary neoplasms of the liver. Arch Path and Lab Med 37:367–382, 1944

Data Form for Cancer Staging

Patient identification
Name _____

Address _____

Hospital or clinic number _____

Age _____ Sex _____ Race _____

Institution identification
Hospital or clinic _____

Address _____

Oncology Record

Anatomic site of cancer _____

Histologic type _____

Grade (G) _____

Date of classification _____

Chronology of classification
[ ] Clinical (use all data prior to first treatment)
[ ] Pathologic (if definitively resected specimen available)

DEFINITIONS

Primary Tumor (T)

Clin	Path		
[ ]	[ ]	TX	Primary tumor cannot be assessed
[ ]	[ ]	T0	No evidence of primary tumor
[ ]	[ ]	T1	Solitary tumor 2 cm or less in greatest dimension without vascular invasion
[ ]	[ ]	T2	Solitary tumor 2 cm or less in greatest dimension with vascular invasion, *or*
[ ]	[ ]		Multiple tumors limited to one lobe none more than 2 cm in greatest dimension without vascular invasion, *or*
[ ]	[ ]		A solitary tumor more than 2 cm in greatest dimension without vascular invasion
[ ]	[ ]	T3	Solitary tumor more than 2 cm in greatest dimension with vascular invasion, *or*
[ ]	[ ]		Multiple tumors limited to one lobe, none more than 2 cm in greatest dimension, with vascular invasion, *or*
[ ]	[ ]		Multiple tumors limited to one lobe, any more than 2 cm in greatest dimension, with or without vascular invasion
[ ]	[ ]	T4	Multiple tumors in more than one lobe *or*
[ ]	[ ]		Tumor(s) involve(s) a major branch of portal or hepatic vein(s)

Lymph Node (N)

Clin	Path		
[ ]	[ ]	NX	Regional lymph nodes cannot be assessed
[ ]	[ ]	N0	No regional lymph node metastasis
[ ]	[ ]	N1	Regional lymph node metastasis

Distant Metastasis (M)

Clin	Path		
[ ]	[ ]	MX	Presence of distant metastasis cannot be assessed
[ ]	[ ]	M0	No distant metastasis
[ ]	[ ]	M1	Distant metastasis

Histopathologic Grade (G)

[ ] GX Grade cannot be assessed
[ ] G1 Well differentiated
[ ] G2 Moderately differentiated
[ ] G3 Poorly differentiated
[ ] G4 Undifferentiated

Illustration

Indicate on diagram primary tumor and regional nodes involved.

Histopathologic Type

The staging system applies to all primary carcinomas of the liver. These include hepatomas or hepatocellular carcinomas and intrahepatic bile duct carcinomas or cholangiocarcinomas and mixed types. Hepatomas are by far the most common. The classification does not apply to sarcomas.

Stage Grouping

Clin	Path				
[ ]	[ ]	I	T1	N0	M0
[ ]	[ ]	II	T2	N0	M0
[ ]	[ ]	III	T1	N1	M0
			T2	N1	M0
			T3	N0	M0
			T3	N1	M0
[ ]	[ ]	IVA	T4	Any N	M0
[ ]	[ ]	IVB	Any T	Any N	M1

Staged by _____ M.D.

_____ Registrar

Date _____

American Joint Committee on Cancer—1992

15
Gallbladder

C23.9 Gallbladder

ANATOMY

Cancers of the gallbladder are staged according to their depth of penetration into the wall and extension to adjacent organs. Distant spread of cancer to the liver is found in 70% of patients at the time of surgical evaluation; tumors that have invaded more than 2 cm usually are nonresectable. Malignant tumors of the gallbladder are insidious in their spread, often metastasizing early before a diagnosis is made. This proclivity for early spread before the appearance of signs and symptoms includes all carcinomas known to occur in the gallbladder. Tumors can also perforate the wall of the gallbladder and cause intra-abdominal metastases, carcinomatosis, and ascites. Unfortunately, because gallbladder cancer is uncommon and usually diagnosed late, physicians have often ignored anatomic staging, even though its importance for survival, management, and prognosis has been emphasized. Many cases are not suspected clinically and are first discovered at laparotomy or incidentally by the pathologist. For carcinomas of the gallbladder, the stage groupings have been further subdivided based on the extent of lymph node involvement.

Primary Site. The gallbladder is a pear-shaped saccular organ located under the liver in the gallbladder fossa. It has three parts: a fundus, a body, and a neck that tapers into the cystic duct. The wall of the gallbladder is much thinner than that of the intestine, lacking a circular and transverse muscle layer. The wall has a mucosa—that is, an epithelial lining and lamina propria, a smooth muscle layer analogous to the muscularis mucosae of the small intestine, perimuscular connective tissue, and serosa. There is no submucosa. Along the attachment to the liver, no serosa exists, and the perimuscular connective tissue is continuous with the interlobular connective tissue of the liver. Tumors arising in the cystic duct are classified according to the scheme for the extrahepatic bile ducts.

Regional Lymph Nodes. The regional lymph nodes include the following:

Cystic duct
Pericholedochal
Hilar
Celiac
Node of foramen of Winslow
Periduodenal
Periportal
Peripancreatic
Superior mesenteric

Peripancreatic nodes located along the body and tail of the pancreas are sites of distant metastasis.

Metastatic Sites. Cancers of the gallbladder usually spread to the lungs, pleura, and diaphragm, and intra-abdominally. Any site can be involved.

RULES FOR CLASSIFICATION

Gallbladder cancers are staged primarily on the basis of surgical exploration or resection. Many in situ and early stage carcinomas are not visible grossly. They are usually staged pathologically after histologic examination of the resected specimen.

The staging classification depends on the depth of tumor penetration into the wall of the gallbladder, the extent of invasion into the liver, and the number of adjacent organs involved with regional spread of the tumor.

Clinical Staging. If only clinical and pathologic data are available without a resected specimen at surgical exploration then staging should be classified as clinical.

Pathologic Staging. Staging is based on imaging, surgical exploration, and examination of the resected specimen.

DEFINITION OF TNM

Primary Tumor (T)

TX   Primary tumor cannot be assessed
T0   No evidence of primary tumor
Tis   Carcinoma *in situ*
T1   Tumor invades mucosa or muscle layer
     T1a   Tumor invades the mucosa
     T1b   Tumor invades the muscle layer
T2   Tumor invades the perimuscular connective tissue; no extension beyond the serosa or into the liver
T3   Tumor perforates the serosa (visceral peritoneum) or directly invades into one adjacent organ, or both (extension 2 cm or less into the liver)
T4   Tumor extends more than 2 cm into the liver and/or into two or more adjacent organs (stomach, duodenum, colon, pancreas, omentum, extrahepatic bile ducts, any involvement of liver)

Regional Lymph Nodes (N)

NX   Regional lymph nodes cannot be assessed
N0   No regional lymph node metastasis
N1   Metastasis in cystic duct, pericholedochal, and/or hilar lymph nodes (i.e., in the hepatoduodenal ligament)
N2   Metastasis in peripancreatic (head only), periduodenal, periportal, celiac, and/or superior mesenteric lymph nodes

Distant Metastasis (M)

MX   Presence of distant metastasis cannot be assessed
M0   No distant metastasis
M1   Distant metastasis

STAGE GROUPING

Stage	T	N	M
Stage 0	Tis	N0	M0
Stage I	T1	N0	M0
Stage II	T2	N0	M0
Stage III	T1	N1	M0
	T2	N1	M0
	T3	N0	M0
	T3	N1	M0
Stage IVA	T4	N0	M0
	T4	N1	M0
Stage IVB	Any T	N2	M0
	Any T	Any N	M1

HISTOPATHOLOGIC TYPE

The staging system applies to all primary carcinomas arising in the gallbladder. Papillary carcinomas have the

SURVIVAL ACCORDING TO AJCC STAGE
GALLBLADDER

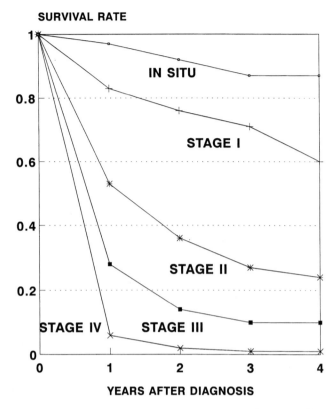

Fig. 15-1. Relative survival rates for 877 patients with gallbladder cancer according to the current AJCC staging classification. Data taken from the Surveillance, Epidemiology, and End Results Program of the National Cancer Institute for the years 1983–1987. Stage 0 includes 40 patients; Stage I, 105; Stage II, 101; Stage III, 132; and Stage IV, 499.

most favorable prognosis. Lymphatic and/or vascular invasion indicates a less favorable prognosis. The staging system does not apply to carcinoid tumors or to sarcomas. Adenocarcinomas are the most common type. The carcinomas are described as follows:

Carcinoma *in situ*
Adenocarcinoma
Papillary adenocarcinoma
Adenocarcinoma, intestinal type
Mucinous adenocarcinoma
Clear cell adenocarcinoma
Signet-ring cell carcinoma
Adenosquamous carcinoma
Squamous cell carcinoma
Small cell (oat cell) carcinoma
Undifferentiated carcinoma
Carcinoma, NOS

HISTOPATHOLOGIC GRADE (G)

GX Grade cannot be assessed
G1 Well differentiated
G2 Moderately differentiated
G3 Poorly differentiated
G4 Undifferentiated

BIBLIOGRAPHY

1. Albores-Saavedra J, Cruz-Ortiz H, Alcantara-Vazquez A, et al: Unusual types of gallbladder carcinoma. Arch Pathol Lab Med 105:287–293, 1981
2. Albores-Saavedra J, Henson DE: Extrahepatic biliary system. In Henson D, Albores-Saavedra J (Eds.), The Pathology of Incipient Neoplasia. Philadelphia, WB Saunders, 1986
3. Albores-Saavedra J, Henson DE: Tumors of the gallbladder and extrahepatic bile ducts. Atlas of Tumor Pathology, Fascicle 22, Second Series. Washington DC, Armed Forces Institute of Pathology, 1986
4. Albores-Saavedra J, Henson DE, Sobin LH: Histological typing of tumors of the gallbladder and extrahepatic bile ducts. WHO International Histological Classification of Tumors. Berlin-New York, Springer-Verlag, 1991
5. Bergdahl L: Gallbladder carcinoma first diagnosed at microscopic examination of gallbladder removed for presumed benign disease. Ann Surg 191:19–22, 1980
6. Bivins BA, Meeker WR Jr, Griffen WO Jr: Importance of histologic classification of carcinoma of the gallbladder. Ann Surg 41:121–124, 1975
7. Fahim RB, McDonald JR, Richards JC, et al: Carcinoma of the gallbladder: A study of its modes of spread. Ann Surg 156:114–124, 1962
8. Henson DE, Albores-Saavedra J, Corle D: Carcinoma of the gallbladder: Histologic types, stage of disease, grade, and survival. Cancer, In Press.
9. Jones RS: Carcinoma of the gallbladder. Surg Clin N Amer 70:1419–1428, 1990
10. Lurie BB, Loewenstein MS, Zamcheck N: Elevated carcinoembryonic antigen levels and biliary tract obstruction. JAMA 233:326–330, 1975
11. Nagorney DM: Management of carcinoma of the gallbladder. Prob Gen Surg 3:170, 1986
12. Nevin JE, Moran TJ, Day S, et al: Carcinoma of the gallbladder: Staging, treatment, and prognosis. Cancer 37:141–148, 1976
13. Ogura Y, Mizumoto R, Isaji S, et al: Radical Operations for carcinoma of the gallbladder: Present status in Japan. World J Surg 15:337–343, 1991
14. Ouchi K, Owada Y, Matsuno S, et al: Prognostic factors in the surgical treatment of gallbladder carcinoma. Surg 101:736–737, 1987
15. Perpetuo MMO, Valdivieso M, Heilbrun LK, et al: Natural history study of gallbladder cancer. Cancer 42:330–335,1978
16. Richard PF, Cantin J: Primary carcinoma of the gallbladder: Study of 108 cases. Can J Surg 19:27–32, 1976
17. Wanebo HJ, Castle WN, Fechner R: Is carcinoma of the gallbladder a curable lesion? Ann Surg 195:624–630, 1982
18. Yamamoto M, Nakajo S, Tahara E: Carcinoma of the gallbladder: The correlation between histogenesis and prognosis. Virchows Arch [A] 414:83–90,1989.

Data Form for Cancer Staging

Patient identification
Name _____
Address _____
Hospital or clinic number _____
Age _____ Sex _____ Race _____

Institution identification
Hospital or clinic _____
Address _____

Oncology Record

Anatomic site of cancer _____
Histologic type _____
Grade (G) _____
Date of classification _____

Chronology of classification
[ ] Clinical (use all data prior to first treatment)
[ ] Pathologic (if definitively resected specimen available)

DEFINITIONS

Primary Tumor (T)

Clin	Path		
[ ]	[ ]	TX	Primary tumor cannot be assessed
[ ]	[ ]	T0	No evidence of primary tumor
[ ]	[ ]	Tis	Carcinoma *in situ*
[ ]	[ ]	T1	Tumor invades mucosa or muscle layer
[ ]	[ ]	T1a	Tumor invades mucosa
[ ]	[ ]	T1b	Tumor invades muscle layer
[ ]	[ ]	T2	Tumor invades perimuscular connective tissue; no extension beyond serosa or into liver
[ ]	[ ]	T3	Tumor perforates the serosa (visceral peritoneum) or directly invades into one adjacent organ, or both (extension 2 cm or less into liver)
[ ]	[ ]	T4	Tumor extends more than 2 cm into liver, and/or into two or more adjacent organs (stomach, duodenum, colon, pancreas, omentum, extrahepatic bile ducts, any involvement of liver)

Lymph Node (N)

Clin	Path		
[ ]	[ ]	NX	Regional lymph nodes cannot be assessed
[ ]	[ ]	N0	No regional lymph node metastasis
[ ]	[ ]	N1	Metastasis in cystic duct, pericholedochal, and/or hilar lymph nodes, *i.e.*, in hepatoduodenal ligament
[ ]	[ ]	N2	Metastasis in peripancreatic (head only), periduodenal, periportal, celiac, and/or superior mesenteric lymph nodes

Distant Metastasis (M)

Clin	Path		
[ ]	[ ]	MX	Presence of distant metastasis cannot be assessed
[ ]	[ ]	M0	No distant metastasis
[ ]	[ ]	M1	Distant metastasis

Stage Grouping

Clin	Path				
[ ]	[ ]	0	Tis	N0	M0
[ ]	[ ]	I	T1	N0	M0
[ ]	[ ]	II	T2	N0	M0
[ ]	[ ]	III	T1	N1	M0
			T2	N1	M0
			T3	N0	M0
			T3	N1	M0
[ ]	[ ]	IVA	T4	N0	M0
			T4	N1	M0
[ ]	[ ]	IVB	Any T	N2	M0
			Any T	Any N	M1

Staged by _____ M.D.
_____Registrar
Date _____

(continued on next page)

Histopathologic Type

The staging system applies to all primary carcinomas arising in the gallbladder. Papillary carcinomas have the most favorable prognosis. Lymphatic and/or vascular invasion indicates a less favorable prognosis. The staging system does not apply to carcinoid tumors or to sarcomas. Adenocarcinomas are the most common type. The carcinomas are described as follows:

Carcinoma *in situ*
Adenocarcinoma
Papillary adenocarcinoma
Adenocarcinoma, intestinal type
Mucinous adenocarcinoma
Clear cell adenocarcinoma
Signet-ring cell carcinoma
Adenosquamous carcinoma
Squamous cell carcinoma
Small cell (oat cell) carcinoma
Undifferentiated carcinoma
Carcinoma, NOS

Histopathologic Grade (G)

[ ] GX   Grade cannot be assessed
[ ] G1   Well differentiated
[ ] G2   Moderately differentiated
[ ] G3   Poorly differentiated
[ ] G4   Undifferentiated

Illustration

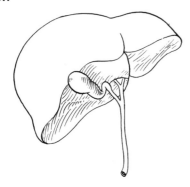

Indicate on diagram primary tumor and regional nodes involved.

16

Extrahepatic Bile Ducts

C24.0 Extrahepatic bile duct
C24.8 Overlapping lesion
C24.9 Biliary tract, NOS

Malignant tumors can develop in any segment of the extrahepatic bile ducts. Nearly 50% occur in the upper third, 25% in the middle third, and 20% in the lower third. In 10% of cases, the ducts are diffusely involved. Tumors that develop near the hilum of the liver are most difficult to resect. As a result, they have the worst prognosis. All malignant tumors inevitably cause partial or complete obstruction of the extrahepatic bile ducts and proximal distention. Clinical symptoms usually occur while the tumor is relatively small, before widespread dissemination has occurred. This staging classification applies only to cancers arising in the extrahepatic bile ducts and in the cystic duct. It does not include those arising in the ampulla of Vater or in the pancreatic ducts. Malignant epithelial tumors originating in the right or left hepatic ducts are often described as hilar carcinomas of the liver.

ANATOMY

Primary Site. Emerging from the transverse fissure of the liver are the right and left hepatic bile ducts, which join to form the common hepatic duct. The cystic duct, which connects to the gallbladder, joins the common hepatic duct to form the common bile duct. The common bile duct passes behind the first part of the duodenum and then traverses the head of the pancreas until it opens into the second part of the duodenum at the ampulla of Vater. The bile ducts are lined by a single layer of tall columnar cells. The mucosa usually forms irregular pleats, or small folds, that run longitudinally. The wall of the bile duct has a layer of subepithelial connective tissue and muscle fibers.

Regional Lymph Nodes. The regional nodes are the same as those listed for the gallbladder, but also include those located near the duodenum and head of the pancreas. They include the following:

Cystic
Hilar
Superior mesenteric
Periduodenal
Node on the anterior border of the foramen of Winslow
Superior retropancreaticoduodenal
Posterior pancreaticoduodenal
Peripancreatic
Periportal
Pericholedochal
Celiac

Involvement of other lymph nodes is considered distant metastasis and should be coded M1. Parapancreatic nodes near the body and tail of the pancreas are also considered sites of distant metastasis.

Metastatic Sites. Carcinomas can extend to the liver, pancreas, ampulla of Vater, duodenum, colon, omentum, stomach, or gallbladder. Tumors arising in the right or left hepatic ducts usually extend proximally into the liver or distal to the common hepatic duct. Neoplasms from the cystic duct invade the gallbladder or the common bile duct, or both. Carcinomas arising in the distal segment of the common duct can spread to the pancreas, duodenum, stomach, colon, or omentum. Distant metastases usually occur late in the course of the disease, most often to the lungs.

RULES FOR CLASSIFICATION

Most cancers are staged following surgery and pathologic examination of the resected specimen. Evaluation of the extent of disease at laparotomy is most important for staging.

Clinical Staging

See Pathologic Staging.

Pathologic Staging. Staging depends on imaging, which often defines the limits of the tumor, and on surgical exploration with pathologic examination of the resected specimen. In many cases, it may be difficult to completely resect the primary tumor.

DEFINITION OF TNM
Primary Tumor (T)

TX   Primary tumor cannot be assessed
T0   No evidence of primary tumor
Tis Carcinoma *in situ*
T1   Tumor invades the mucosa or muscle layer
    T1a   Tumor invades the mucosa
    T1b   Tumor invades the muscle layer
T2   Tumor invades the perimuscular connective tissue
T3   Tumor invades adjacent structures: liver, pancreas, duodenum, gallbladder, colon, stomach

Regional Lymph Nodes (N)

NX   Regional lymph nodes cannot be assessed
N0   No regional lymph node metastasis
N1   Metastasis in the cystic duct, pericholedochal and/or hilar lymph nodes (i.e., in the hepatoduodenal ligament)
N2   Metastasis in the peripancreatic (head only), periduodenal, periportal, celiac, superior mesenteric, and/or posterior pancreaticoduodenal lymph nodes

Distant Metastasis (M)

MX   Presence of distant metastasis cannot be assessed
M0   No distant metastasis
M1   Distant metastasis

STAGE GROUPING

Stage 0	Tis	N0	M0
Stage I	T1	N0	M0
Stage II	T2	N0	M0
Stage III	T1	N1	M0
	T1	N2	M0
	T2	N1	M0
	T2	N2	M0
Stage IVA	T3	Any N	M0
Stage IVB	Any T	Any N	M1

HISTOPATHOLOGIC TYPE

The staging system applies to all primary carcinomas arising in the extrahepatic bile ducts or in the cystic duct. Sarcomas and carcinoid tumors are excluded. Adenocarcinomas are the most common type. The histologic types are as follows:

Carcinoma *in situ*
Adenocarcinoma
Papillary adenocarcinoma
Adenocarcinoma, intestinal type
Mucinous adenocarcinoma
Clear cell adenocarcinoma
Signet-ring cell carcinoma
Adenosquamous carcinoma
Squamous cell carcinoma
Small cell (oat cell) carcinoma
Undifferentiated carcinoma
Carcinoma, NOS

SITE-SPECIFIC INFORMATION

Recording the location of the primary tumor is important for prognosis. However, it is often difficult to establish with certainty the origin of these tumors when the pathologic process is far advanced.

Location of tumor: Upper third
                         Middle third
                         Lower third
                         Diffuse

HISTOPATHOLOGIC GRADE (G)

GX   Grade cannot be assessed
G1   Well differentiated
G2   Moderately differentiated
G3   Poorly differentiated
G4   Undifferentiated

BIBLIOGRAPHY

1. Albores-Saavedra J, Henson DE: Tumors of the gallbladder and extrahepatic bile ducts. Atlas of Tumor Pathology, Fascicle 22, Second Series. Washington DC, Armed Forces Institute of Pathology, 1986
2. Albores-Saavedra J, Henson DE, Sobin LH: Histological typing of tumors of the gallbladder and extrahepatic bile ducts. WHO International Histological Classification of Tumors. Berlin-New York, Springer-Verlag, 1991
3. Braasch JW, Warren KW, Kune GA: Malignant neoplasms of the bile ducts. Surg Clin North Am 47:627–638, 1967
4. Henson DE, Albores-Saavedra J, Corle D: Carcinoma of the extrahepatic bile ducts: Histologic

types, stage of disease, grade, and survival. Submitted to Cancer

5. Krain LS: Gallbladder and extrahepatic bile duct carcinoma. Geriatrics 27:111–117, 1972

6. Longmire WP Jr, McArthur MS, Bastounis EA, et al: Carcinoma of the extrahepatic biliary tract. Ann Surg 178:333–343, 1973

7. Tompkins RK, Saunders K, Roslyn JJ, et al: Changing patterns in diagnosis and management of bile duct cancer. Ann Surg 211:614–620, 1990

8. Tompkins RK, Thomas D, Wile A, et al: Prognostic factors in bile duct carcinoma. Ann Surg 194:447–455, 1981

9. Tio TL, Cheng J, Wijers OB, et al: Endosonographic TNM staging of extrahepatic bile duct cancer: Comparison with pathological staging. Gastroenterol 100:1351–1361, 1991

10. Tio TL, Wijers OB, Sars PR, et al: Preoperative TNM classification of proximal extrahepatic bile duct carcinoma by endosonography. Semin Liver Dis 10:114–120, 1990

11. Tsunoda T, Eto T, Koga M, et al: Early carcinoma of the extrahepatic bile duct. Jpn J Surg 19:691–698, 1989

12. Wanebo JH, Grimes OF: Cancer of the bile duct: The occult malignancy. Am J Surg 130:262–268, 1975

Data Form for Cancer Staging

Patient identification
Name _____
Address _____
Hospital or clinic number _____
Age _____ Sex _____ Race _____

Institution identification
Hospital or clinic _____
Address _____

Oncology Record

Anatomic site of cancer _____
Histologic type _____
Grade (G) _____
Date of classification _____

Chronology of classification
[ ] Clinical (use all data prior to first treatment)
[ ] Pathologic (if definitively resected specimen available)

DEFINITIONS

Primary Tumor (T)

Clin	Path		
[ ]	[ ]	TX	Primary tumor cannot be assessed
[ ]	[ ]	T0	No evidence of primary tumor
[ ]	[ ]	Tis	Carcinoma *in situ*
[ ]	[ ]	T1	Tumor invades mucosa or muscle layer
[ ]	[ ]	T1a	Tumor invades mucosa
[ ]	[ ]	T1b	Tumor invades muscle layer
[ ]	[ ]	T2	Tumor invades perimuscular connective tissues
[ ]	[ ]	T3	Tumor invades adjacent structure(s), liver, pancreas, duodenum, gallbladder, colon, stomach

Lymph Node (N)

Clin	Path		
[ ]	[ ]	NX	Regional lymph nodes cannot be assessed
[ ]	[ ]	N0	No regional lymph node metastasis
[ ]	[ ]	N1	Metastasis in cystic duct, pericholedochal and/or hilar lymph nodes
[ ]	[ ]	N2	Metastasis in peripancreatic (head only), periduodenal, periportal, celiac, and/or superior mesenteric and/or posterior pancreatic duodenal lymph nodes

Distant Metastasis (M)

Clin	Path		
[ ]	[ ]	MX	Presence of distant metastasis cannot be assessed
[ ]	[ ]	M0	No distant metastasis
[ ]	[ ]	M1	Distant metastasis

Stage Grouping

Clin	Path				
[ ]	[ ]	0	Tis	N0	M0
[ ]	[ ]	I	T1	N0	M0
[ ]	[ ]	II	T2	N0	M0
[ ]	[ ]	III	T1	N1	M0
			T1	N2	M0
			T2	N1	M0
			T2	N2	M0
[ ]	[ ]	IVA	T3	Any N	M0
[ ]	[ ]	IVB	Any T	Any N	M1

Histopathologic Grade (G)

[ ] GX Grade cannot be assessed
[ ] G1 Well differentiated
[ ] G2 Moderately differentiated
[ ] G3 Poorly differentiated
[ ] G4 Undifferentiated

Illustration

Upper third
Middle third
Lower third
Diffuse

Indicate on diagram primary tumor and regional nodes involved.

Histopathologic Types

The staging system applies to all primary carcinomas arising in the extrahepatic bile ducts or in the cystic duct. Sarcomas and carcinoid tumors are excluded. Adenocarcinomas are the most common type. The histologic types are as follows:

Carcinoma *in situ*
Adenocarcinoma
Papillary adenocarcinoma
Adenocarcinoma, intestinal type
Mucinous adenocarcinoma
Clear cell adenocarcinoma
Signet-ring cell carcinoma
Adenosquamous carcinoma
Squamous cell carcinoma
Small cell (oat cell) carcinoma
Undifferentiated carcinoma
Carcinoma, NOS

Staged by _____ M.D.
_____ Registrar
Date _____

17

Ampulla of Vater

C24.1 Ampulla of Vater

The importance of the ampulla of Vater lies in its strategic location. Most tumors arising in this small structure will obstruct the common bile duct, causing severe jaundice. Clinically, cancers of the ampulla may be difficult to differentiate from those arising in the head of the pancreas or even in the distal segment of the common bile duct, especially if they become large and bulky. Primary cancers of the ampulla are not common, although they comprise a high proportion of malignant tumors found in the duodenum.

ANATOMY

Primary Site. A small dilated duct, less than 1.5 cm long, the ampulla is formed in most individuals by the union of the terminal segments of the pancreatic and common bile ducts. In 25% of individuals, however, the ampulla is the termination of the common duct only, the pancreatic duct having its own entrance into the duodenum adjacent to the ampulla. In these individuals, the ampulla may be difficult to locate or even nonexistent. The ampulla opens into the duodenum, usually on the posterior-medial wall, through a small mucosal elevation—the duodenal papilla, also called the papilla of Vater. Although carcinomas can arise in either the ampulla or on the papilla, they most commonly arise near the junction of the mucosa of the ampulla with that of the papilla. Nearly all cancers arising in this area are well-differentiated adenocarcinomas. They have various designations; for example, carcinoma of the ampulla of Vater, carcinoma of the periampullary portion of the duodenum, or carcinoma of the peripapillary portion of the duodenum. It may not be possible to determine the exact site of origin for large tumors.

Regional Lymph Nodes. The regional lymph nodes of the ampulla of Vater are:

Superior: Lymph nodes superior to the head and body of the pancreas
Inferior: Lymph nodes inferior to the head and body of the pancreas
Anterior: Anterior pancreaticoduodenal, pyloric, and proximal mesenteric
Posterior: Posterior pancreaticoduodenal, common bile duct, and proximal mesenteric

Other Regional Nodes:

Pancreaticoduodenal NOS
Peripancreatic
Infrapyloric
Hepatic
Subpyloric
Celiac
Superior mesenteric
Retroperitoneal
Lateral aortic

The splenic lymph nodes and those at the tail of the pancreas are not regional nodes; metastases to these lymph nodes are coded as M1.

Metastatic Sites. Tumors of the ampulla can spread to almost any site. However, they usually infiltrate adjacent structures, such as the wall of the duodenum, the head of the pancreas, and the extrahepatic bile ducts, at an early stage. Spread to distant sites usually occurs late in the course of the disease.

RULES FOR CLASSIFICATION

Most patients are staged pathologically after examination of the surgically resected specimen. Classification is based primarily on size and local extension.

Clinical Staging. See Pathologic Staging.

Pathologic Staging. Staging depends on surgical resection and pathologic examination of the specimen and associated lymph nodes.

DEFINITION OF TNM

Primary Tumor (T)

TX   Primary tumor cannot be assessed
T0   No evidence of primary tumor
Tis Carcinoma *in situ*
T1   Tumor limited to the ampulla of Vater
T2   Tumor invades the duodenal wall
T3   Tumor invades 2 cm or less into the pancreas
T4   Tumor invades more than 2 cm into the pancreas and/or into other adjacent organs

Regional Lymph Nodes (N)

NX   Regional lymph nodes cannot be assessed
N0   No regional lymph node metastasis
N1   Regional lymph node metastasis

Distant Metastasis (M)

MX   Presence of distant metastasis cannot be assessed
M0   No distant metastasis
M1   Distant metastasis

STAGE GROUPING

Stage 0	Tis	N0	M0
Stage I	T1	N0	M0
Stage II	T2	N0	M0
	T3	N0	M0
Stage III	T1	N1	M0
	T2	N1	M0
	T3	N1	M0
Stage IV	T4	Any N	M0
	Any T	Any N	M1

HISTOPATHOLOGIC TYPE

The staging system applies to all primary carcinomas arising in the ampulla or on the papilla. Adenocarcinomas are the most common type. The classification does not apply to carcinoid tumors or to lymphomas.

HISTOPATHOLOGIC GRADE (G)

GX   Grade cannot be assessed
G1   Well differentiated
G2   Moderately differentiated
G3   Poorly differentiated
G4   Undifferentiated

BIBLIOGRAPHY

1. Braasch JW, Camer SJ: Periampullary carcinoma. Med Clin North Am 59:309–314, 1975
2. Delcore R Jr, Connor CS, Thomas JH, et al: Significance of tumor spread in adenocarcinoma of the ampulla of Vater. Am J Surg 158:593–596, 1989
3. Edmondson HA: Tumors of the gallbladder and extrahepatic bile ducts. Atlas of Tumor Pathology, Fascicle 26, Section 7. Washington DC, Armed Forces Institute of Pathology, 1967
4. Knox RA, Kingston RD. Carcinoma of the ampulla of Vater. Br J Surg 73:72–73, 1986
5. Makipour H, Cooperman A, Danzi JT, et al: Carcinoma of the ampulla of Vater. Ann Surg 183:341–344, 1976
6. Monson JRT, Donohue JH, McEntee GP, et al: Radical resection for carcinoma of the ampulla of Vater. Arch Surg 126:353–357, 1991
7. Mori K, Ikei S, Yamane T, et al: Pathological factors influencing survival of carcinoma of the ampulla of Vater. Eur J Surg Oncol 16:183–188, 1990
8. Yamaguchi K, Enjoji M: Carcinoma of the ampulla of Vater: A clinicopathologic study and pathologic staging of 109 cases of carcinoma and 5 cases of adenoma. Cancer 59:506–515, 1987
9. Yasuda K, Mukai H, Cho E, et al: The use of endoscopic ultrasonography in the diagnosis and staging of carcinoma of the papilla of Vater. Endoscopy 20: Suppl 218–222, 1988.
10. Wise L, Pizzimbono C, Dehner IP: Periampullary cancer. Am J Surg 131:141–148, 1976

Data Form for Cancer Staging

Patient identification
Name _____
Address _____
Hospital or clinic number _____
Age _____ Sex _____ Race _____

Institution identification
Hospital or clinic _____
Address _____

Oncology Record

Anatomic site of cancer _____
Histologic type _____
Grade (G) _____
Date of classification _____

Chronology of classification
[ ] Clinical (use all data prior to first treatment)
[ ] Pathologic (if definitively resected specimen available)

DEFINITIONS

Primary Tumor (T)

Clin	Path		
[ ]	[ ]	TX	Primary tumor cannot be assessed
[ ]	[ ]	T0	No evidence of primary tumor
[ ]	[ ]	Tis	Carcinoma *in situ*
[ ]	[ ]	T1	Tumor limited to ampulla of Vater
[ ]	[ ]	T2	Tumor invades duodenal wall
[ ]	[ ]	T3	Tumor invades 2 cm or less into pancreas
[ ]	[ ]	T4	Tumor invades more than 2.0 cm into pancreas and/or into other adjacent organs

Lymph Node (N)

[ ]	[ ]	NX	Regional lymph nodes cannot be assessed
[ ]	[ ]	N0	No regional lymph node metastasis
[ ]	[ ]	N1	Regional lymph node metastasis

Distant Metastasis (M)

[ ]	[ ]	MX	Presence of distant metastasis cannot be assessed
[ ]	[ ]	M0	No distant metastasis
[ ]	[ ]	M1	Distant metastasis

Histopathologic Grade (G)

[ ] GX Grade cannot be assessed
[ ] G1 Well differentiated
[ ] G2 Moderately differentiated
[ ] G3 Poorly differentiated
[ ] G4 Undifferentiated

Illustration

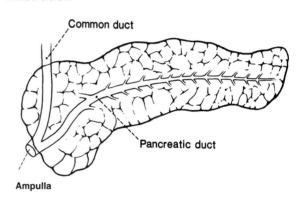

Common duct

Pancreatic duct

Ampulla

Indicate on diagram primary tumor and regional nodes involved.

Stage Grouping

Clin	Path				
[ ]	[ ]	0	Tis	N0	M0
[ ]	[ ]	I	T1	N0	M0
[ ]	[ ]	II	T2	N0	M0
			T3	N0	M0
[ ]	[ ]	III	T1	N1	M0
			T2	N1	M0
			T3	N1	M0
[ ]	[ ]	IV	T4	Any N	M0
			Any T	Any N	M1

Histopathologic Type

The staging system applies to all primary carcinomas that arise in the ampulla or on the papilla. Adenocarcinomas are the most common type. The classification does not apply to the carcinoid tumors or to lymphomas.

Staged by _____ M.D.
_____ Registrar
Date _____

18

Exocrine Pancreas

C25.0 Head
C25.1 Body
C25.2 Tail
C25.3 Pancreatic duct
C25.7 Other specified parts
C25.8 Overlapping lesion
C25.9 Pancreas, NOS

In the United States, pancreatic cancer is the third most common malignancy of the gastrointestinal tract. The disease is often difficult to diagnose, especially in its early stages. Cancers of the exocrine pancreas are almost always fatal; nearly all patients die within 2 years following diagnosis. Most cancers arise in the head of the pancreas, eventually causing extrahepatic bile duct obstruction and clinical jaundice. Cancers arising in either the body or tail of the pancreas are insidious in their development and often far advanced when first detected. Most cancers are adenocarcinomas that can originate either from the pancreatic ducts or from the acini. Most cancers, however, arise from the ducts. This staging classification does not apply to endocrine tumors or to tumors arising in the islets of Langerhans. Staging depends on the size and extent of the primary tumor.

ANATOMY

Primary Site. The exocrine pancreas is a long, coarsely lobulated gland that lies transversely in the posterior abdomen. It lies retroperitoneally in the concavity of the duodenum on its right and touches the spleen with its tail. The shape of the pancreas is often compared to the letter "J" placed sideways. The organ is divided into a head with a small uncinate process, a neck, a body, and a tail that is usually in contact with the spleen. The body is in direct relation anteriorly with the stomach and posteriorly with the aorta, splenic veins, and left kidney.

Regional Lymph Nodes. A rich lymphatic network surrounds the pancreas, with left splenic and superior and inferior right side truncal drainage. The regional lymph nodes are the peripancreatic nodes, which may be subdivided as follows:

Superior: Lymph nodes superior to the head and body of the pancreas
Inferior: Lymph nodes inferior to the head and body of the pancreas
Anterior: Anterior pancreaticoduodenal, pyloric, and proximal mesenteric lymph nodes
Posterior: Posterior pancreaticoduodenal, common bile duct or pericholedochal, and proximal mesenteric nodes
Splenic: Hilum of the spleen and tail of the pancreas (for tumors in the body and tail only)

The following lymph nodes are considered regional:

Peripancreatic (superior, inferior, anterior, posterior)
Hepatic artery
Infrapyloric (for tumors in the head only)
Subpyloric (for tumors in the head only)
Celiac (for tumors in the head only)
Superior mesenteric
Pancreaticolienal (for tumors in the body and tail only)
Splenic (for tumors in the body and tail only)
Retroperitoneal
Lateral aortic

Tumor involvement of other nodal groups is considered distant metastasis.

Metastatic Sites. Distant spread occurs mainly to the liver and the lungs. Other sites can also be involved, including the bones.

RULES FOR CLASSIFICATION

Clinical Staging. Imaging procedures such as ultrasonic scanning and computed tomography, along with cytology and laparoscopy, are available. Laparotomy and surgical exploration of the pancreas with biopsy can accurately assess the extent of the tumor for staging the patient.

Pathologic Staging. Complete or subtotal resection of the pancreas along with the tumor and associated regional lymph nodes provides the information necessary for staging. A single TNM classification serves both clinical and pathologic staging. The anatomic subdivisions are as follows:

1. Tumors of the head of the pancreas are those arising to the right of the left border of the superior mesenteric vein. The uncinate process is part of the head.
2. Tumors of the body of the pancreas are those arising between the left border of the superior mesenteric vein and the left border of the aorta.
3. Tumors of the tail of the pancreas are those arising between the left border of the aorta and the hilum of the spleen.

For the T3 classification, the adjacent large vessels are the portal vein and the mesenteric and common hepatic arteries and veins (not the splenic vessels). Direct extension to an organ or structure not listed in T1–T3 is M1. For example, extension to the liver is coded as M1. Peritoneal seeding is also considered M1.

For T2, peripancreatic tissues include soft tissues adjacent to the pancreas in addition to the common bile duct and duodenum. Specifically, peripancreatic tissues include the surrounding retroperitoneal fat (retroperitoneal soft tissue), including mesentery (mesenteric fat), mesocolon, greater and lesser omentum, and peritoneum.

DEFINITION OF TNM

Primary Tumor (T)

TX	Primary tumor cannot be assessed
T0	No evidence of primary tumor
T1	Tumor limited to the pancreas
	T1a Tumor 2 cm or less in greatest dimension
	T1b Tumor more than 2 cm in greatest dimension
T2	Tumor extends directly to any of the following: duodenum, bile duct, or peripancreatic tissues
T3	Tumor extends directly to any of the following: stomach, spleen, colon, or adjacent large vessels

Regional Lymph Nodes (N)

NX	Regional lymph nodes cannot be assessed
N0	No regional lymph node metastasis
N1	Regional lymph node metastasis

Distant Metastasis (M)

MX	Presence of distant metastasis cannot be assessed
M0	No distant metastasis
M1	Distant metastasis

STAGE GROUPING

Stage I	T1	N0	M0
	T2	N0	M0
Stage II	T3	N0	M0
Stage III	Any T	N1	M0
Stage IV	Any T	Any N	M1

HISTOPATHOLOGIC TYPE

The staging system applies to all carcinomas arising in pancreas. It does not apply to the endocrine cell tumors arising in the islets of Langerhans. Carcinoid tumors are excluded. The following carcinomas are included:

Duct cell carcinoma
Pleomorphic giant cell carcinoma
Giant cell carcinoma, osteoclastoid type
Adenocarcinoma
Adenosquamous carcinoma
Mucinous (colloid) carcinoma
Cystadenocarcinoma
Acinar cell carcinoma
Papillary carcinoma
Small cell (oat cell) carcinoma
Mixed cell types
Carcinoma, NOS
Undifferentiated carcinoma

HISTOPATHOLOGIC GRADE (G)

GX	Grade cannot be assessed
G1	Well differentiated
G2	Moderately differentiated
G3	Poorly differentiated
G4	Undifferentiated

BIBLIOGRAPHY

1. Albores-Saavedra J, Gould EW, Angeles-Angeles A, et al: Cystic tumors of the pancreas (Part 2). Pathol Ann 25:19–50, 1990

2. Baisch H, Klppel G, Reinke B: DNA ploidy and cell-cycle analysis in pancreatic and ampullary carcinoma: Flow cytometric study of formalin-fixed paraffin-embedded tissue. Virchows Arch [A] 417:145–150, 1990

3. Cubilla AL, Fitzgerald PJ: Tumors of the exocrine pancreas. Atlas of Tumor Pathology, Second Series, Fascicle 19. Washington DC, Armed Forces Institute of Pathology, 1984

4. Cubilla AL, Fortner J, Fitzgerald PJ: Lymph node involvement in carcinoma of the head of the pancreas area. Cancer 41:880–887, 1978

5. Fugazzola C, Procacci C, Bergamo Andreis IA, et al: Cystic tumors of the pancreas: evaluation by ultrasonography and computed tomography. Gastrointest Radiol 16:53–61, 1991

6. Hermanek P, Staging of exocrine pancreatic carcinoma. Eur J Surg Oncol 17:167–172, 1991

7. Lack EE: Primary tumors of the exocrine pancreas: Classification, overview, and recent contributions by immunohistochemistry and electron microscopy. Am J Surg Pathol 13 Suppl 1:66–88, 1989

8. Levison DA: Carcinoma of the pancreas. J Pathol 129:203–223, 1979

9. Manabe T, Ohshio G, Baba N, et al: Factors influencing prognosis and indications for curative pancreatectomy for ductal adenocarcinoma of the head of the pancreas. Int J Pancreatol 7:187–193, 1990

10. Moossa AR, Levin B: The diagnosis of "early" pancreatic cancer. Cancer 47:1688–1697, 1981

11. Nix GA, Dubbelman C, Wilson JH, et al: Prognostic implications of tumor diameter in carcinoma of the head of the pancreas. Cancer 67:529–535, 1991

12. Pollard HM, et al: Staging of cancer of the pancreas. Cancer 47:1631–1637, 1981

13. Safi F, Roscher R, Beger HG: The clinical relevance of the tumor marker CA 19-9 in the diagnosing and monitoring of pancreatic carcinoma. Bull Cancer (Paris) 77:83–91, 1990

14. Sugarbaker EV: Patterns of metastasis in human malignancies. In Fidler IJ (ed), Cancer Metastases. New York, Marcel Dekker, 1977

15. Trapnell JE: Staging of cancer of the pancreas. Int J Pancreatol 7:109–116, 1990

Data Form for Cancer Staging

Patient identification
Name _____
Address _____
Hospital or clinic number _____
Age _____ Sex _____ Race _____

Institution identification
Hospital or clinic _____
Address _____

Oncology Record

Anatomic site of cancer _____
Histologic type _____
Grade (G) _____
Date of classification _____

Chronology of classification
[ ] Clinical (use all data prior to first treatment)
[ ] Pathologic (if definitively resected specimen available)

DEFINITIONS

Primary Tumor (T)

Clin	Path		
[ ]	[ ]	TX	Primary tumor cannot be assessed
[ ]	[ ]	T0	No evidence of primary tumor
[ ]	[ ]	T1	Tumor limited to the pancreas
[ ]	[ ]	T1a	Tumor 2 cm or less in greatest dimension
[ ]	[ ]	T1b	Tumor more than 2 cm in greatest dimension
[ ]	[ ]	T2	Tumor extends directly to any of the following: duodenum, bile duct, or peripancreatic tissues
[ ]	[ ]	T3	Tumor extends directly to any of the following: stomach, spleen, colon, or adjacent large vessels

Lymph Node (N)

Clin	Path		
[ ]	[ ]	NX	Regional lymph nodes cannot be assessed
[ ]	[ ]	N0	No regional lymph node metastasis
[ ]	[ ]	N1	Regional lymph node metastasis

Distant Metastasis (M)

Clin	Path		
[ ]	[ ]	MX	Presence of distant metastasis cannot be assessed
[ ]	[ ]	M0	No distant metastasis
[ ]	[ ]	M1	Distant metastasis

Stage Grouping

Clin	Path				
[ ]	[ ]	I	T1	N0	M0
			T2	N0	M0
[ ]	[ ]	II	T3	N0	M0
[ ]	[ ]	III	Any T	N1	M0
[ ]	[ ]	IV	Any T	Any N	M1

Staged by _____ M.D.
_____ Registrar
Date _____

Histopathologic Grade (G)

[ ] GX   Grade cannot be assessed
[ ] G1   Well differentiated
[ ] G2   Moderately differentiated
[ ] G3   Poorly differentiated
[ ] G4   Undifferentiated

Location in Pancreas

[ ] Head
[ ] Body
[ ] Tail
[ ] Diffuse
Size (largest diameter) _____ cm

Illustration

Indicate on diagram primary tumor and regional nodes involved.

Histopathologic Type

The staging system applies to all carcinomas arising in the pancreas. It does not apply to the endocrine cell tumors arising in the islets of Langerhans. Carcinoid tumors are excluded. The following carcinomas are included:

Duct cell carcinoma
Pleomorphic giant cell carcinoma
Giant cell carcinoma, osteoclastoid type
Adenocarcinoma
Adenosquamous carcinoma
Mucinous (colloid) carcinoma
Cystadenocarcinoma
Acinar cell carcinoma
Papillary carcinoma
Small cell (oat cell) carcinoma
Mixed cell types
Carcinoma, NOS
Undifferentiated carcinoma

American Joint Committee on Cancer—1992

THORAX

19

Lung

C34.0 Main bronchus
C34.1 Upper lobe
C34.2 Middle lobe
C34.3 Lower lobe
C34.8 Overlapping lesion
C34.9 Lung, NOS

Lung cancers are among the few cancers with a known etiology. If trends continue, lung cancer will become the leading cause of cancer deaths in women, surpassing breast cancer. The disease is difficult to treat, and the 5-year survival rate is under 15%. The staging of lung cancer depends on the extent of disease, location of the primary tumor, and associated clinical complications. Important for staging and patient evaluation is the assessment of both extrapulmonic and extrathoracic metastasis.

ANATOMY

Primary Site

The mucosa lining the bronchus is the usual site of origin for lung carcinomas. Lying in the anterior mediastinum, the trachea divides into the right and left main bronchi, which extend into the right and left lungs, respectively. The bronchi then subdivide into the lobar bronchi for the upper, middle, and lower lobes on the right and for the upper and lower lobes on the left. The lungs are encased in membranes called the visceral pleura. The inside of the chest cavity is lined by a similar membrane called the parietal pleura. The potential space between these two membranes is the pleural space. The mediastinum, which contains the heart, thymus, great vessels, and other structures, separates the lungs in the midline.

The great vessels (T4) are:

Aorta
Superior caval vein
Inferior caval vein
Main pulmonary artery

Intrapericardial segments of the trunk of the right and left pulmonary artery
Interpericardial segments of the superior or inferior right or left pulmonary veins

Regional Lymph Nodes. All regional nodes are above the diaphragm. They include the intrathoracic, scalene, and supraclavicular nodes. The intrathoracic nodes are as follows:

Mediastinal:
  Peritracheal (including those that may be designated tracheobronchial, e.g., lower peritracheal, including azygos)
  Pretracheal and retrotracheal (including precarinal)
  Aortic (including subaortic, aorticopulmonary window, and periaortic, including ascending aorta or phrenic)
  Carinal
  Subcarinal
  Periesophageal
  Pulmonary ligament
  Anterior mediastinal
  Posterior mediastinal

Intrapulmonic:
  Hilar (proximal lobar)
  Peribronchial
  Intrapulmonic (including interlobar, lobar, segmental)

Metastatic Sites. The most common metastatic sites are the cervical lymph nodes, liver, brain, bones, adrenal glands, kidneys, and contralateral lung. No organ is safe.

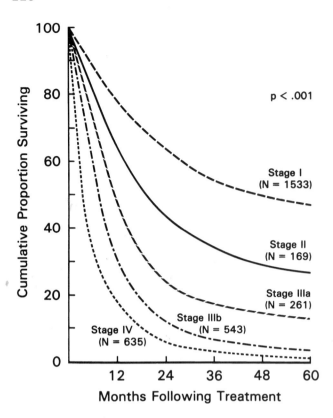

Fig. 19-1. Cumulative proportion of patients expected to survive following treatment according to CLINICAL estimates of the stage of disease (Mountain, 1986: with permission).

RULES FOR CLASSIFICATION

Clinical Staging. Clinical staging is based on the assessment of the anatomic extent of disease before instituting definitive therapy. This includes a medical history, physical examination, various imaging procedures, endoscopic studies (including bronchoscopy, esophagoscopy, mediastinoscopy, mediastinotomy, thoracentesis, and thoracoscopy), and other tests designed to demonstrate extrathoracic metastasis and regional extension. Clinical assignment of N2 disease in patients who are not appropriate candidates for mediastinoscopy or mediastinotomy is often made according to the assessment and judgment of the radiologist.

For the classification of pleural effusion, a footnote has been added to the T categories regarding the implications of pleural fluid as a staging variable. Patients with a malignant pleural effusion—that is, either cytologically positive for cancer cells or clinically related to the underlying malignancy—are coded as T4. Pericardial effusion is classified the same as pleural effusion.

Lung cancer detected by sputum cytology but not seen radiographically or during bronchoscopy is known as "occult" carcinoma and is coded as TX.

Occult cancers without evidence of regional lymph node involvement or distant metastasis are coded as TX, N0, M0. Any tumor that cannot be assessed— that is, lung cancer proved, no tumor mass present, or evaluable—is designated as TX.

Vocal cord paralysis (resulting from involvement of the recurrent branch of the vagus nerve), superior vena caval obstruction, or compression of the trachea or esophagus may be related to direct extension of the primary tumor or to lymph node involvement. The treatment options and prognosis associated with these manifestations of disease extent fall within the T4-Stage IIIB category; therefore, a classification of T4 is recommended. If the primary tumor is peripheral and clearly unrelated to vocal cord paralysis, vena caval obstruction, or compression of the trachea and esophagus, then the nodal classification according to the established rules is appropriate.

Invasion of the phrenic nerve, which invariably indicates direct extension of the primary tumor, is classified as T3.

T2 is used when there is direct extension into the visceral pleura. T3 is used if the lesion directly invades the parietal pleura covering the mediastinum and pericardium, as well as that lining the chest wall and covering the diaphragm.

Pleural tumor foci that are discontinuous from direct pleural invasion by the primary tumor should be listed as T4. A discontinuous lesion outside the parietal pleura in the chest wall or in the diaphragm should be designated as M1. Peripheral tumors directly invading the chest wall and ribs are classified as T3.

Intrapulmonic ipsilateral metastasis in the non-primary tumor lobe should be classified as T4; if contralateral, as M1. Multiple tumor masses in the same lobe meeting the criteria for T1 should be designated as T2; a T2 primary tumor with another (non-lymph node) mass in the same lobe should be designated as T3 and all other multiple ipsilateral masses as T4. Discontinuous tumor foci only histologically detectable do not affect the clinical TNM classification, but would be reflected in the pathologic staging.

The designation of "Pancoast" tumors relates to the symptom complex or syndrome caused by a tumor arising in the superior sulcus of the lung that involves the sympathetic nerve trunks, including the stellate ganglion. The extent of disease varies in these tumors, and they should be classified according to the established rules. If there is evidence of invasion of the vertebral body or extension into the neural foramina, the "Pancoast" tumor would be classified as T4. If no criteria for T4 disease pertain, the tumor would be classified as T3.

Pathologic Staging. Pathologic staging is based on the information obtained from clinical staging, from thoracotomy, and from examination of the resected specimen, including lymph nodes. The same classification applies to both clinical and pathologic staging. The histologic type of cancer should be recorded, because it also has a bearing on prognosis.

Multiple synchronous tumors of different histologic cell types should be considered separate primary lung cancers and each staged separately. For data analysis, the highest stage of disease should be recorded.

DEFINITION OF TNM

Primary Tumor (T)

TX Primary tumor cannot be assessed, or tumor proven by the presence of malignant cells in sputum or bronchial washings but not visualized by imaging or bronchoscopy

T0 No evidence of primary tumor

Tis Carcinoma *in situ*

T1 Tumor 3 cm or less in greatest dimension, surrounded by lung or visceral pleura, without bronchoscopic evidence of invasion more proximal than the lobar bronchus (i.e., not in the main bronchus)*

T2 Tumor with any of the following features of size or extent:
   More than 3 cm in greatest dimension
   Involving main bronchus, 2 cm or more distal to the carina
   Invading the visceral pleura
   Associated with atelectasis or obstructive pneumonitis that extends to the hilar region but does not involve the entire lung

T3 Tumor of any size that directly invades any of the following: chest wall (including superior sulcus tumors), diaphragm, mediastinal pleura, or parietal pericardium; or tumor in the main bronchus less than 2 cm distal to the carina but without involvement of the carina; or associated atelectasis or obstructive pneumonitis of the entire lung

T4 Tumor of any size that invades any of the following: mediastinum, heart, great vessels, trachea, esophagus, vertebral body, carina; or tumor with a malignant pleural effusion**

*Note: The uncommon superficial tumor of any size with its invasive component limited to the bronchial wall, which may extend proximal to the main bronchus, is also classified as T1.

**Note: Most pleural effusions associated with lung cancer are due to tumor. However, there are a few patients in whom multiple cytopathologic examinations of pleural fluid are negative for tumor. In these cases, fluid is non-bloody and is not an exudate. When these elements

and clinical judgment dictate that the effusion is not related to the tumor, the effusion should be excluded as a staging element and the patient should be staged as T1, T2, or T3.

Regional Lymph Nodes (N)

NX Regional lymph nodes cannot be assessed

N0 No regional lymph node metastasis

N1 Metastasis in ipsilateral peribronchial and/or ipsilateral hilar lymph nodes, including direct extension

N2 Metastasis in ipsilateral mediastinal and/or subcarinal lymph node(s)

N3 Metastasis in contralateral mediastinal, contralateral hilar, ipsilateral or contralateral scalene, or supraclavicular lymph node(s)

Distant Metastasis (M)

MX Presence of distant metastasis cannot be assessed

M0 No distant metastasis

M1 Distant metastasis

STAGE GROUPING

Occult	TX	N0	M0
Stage 0	Tis	N0	M0
Stage I	T1	N0	M0
	T2	N0	M0
Stage II	T1	N1	M0
	T2	N1	M0
Stage IIIA	T1	N2	M0
	T2	N2	M0
	T3	N0	M0
	T3	N1	M0
	T3	N2	M0
Stage IIIB	Any T	N3	M0
	T4	Any N	M0
Stage IV	Any T	Any N	M1

PROGNOSIS OF 1479 PATIENTS WITHOUT
DISTANT METASTASIS ANALYZED
ACCORDING TO T AND N FACTORS*

TNM STAGE			NUMBER OF PATIENTS	5-YEAR SURVIVAL RATES
T1	N0	M0	245	75.5
T2	N0	M0	291	57.0
T1	N1	M0	66	52.5
T2	N1	M0	153	38.4
T3	N0	M0	106	33.3
T3	N1	M0	85	39.0
T1-3	N2	M0	368	15.1
T1-3	N3	M0	55	0
T4	ANY	N	104	8.2

* Data from Naruke et al, 1988.

HISTOPATHOLOGIC TYPE

There are four common types of lung cancer:

1. Squamous cell carcinoma (epidermoid carcinoma)
     Variant: Spindle cell
2. Small cell carcinoma
     Oat cell carcinoma
     Intermediate cell type
     Combined oat cell carcinoma
3. Adenocarcinoma
     Acinar adenocarcinoma
     Papillary adenocarcinoma
     Bronchiolo-alveolar carcinoma
     Solid carcinoma with mucus formation
4. Large cell carcinoma
     Variants: Giant cell carcinoma
                        Clear cell carcinoma

This classification applies only to carcinomas. The classification may be applied to those tumors classified as "undifferentiated carcinomas" with no special cell types identified. Sarcomas and other rare tumors are excluded, because the relationship between disease extent and prognosis has not been established or does not pertain.

HISTOPATHOLOGIC GRADE (G)

GX   Grade cannot be assessed
G1   Well differentiated
G2   Moderately differentiated
G3   Poorly differentiated
G4   Undifferentiated

BIBLIOGRAPHY

1. Angeletti CA, Macchiarini P, Mussi A, et al: Influence of T and N stages on long-term survival in resectable small cell lung cancer. Eur J Surg Oncol 15:337–340, 1989
2. Byhardt RW, Hartz A, Libnoch JA, et al: Prognostic influence of TNM staging and LDH levels in small cell carcinoma of the lung (SCCL). Int J Radiat Oncol Biol Phys 12:771–777, 1986
3. Capewell S, Sudlow MF: Performance and prognosis in patients with lung cancer. Thorax 45:951–956, 1990
4. Carr DT, Mountain CF: The staging of lung cancer. Semin Oncol 1:229–234, 1974
5. Carter D, Eggleston JC: Tumors of the lower respiratory tract. Atlas of Tumor Pathology. Washington DC, Armed Forces Institute of Pathology, 1980
6. Dearing MP, Steinberg SM, Phelps R, et al: Outcome of patients with small-cell lung cancer: Effect of changes in staging procedures and imaging technology on prognostic factors over 14 years. J Clin Oncol 8:1042–1049, 1990
7. Gail MH, Eagan RT, Feld R, et al: Prognostic factors in patients with resected stage I non-small cell lung cancer. Cancer 54:1802–1813, 1984
8. Feinstein AR, Wells CK: Lung cancer staging: A critical evaluation. Clin Chest Med 3:291–305, 1982
9. Harper PG, Souhami RL, Spiro SG, et al: Tumor size, response rate, and prognosis in small cell carcinoma of the bronchus treated by combination chemotherapy. Cancer Treat Rep 66:463–470, 1982
10. Ishikawa S: Staging system on TNM classification for lung cancer. Jpn J Clin Oncol 6:19–30, 1973
11. Libshitz HI, Computed tomography in bronchogenic carcinoma. Semin Roentgenol 25:64–72, 1990
12. Little AG, DeMeester TR, MacMahon H: The staging of lung cancer. Semin Oncol 10:56–70, 1983
13. McKenna RJ, Libshitz HI, Mountain CF, et al: Roentgenographic evaluation of mediastinal nodes for preoperative assessment in lung cancer. Chest 88:206–210, 1985.
14. Mountain CF: A method for the assessment of operation in the control of lung cancer. Ann Thorac Surg 24:365–373, 1977
15. Mountain CF: A new international staging system for lung cancer. Chest (Suppl) 225S–233S, 1986
16. Mountain CF Prognostic implication of the international staging system for lung cancer. Semin Oncol 15:236–245, 1988
17. Naruke T, Goya T, Tsuchiya R, et al: Prognosis and survival in resected lung carcinoma based on the new international staging system. J Thorac Cardiovas Surg 96:440–447, 1988.
18. Naruke T, Suemasu K, Ishikawa S: Lymph node mapping and curability at various levels of metastasis in resected lung cancer. J Thorac Cardiovas Surg 76:832–839, 1978
19. Ogawa J, Iwazaki M, Tsurumi T, et al: Prognostic implications of DNA histogram, DNA content, and histologic changes of regional lymph nodes in patients with lung cancer. Cancer 67:1370–1376, 1991
20. Pater JL, Loeb M: Nonanatomic prognostic factors in carcinoma of the lung. Cancer 50:326–331, 1982
21. Rawson NS, Peto J: An overview of prognostic factors in small cell lung cancer. A report from the Subcommittee for the Management of Lung. Br J Cancer 61:597–604, 1990
22. Sagawa M, Saito Y, Takahashi S, et al: Clinical and prognostic assessment of patients with resected small peripheral lung cancer lesions. Cancer 66:2653–2657, 1990
23. Sandler HM, Curran WJ Jr, Turrisi AT 3d: The influence of tumor size and pre-treatment staging on outcome following radiation therapy alone for stage I non-small cell lung cancer. Int J Radiat Oncol Biol Phys 19:9–13, 1990
24. Sano T, Naruke T, Kondo H, et al: Prognosis for resected lung cancer patients with tumors greater than ten centimeters in diameter. Jpn J Clin Oncol 20:369–373, 1990
25. Sheehan RG, Balaban EP, Cox JV, et al: The relative value of conventional staging procedures for develop-

ing prognostic models in extensive-stage small-cell lung cancer. J Clin Oncol 8:2047–2053, 1990

26. Stanley KD: Prognostic factors for survival in patients with inoperable lung cancer. J Natl Cancer Inst 65:25–32, 1980

27. Templeton PA, Caskey CI, Zerhouni EA: Current uses of CT and MR imaging in the staging of lung cancer. Radiol Clin North Am 28:631–46, 1990

28. World Health Organization. Histological Typing of Lung Tumors, 2nd ed. Geneva, WHO, 1981

Data Form for Cancer Staging

Patient identification
Name _____
Address _____
Hospital or clinic number _____
Age _____ Sex _____ Race _____

Institution identification
Hospital or clinic _____
Address _____

Oncology Record

Anatomic site of cancer _____
Histologic type _____
Grade (G) _____
Date of classification _____

Chronology of classification
[ ] Clinical (use all data prior to first treatment)
[ ] Pathologic (if definitively resected specimen available)

DEFINITIONS

Clin	Path	

Primary Tumor (T)

Clin	Path		
[ ]	[ ]	TX	Primary tumor cannot be assessed, or tumor proven by presence of malignant cells in sputum or bronchial washings but not visualized by imaging or bronchoscopy
[ ]	[ ]	T0	No evidence of primary tumor
[ ]	[ ]	Tis	Carcinoma *in situ*
[ ]	[ ]	T1	Tumor 3 cm or less in greatest dimension, surrounded by lung or visceral pleura, without bronchoscopic evidence of invasion more proximal than the lobar bronchus (*i.e.* not in main bronchus)
[ ]	[ ]	T2	Tumor with *any* of the following features of size or extent: More than 3 cm in greatest dimension Involves main bronchus, 2 cm or more distal to the carina Invades the visceral pleura Associated with atelectasis or obstructive pneumonitis which extends to the hilar region but does not involve the entire lung
[ ]	[ ]	T3	Tumor of any size that directly invades any of the following: chest wall (including superior sulcus tumors), diaphragm, mediastinal pleura, parietal pericardium; or tumor in the main bronchus less than 2 cm distal to the carina but without involvement of the carina; or associated atelectasis or obstructive pneumonitis of the entire lung
[ ]	[ ]	T4	Tumor of any size that invades any of the following: mediastinum, heart, great vessels, trachea, esophagus, vertebral body, carina; or tumor with a malignant pleural effusion

Lymph Node (N)

Clin	Path		
[ ]	[ ]	NX	Regional lymph nodes cannot be assessed
[ ]	[ ]	N0	No regional lymph node metastasis
[ ]	[ ]	N1	Metastasis in ipsilateral peribronchial and/or ipsilateral hilar lymph nodes, including direct extension
[ ]	[ ]	N2	Metastasis in ipsilateral mediastinal and/or subcarinal lymph node(s)
[ ]	[ ]	N3	Metastasis in contralateral mediastinal, contralateral hilar, ipsilateral or contralateral scalene or supraclavicular lymph node(s)

Distant Metastasis (M)

Clin	Path		
[ ]	[ ]	MX	Presence of distant metastasis cannot be assessed
[ ]	[ ]	M0	No distant metastasis
[ ]	[ ]	M1	Distant metastasis

Stage Grouping

Clin	Path				
[ ]	[ ]	Occult	TX	N0	M0
[ ]	[ ]	0	Tis	N0	M0
[ ]	[ ]	I	T1	N0	M0
			T2	N0	M0
[ ]	[ ]	II	T1	N1	M0
			T2	N1	M0
[ ]	[ ]	IIIA	T1	N2	M0
			T2	N2	M0
			T3	N0	M0
			T3	N1	M0
			T3	N2	M0
[ ]	[ ]	IIIB	Any T	N3	M0
			T4	Any N	M0
[ ]	[ ]	IV	Any T	Any N	M1

Staged by _____ M.D.
_____ Registrar
Date _____

(continued on next page)

American Joint Committee on Cancer—1992

Histopathologic Grade (G)

[ ] GX   Grade cannot be assessed
[ ] G1   Well differentiated
[ ] G2   Moderately differentiated
[ ] G3   Poorly differentiated
[ ] G4   Undifferentiated

Lymph Nodes

Mediastinal:

Peritracheal (including those that may be designated tracheobronchial, *e.g.*, lower peritracheal, including azygos)

Pretracheal and retrotracheal (including precarinal)

Aortic (including subaortic, aorticopulmonary window, and periaortic, including ascending aorta or phrenic)

Carinal

Subcarinal

Periesophageal

Pulmonary ligament

Anterior mediastinal

Posterior mediastinal

Intrapulmonic:

Hilar (proximal lobar)

Peribronchial

Intrapulmonic (including interlobar, lobar, segmental)

Histopathologic Type

There are four common types of lung cancer, or bronchogenic carcinoma:

Squamous cell carcinoma (epidermoid carcinoma)

Variant: Spindle cell

Small cell carcinoma

Oat cell carcinoma

Intermediate cell type

Combined oat cell carcinoma

Adenocarcinoma

Acinar adenocarcinoma

Papillary adenocarcinoma

Bronchiolo-alveolar carcinoma

Solid carcinoma with mucus formation

Large cell carcinoma

Variants: Giant cell carcinoma

Clear cell carcinoma

This staging system applies only to the carcinomas. Sarcomas and other rare tumors are excluded.

Illustrations

Show primary tumor, indicating size in cm (greatest diameter) and measurability:

EV = evaluable
ME = measurable
NE = nonevaluable

Show lymph node metastasis.

N-Regional nodes

Indicate on diagrams primary tumor and regional nodes involved.

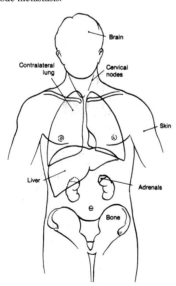

Distant metastasis beyond hemithorax

Indicate all known metastases.

American Joint Committee on Cancer—1992

20

Pleural Mesothelioma

C38.4 Pleura

Mesotheliomas are relatively rare tumors arising from the mesothelium lining the pleural cavities. They represent less than 2% of all malignant tumors. Highly virulent, mesotheliomas are usually associated with long-term exposure to asbestos. Although similar tumors can arise along the mesothelial surfaces in the abdomen or pericardial cavity, this staging system applies only to tumors arising in the pleural cavities. Because these tumors are not common, a staging system was not published previously by the International Union Against Cancer or by the American Joint Committee on Cancer. For staging, the disease should be histologically confirmed. The initial symptoms may be nonspecific.

ANATOMY

The mesothelium covers the external surface of the lungs and the inside of the chest wall. It is usually composed of flat, tightly connected cells no more than one layer thick.

Regional Lymph Nodes. The regional lymph nodes include:

Intrathoracic
Scalene
Supraclavicular

See Chapter 19, Lung, for a detailed list of intrathoracic lymph nodes.

RULES FOR CLASSIFICATION

This staging system serves both clinical and pathological staging. Clinical staging depends on imaging, especially computed tomography scanning. Pathologic staging is based on surgical resection. The extent of disease before and after resection should be carefully documented. In some cases, complete N staging may not be possible, especially if tumor has encompassed the hilar and mediastinal structures.

TNM CLASSIFICATION

Primary Tumor (T)

TX   Primary tumor cannot be assessed
T0   No evidence of primary tumor
T1   Tumor limited to ipsilateral parietal and/or visceral pleura
T2   Tumor invades any of the following: ipsilateral lung, endothoracic fascia, diaphragm, or pericardium
T3   Tumor invades any of the following: ipsilateral chest wall muscle, ribs, or mediastinal organs or tissues
T4   Tumor directly extends to any of the following: contralateral pleura, lung, peritoneum, intraabdominal organs, or cervical tissues

Regional Lymph Nodes (N)

NX   Regional lymph nodes cannot be assessed
N0   No regional lymph node metastasis
N1   Metastasis in ipsilateral peribronchial and/or ipsilateral hilar lymph nodes, including direct extension
N2   Metastasis in ipsilateral mediastinal and/or subcarinal lymph node(s)
N3   Metastasis in contralateral mediastinal, contralateral hilar, ipsilateral or contralateral scalene, or supraclavicular lymph node(s)

Distant Metastasis (M)

MX   Distant metastasis cannot be assessed
M0   No evidence of distant metastasis
M1   Distant metastasis

STAGE GROUPING

Stage I	T1	N0	M0
	T2	N0	M0
Stage II	T1	N1	M0
	T2	N1	M0
Stage III	T1	N2	M0
	T2	N2	M0
	T3	N0	M0
	T3	N1	M0
	T3	N2	M0
Stage IV	Any T	N3	M0
	T4	Any N	M0
	Any T	Any N	M1

HISTOPATHOLOGIC TYPE

This staging classification applies only to primary pleural mesotheliomas. It does not apply to metastatic tumors or to lung tumors that have extended to the pleural surfaces.

BIBLIOGRAPHY

1. Bignon J, Brochard P, de Cremous H, et al: Contribution of epidemiology and biology to the comprehension of causes and mechanisms of mesothelioma. Int Trends in Gen Thoracic Surg 327–335, 1990
2. Brunner J, Sordillo PP, Magill GB, et al: Malignant mesothelioma of the pleura. Review of 123 patients. Cancer 49:2431–2435, 1982
3. Borden EC: Mesothelioma: Natural history and current therapeutic approaches. Curr Conc Oncol 5:3–8, 1983
4. Dimitrov NV, McMahon SM, Carr DT: Multidisciplinary approach to management of patients with mesothelioma. Cancer Res 43:3974, 1983
5. Rusch V, Ginsberg RJ: New concepts in the staging of mesotheliomas. Int Trends in Gen Thoracic Surg 336–343, 1990

Data Form for Cancer Staging

Patient identification
Name _____

Address _____

Hospital or clinic number _____

Age _____ Sex _____ Race _____

Institution identification
Hospital or clinic _____

Address _____

Oncology Record

Anatomic site of cancer _____

Histologic type _____

Grade (G) _____

Date of classification _____

Chronology of classification

[ ] Clinical (use all data prior to first treatment)

[ ] Pathologic (if definitively resected specimen available)

DEFINITIONS

Primary Tumor (T)

Clin	Path		
[ ]	[ ]	TX	Primary tumor cannot be assessed
[ ]	[ ]	T0	No evidence of primary tumor
[ ]	[ ]	T1	Tumor limited to ipsilateral parietal and/or visceral pleura
[ ]	[ ]	T2	Tumor invades any of the following: ipsilateral lung, endothoracic fascia, diaphragm, or pericardium
[ ]	[ ]	T3	Tumor invades any of the following: ipsilateral chest wall muscle, ribs, or mediastinal organs or tissues
[ ]	[ ]	T4	Tumor directly extends to any of the following: contralateral pleura, lung, peritoneum, intraabdominal organs, or cervical tissues

Lymph Node (N)

Clin	Path		
[ ]	[ ]	NX	Regional lymph nodes cannot be assessed
[ ]	[ ]	N0	No regional lymph node metastasis
[ ]	[ ]	N1	Metastasis in ipsilateral peribronchial and/or ipsilateral hilar lymph nodes, including direct extension
[ ]	[ ]	N2	Metastasis in ipsilateral mediastinal and/or subcarinal lymph node(s)
[ ]	[ ]	N3	Metastasis in contralateral mediastinal, contralateral hilar, ipsilateral or contralateral scalene, or supraclavicular lymph node(s)

Distant Metastasis (M)

Clin	Path		
[ ]	[ ]	MX	Distant metastasis cannot be assessed
[ ]	[ ]	M0	No evidence of distant metastasis
[ ]	[ ]	M1	Distant metastasis

Stage Grouping

Clin	Path				
[ ]	[ ]	Stage I	T1	N0	M0
			T2	N0	M0
[ ]	[ ]	Stage II	T1	N1	M0
			T2	N1	M0
[ ]	[ ]	Stage III	T1	N2	M0
			T2	N2	M0
			T3	N0	M0
			T3	N1	M0
			T3	N2	M0
[ ]	[ ]	Stage IV	Any T	N3	M0
			T4	Any N	M0
			Any T	Any N	M1

Histopathologic Type

This staging classification applies only to primary pleural mesotheliomas. It does not apply to metastatic tumors or to lung tumors that have extended to the pleural surfaces.

Staged by _____ M.D.

_____ Registrar

Date _____

American Joint Committee on Cancer—1992

MUSCULOSKELETAL

21

Bone

C40.0 Long bones of upper limb, scapula, and associated joints	C40.9 Bone of limb, NOS
C40.1 Short bones of upper limb and associated joints	C41.0 Bones of skull and face and associated joints
	C41.1 Mandible
C40.2 Long bones of lower limb and associated joints	C41.2 Vertebral column
	C41.3 Rib, sternum, clavicle, and associated joints
C40.3 Short bones of lower limb and associated joints	C41.4 Pelvic bones, sacrum, coccyx, and associated joints
C40.8 Overlapping lesion of bones, joints, and articular cartilage of limbs	C41.8 Overlapping lesion of bones, joints, and articular cartilage
	C41.9 Bone, NOS

This classification is used for all primary malignant tumors of bone except for primary malignant lymphoma, multiple myeloma, juxtacortical osteosarcoma, and juxtacortical chondrosarcoma. There should be histologic confirmation of the disease to permit division of cases by histologic type.

ANATOMY

Primary Site. Primary sites include all skeletal bones.

Regional Lymph Nodes. The regional lymph nodes are those appropriate to the site of the primary tumor.

Metastatic Sites. A metastatic site includes any site beyond the regional lymph nodes of the primary site. Spread to the lungs is frequent.

RULES FOR CLASSIFICATION

Clinical Staging. All data available prior to definitive treatment are to be used for staging.

Pathologic Staging. All clinical and pathologic data obtained on examination of the resected tissue are to be used for staging.

HISTOPATHOLOGIC GRADE (G)

GX   Grade cannot be assessed
G1   Well differentiated
G2   Moderately differentiated
G3   Poorly differentiated
G4   Undifferentiated

Note: Ewing's sarcoma is classified as G4.

DEFINITION OF TNM

Primary Tumor (T)

TX   Primary tumor cannot be assessed
T0   No evidence of primary tumor
T1   Tumor confined within the cortex
T2   Tumor invades beyond the cortex

Regional Lymph Nodes (N)

NX   Regional lymph nodes cannot be assessed
N0   No regional lymph node metastasis
N1   Regional lymph node metastasis

Distant Metastasis (M)

MX   Presence of distant metastasis cannot be assessed
M0   No distant metastasis
M1   Distant metastasis

STAGE GROUPING				
Stage IA	G1,2	T1	N0	M0
Stage IB	G1,2	T2	N0	M0
Stage IIA	G3,4	T1	N0	M0
Stage IIB	G3,4	T2	N0	M0
Stage III	Not defined			
Stage IVA	Any G	Any T	N1	M0
Stage IVB	Any G	Any T	Any N	M1

HISTOPATHOLOGIC TYPE

See bibliography for reference material.

A. Bone-forming
   1. Osteosarcoma (osteogenic sarcoma)

B. Cartilage-forming
   1. Chondrosarcoma
   2. Mesenchymal chondrosarcoma
C. Giant cell tumor, malignant
D. Ewing's sarcoma
E. Vascular tumors
   1. Hemangioendothelioma
   2. Hemangiopericytoma
   3. Angiosarcoma
F. Connective tissue tumors
   1. Fibrosarcoma
   2. Liposarcoma
   3. Malignant mesenchymoma
   4. Undifferentiated sarcoma
G. Other tumors
   1. Chordoma
   2. Adamantinoma of long bones

BIBLIOGRAPHY

1. World Health Organization: Histological typing of bone tumors. International Histological Classification of Tumors, No. 6. Geneva, WHO, 1972

Data Form for Cancer Staging

Patient identification
Name _____
Address _____
Hospital or clinic number _____
Age _____ Sex _____ Race _____

Institution identification
Hospital or clinic _____
Address _____

Oncology Record

Anatomic site of cancer _____
Histologic type _____
Grade (G) _____
Date of classification _____

Chronology of classification
[ ] Clinical (use all data prior to first treatment)
[ ] Pathologic (if definitively resected specimen available)

Clin	Path	
		DEFINITIONS

Primary Tumor (T)

Clin	Path		
[ ]	[ ]	TX	Primary tumor cannot be assessed
[ ]	[ ]	T0	No evidence of primary tumor
[ ]	[ ]	T1	Tumor confined within the cortex
[ ]	[ ]	T2	Tumor invades beyond the cortex

Lymph Node (N)

Clin	Path		
[ ]	[ ]	NX	Regional lymph nodes cannot be assessed
[ ]	[ ]	N0	No regional lymph node metastasis
[ ]	[ ]	N1	Regional lymph node metastasis

Distant Metastasis (M)

Clin	Path		
[ ]	[ ]	MX	Presence of distant metastasis cannot be assessed
[ ]	[ ]	M0	No distant metastasis
[ ]	[ ]	M1	Distant metastasis

Histopathologic Grade (G)

Clin	Path		
[ ]	[ ]	GX	Grade cannot be assessed
[ ]	[ ]	G1	Well differentiated
[ ]	[ ]	G2	Moderately differentiated
[ ]	[ ]	G3	Poorly differentiated
[ ]	[ ]	G4	Undifferentiated

Histopathologic Type

A. Bone-forming
  1. Osteosarcoma (osteogenic sarcoma)
B. Cartilage-forming
  1. Chondrosarcoma
  2. Mesenchymal chondrosarcoma
C. Giant cell tumor, malignant
D. Ewing's sarcoma
E. Vascular tumors
  1. Hemangioendothelioma
  2. Hemangiopericytoma
  3. Angiosarcoma
F. Connective tissue tumors
  1. Fibrosarcoma
  2. Liposarcoma
  3. Malignant mesenchymoma
  4. Undifferentiated sarcoma
G. Other tumors
  1. Chordoma
  2. Adamantinoma of long bones

Stage Grouping

Clin	Path	Stage	G	T	N	M
[ ]	[ ]	IA	G1	T1	N0	M0
			G2	T1	N0	M0
[ ]	[ ]	IB	G1	T2	N0	M0
			G2	T2	N0	M0
[ ]	[ ]	IIA	G3	T1	N0	M0
			G4	T1	N0	M0
[ ]	[ ]	IIB	G3	T2	N0	M0
			G4	T2	N0	M0
[ ]	[ ]	III	Not defined			
[ ]	[ ]	IVA	Any G	Any T	N1	M0
[ ]	[ ]	IVB	Any G	Any T	Any N	M1

Staged by _____ M.D.
_____ Registrar
Date _____

22

Soft Tissues

C38.0 Heart
C38.1 Anterior mediastinum
C38.2 Posterior mediastinum
C38.3 Mediastinum, NOS
C38.8 Overlapping lesion of heart, mediastinum, and pleura

C47.0 Peripheral nerves and autonomic nervous system of head, face, and neck
C47.1 Peripheral nerves and autonomic nervous system of upper limb and shoulder
C47.2 Peripheral nerves and autonomic nervous system of lower limb and hip
C47.3 Peripheral nerves and autonomic nervous system of thorax
C47.4 Peripheral nerves and autonomic nervous system of abdomen
C47.5 Peripheral nerves and autonomic nervous system of pelvis
C47.6 Peripheral nerves and autonomic nervous system of trunk, NOS
C47.8 Overlapping lesion of peripheral nerves and autonomic nervous system
C47.9 Autonomic nervous system, NOS

C48.0 Retroperitoneum
C48.1 Specified parts of peritoneum
C48.2 Peritoneum, NOS
C48.8 Overlapping lesion of retroperitoneum and peritoneum

C49.0 Connective, subcutaneous, and other soft tissues of head, face, and neck
C49.1 Connective, subcutaneous, and other soft tissues of upper limb and shoulder
C49.2 Connective, subcutaneous, and other soft tissues of lower limb and hip
C49.3 Connective, subcutaneous, and other soft tissues of thorax
C49.4 Connective, subcutaneous, and other soft tissues of abdomen
C49.5 Connective, subcutaneous, and other soft tissues of pelvis
C49.6 Connective, subcutaneous, and other soft tissues of trunk, NOS

C49.8 Overlapping lesion of connective, subcutaneous, and other soft tissues
C49.9 Connective, subcutaneous, and other soft tissues, NOS

The staging system applies to all soft-tissue sarcomas except Kaposi's sarcoma, dermatofibrosarcoma, and desmoid type of fibrosarcoma grade 1. Excluded from the staging system are those sarcomas arising within the confines of the dura mater, including the brain, and sarcomas arising in parenchymatous organs and from hollow viscera. The system is based on an analysis of 1,215 cases obtained from 13 institutions. Cases were collected on the basis of histology, diagnosis, and type of soft tissue and include all age groups. For the most part, recommendations regarding staging of soft-tissue sarcomas in children are the same as the AJCC staging system for adults.

Grading of soft-tissue sarcomas has not been used in the stage grouping for pediatric tumors, however.

In the analysis, it was determined that in addition to clinical information, the histologic type, grade, and tumor size are essential for a meaningful staging system. The histologic diagnosis identifying the type of tumor and the pathologist's assessment of the inherent extent of malignancy (tumor differentiation) are fundamentals on which the staging is based.

Determination of the histologic grade and type of tumor is required for staging soft-tissue sarcomas and must be established by a qualified pathologist working with an adequate sample of the tumor.

ANATOMY

Primary Site. Various soft tissues can give rise to these sarcomas, including fibrous connective tissue, fat, smooth and striated muscle, vascular tissue, and peripheral neural tissue, as well as undifferentiated mesenchyma.

Connective, subcutaneous, and other soft tissues, and
    peripheral nerves
Retroperitoneum
Mediastinum

Regional Lymph Nodes. The regional lymph nodes are those appropriate to the site of the primary tumor.

Unilateral Tumors

Head and neck	Ipsilateral preauricular, submandibular, cervical, and supraclavicular lymph nodes
Thorax	Ipsilateral axillary lymph nodes
Arm	Ipsilateral epitrochlear and axillary lymph nodes
Abdomen, loins, and buttocks	Ipsilateral inguinal lymph nodes
Leg	Ipsilateral popliteal and inguinal lymph nodes
Anal margin and perianal skin	Ipsilateral inguinal lymph nodes

Metastatic Sites. The lung is the most common site, but any body site may be involved.

RULES FOR CLASSIFICATION

Clinical Staging. Clinical staging includes physical examination, imaging, clinical laboratory tests, and biopsy of the sarcoma for microscopic diagnosis and grading.

Pathologic Staging. Pathologic (pTNM) staging consists of the removal and pathologic evaluation of the primary tumor, histopathologic grade, and, if submitted, regional lymph nodes or distant metastases.

HISTOPATHOLOGIC GRADE (G)

After the histologic type has been determined, the tumor should be graded according to the accepted criteria of malignancy, including cellularity, cellular pleomorphism, mitotic activity, and necrosis. The amount of intercellular substance, such as collagen or mucoid material, should be considered as favorable in assessing grade.

GX Grade cannot be assessed
G1 Well differentiated
G2 Moderately differentiated
G3 Poorly differentiated
G4 Undifferentiated

DEFINITION OF TNM

Primary Tumor (T)

TX Primary tumor cannot be assessed
T0 No evidence of primary tumor
T1 Tumor 5 cm or less in greatest dimension
T2 Tumor more than 5 cm in greatest dimension

Regional Lymph Nodes (N)

NX Regional lymph nodes cannot be assessed
N0 No regional lymph node metastasis
N1 Regional lymph node metastasis

Distant Metastasis (M)

MX Presence of distant metastasis cannot be assessed
M0 No distant metastasis
M1 Distant metastasis

STAGE GROUPING

Stage IA	G1	T1	N0	M0
Stage IB	G1	T2	N0	M0
Stage IIA	G2	T1	N0	M0
Stage IIB	G2	T2	N0	M0
Stage IIIA	G3,4	T1	N0	M0
Stage IIIB	G3,4	T2	N0	M0
Stage IVA	Any G	Any T	N1	M0
Stage IVB	Any G	Any T	Any N	M1

HISTOPATHOLOGIC TYPE

Tumors included in the analysis are listed below:

Alveolar soft-part sarcoma
Angiosarcoma
Epithelioid sarcoma
Extraskeletal chondrosarcoma

Extraskeletal osteosarcoma
Fibrosarcoma
Leiomyosarcoma
Liposarcoma
Malignant fibrous histiocytoma
Malignant hemangiopericytoma
Malignant mesenchymoma
Malignant schwannoma
Rhabdomyosarcoma
Synovial sarcoma
Sarcoma, NOS

BIBLIOGRAPHY

1. Castro EB, Hajdu SI, Fortner JG: Surgical therapy of fibrosarcoma of extremities. Arch Surg 107:284–286, 1973

2. Enzinger FM, Lattes R, Torloni H: Histological typing of soft tissue tumors. WHO International Histological Classification of Tumors, No. 3. Geneva, WHO, 1969

3. Enzinger FM, Shiraki M: Alveolar rhabdomyosarcoma: An analysis of 110 cases. Cancer 24:18–31, 1969

4. Enzinger FM, Weiss SW: Soft Tissue Tumors, 2nd ed. St. Louis, C.V. Mosby, 1988

5. Hajdu SI: Pathology of Soft Tissue Tumors. Philadelphia, Lea & Febiger, 1979

6. Heise HW, Myers MH, Russell WO, et al: Recurrence-free survival time for surgically-treated soft tissue sarcoma patients. Cancer 57:172–177, 1986

7. Pritchard J, Soule EH, Taylor WF, et al: Fibrosarcoma: A clinicopathologic and statistical study of 1,969 tumors of the soft tissues of the extremities and trunk. Cancer 33:888–897, 1974

8. Russell WO, Cohen J, Enzinger F, et al: A clinical and pathological staging system for soft tissue sarcomas. Cancer 40:1562–1570, 1977

9. Soule EH, Geitz M, Henderson ED: Embryonal rhabdomyosarcoma of the limbs and the limb-girdles. Cancer 23:1336–1346, 1969

10. Suit HD, Russell WO, Martin RG: Sarcoma of soft tissue: Clinical and histopathologic parameters and response to treatment. Cancer 35:1478–1483, 1975

11. Sutow WW, Sullivan MP, Ried HL, et al: Prognosis in childhood rhabdomyosarcoma. Cancer 35:1384–1390, 1970

12. Van der Werf-Messing B, van Unnik JAM: Fibrosarcoma of the soft tissues: A clinicopathologic study. Cancer 18:1113–1123, 1965

Data Form for Cancer Staging

Patient identification
Name _____
Address _____
Hospital or clinic number _____
Age _____ Sex _____ Race _____

Institution identification
Hospital or clinic _____
Address _____

Oncology Record

Anatomic site of cancer _____
Histologic type _____
Grade (G) _____
Date of classification _____

Chronology of classification
[ ]   Clinical (use all data prior to first treatment)
[ ]   Pathologic (if definitively resected specimen available)

DEFINITIONS

Clin	Path		

Primary Tumor (T)

Clin	Path		
[ ]	[ ]	TX	Primary tumor cannot be assessed
[ ]	[ ]	T0	No evidence of primary tumor
[ ]	[ ]	T1	Tumor 5 cm or less in greatest dimension
[ ]	[ ]	T2	Tumor more than 5 cm in greatest dimension

Lymph Node (N)

Clin	Path		
[ ]	[ ]	NX	Regional lymph nodes cannot be assessed
[ ]	[ ]	N0	No regional lymph node metastasis
[ ]	[ ]	N1	Regional lymph node metastasis

Distant Metastasis (M)

Clin	Path		
[ ]	[ ]	MX	Presence of distant metastasis cannot be assessed
[ ]	[ ]	M0	No distant metastasis
[ ]	[ ]	M1	Distant metastasis

Histopathologic Grade (G)

Clin	Path		
[ ]	[ ]	GX	Grade cannot be assessed
[ ]	[ ]	G1	Well differentiated
[ ]	[ ]	G2	Moderately differentiated
[ ]	[ ]	G3	Poorly differentiated
[ ]	[ ]	G4	Undifferentiated

Histopathologic Type

Tumors included in the analysis are listed below:

Alveolar soft-part sarcoma
Angiosarcoma
Epithelioid sarcoma
Extraskeletal chondrosarcoma
Extraskeletal osteosarcoma
Fibrosarcoma
Leiomyosarcoma
Liposarcoma
Malignant fibrous histiocytoma
Malignant hemangiopericytoma
Malignant mesenchymoma
Malignant schwannoma
Rhabdomyosarcoma
Synovial sarcoma
Sarcoma, NOS (not otherwise specified)

Stage Grouping

Clin	Path					
[ ]	[ ]	IA	G1	T1	N0	M0
[ ]	[ ]	IB	G1	T2	N0	M0
[ ]	[ ]	IIA	G2	T1	N0	M0
		IIB	G2	T2	N0	M0
[ ]	[ ]	IIIA	G3	T1	N0	M0
			G4	T1	N0	M0
[ ]	[ ]	IIIB	G3	T2	N0	M0
			G4	T2	N0	M0
[ ]	[ ]	IVA	Any G	Any T	N1	M0
[ ]	[ ]	IVB	Any G	Any T	Any N	M1

Staged by _____ M.D.
_____ Registrar
Date _____

SKIN

23

Carcinoma of the Skin (Excluding Eyelid, Vulva, and Penis)

C44.0 Skin of lip, NOS
C44.2 External ear
C44.3 Skin of other and unspecified parts of face
C44.4 Skin of scalp and neck
C44.5 Skin of trunk
C44.6 Skin of upper limb and shoulder
C44.7 Skin of lower limb and hip
C44.8 Overlapping lesion
C44.9 Skin, NOS

C63.2 Scrotum

This chapter applies to carcinomas of the skin, predominantly squamous cell carcinomas and basal cell carcinomas. Skin cancers are relatively common and for the most part have a good prognosis. Basal cell carcinomas, the most common cancers in humans, are easily treated with surgery. Staging of skin cancer depends on the size of the primary tumor. Refer to Chapter 38 for lesions on the eyelid and Chapter 24 for melanomas.

ANATOMY

Primary Site. The skin has two layers: an outer epidermis and the inner dermis. The epidermis consists predominantly of stratified squamous epithelium, the external layer of which is keratinized. The dermis contains connective tissue and elastic fibers. Immediately below the dermis is the subcutaneous tissue. The sebaceous glands and other glands of the skin are found in the dermis and adjacent subcutaneous tissue. All skin components—epidermis, dermis, and adnexal structures—can give rise to malignant neoplasms.

Cancers can arise from any area of the skin. They are most common on those surfaces exposed to sunlight, including the face, ears, hands, and scalp. Cancers can also arise on the truncal regions and on the extremities. Basal cell carcinomas often occur on the face.

This classification also includes tumors arising in the anal margin.

Regional Lymph Nodes. The regional lymph nodes are those appropriate to the location of the primary tumor.

Unilateral Tumors

Head, neck	Ipsilateral preauricular, submandibular, cervical, and supraclavicular lymph nodes
Thorax	Ipsilateral axillary lymph nodes
Arm	Ipsilateral epitrochlear and axillary lymph nodes
Abdomen, loins and buttocks	Ipsilateral inguinal lymph nodes
Leg	Ipsilateral popliteal and inguinal lymph nodes
Anal margin and perianal skin	Ipsilateral inguinal lymph nodes

With tumors in the boundary zones between the above, the lymph nodes pertaining to the regions on both sides of the boundary zone are considered to be regional lymph nodes. The following 4 cm-wide bands are considered boundary zones:

Between (Right/left)	*Along* (Midline)
Head and neck/thorax	Claviculo-acromion-upper shoulder blade edge
Thorax/arm	Shoulder-axilla-shoulder
Thorax/abdomen, loins, buttocks	Front: Middle between navel and costal arch
	Back: Lower border of thoracic vertebrae (midtransverse-axis)
Abdomen, loins, and buttock/leg	Groin-trochanter-gluteal sulcus

For tumors arising on the leg, the iliac nodes are considered sites of distant metastasis and should be coded as M1.

Metastatic Sites. The most common metastatic site is the lung, especially for the squamous cell carcinomas. Other sites of distant spread are unusual. Basal cell carcinomas tend to erode locally, although rarely they may metastasize.

RULES FOR CLASSIFICATION

The clinical and pathologic classifications are identical. However, pathologic staging uses the symbol "p" as a prefix.

The classification applies only to carcinomas. There should be microscopic verification of the disease to permit division of cases by histologic type. The following are suggested procedures for assessing the T, N, and M categories.

Clinical Staging. Assessment of skin cancer is based on inspection and palpation of the involved area and the regional lymph nodes. Imaging studies of the underlying bony structures is important, especially in the scalp, if the lesion is fixed.

T categories: Clinical examination
N categories: Clinical examination
M categories: Examination and imaging

Pathologic Staging. Complete resection of the entire site is indicated. Confirmation of lymph node involvement is also required.

DEFINITION OF TNM

Definitions for clinical (cTNM) and pathologic (pTNM) classifications are the same.

Primary Tumor (T)

TX   Primary tumor cannot be assessed
T0   No evidence of primary tumor
Tis Carcinoma *in situ*
T1   Tumor 2 cm or less in greatest dimension
T2   Tumor more than 2 cm but not more than 5 cm in greatest dimension
T3   Tumor more than 5 cm in greatest dimension
T4   Tumor invades deep extradermal structures (e.g., cartilage, skeletal muscle, or bone)

Note: In the case of multiple simultaneous tumors, the tumor with the highest T category will be classified and the number of separate tumors will be indicated in parentheses; e.g., T2 (5).

Regional Lymph Nodes (N)

NX   Regional lymph nodes cannot be assessed
N0   No regional lymph node metastasis
N1   Regional lymph node metastasis

Distant Metastasis (M)

MX   Presence of distant metastasis cannot be assessed
M0   No distant metastasis
M1   Distant metastasis

STAGE GROUPING

Stage 0	Tis	N0	M0
Stage I	T1	N0	M0
Stage II	T2	N0	M0
	T3	N0	M0
Stage III	T4	N0	M0
	Any T	N1	M0
Stage IV	Any T	Any N	M1

HISTOPATHOLOGIC TYPE

The staging system is used primarily for squamous cell and basal cell carcinomas of the skin. It also applies to adenocarcinomas developing from sweat or sebaceous glands and a spindle cell variant of squamous cell carcinoma. Squamous cell tumors may also be described as verrucous.

A form of *in situ* carcinoma or intraepidermal carcinoma is often referred to as Bowen's disease. This lesion should be coded as Tis.

HISTOPATHOLOGIC GRADE (G)

GX Grade cannot be assessed
G1 Well differentiated
G2 Moderately differentiated
G3 Poorly differentiated
G4 Undifferentiated

BIBLIOGRAPHY

1. Edmundson WF: Microscopic grading of cancer and its practical implications. Arch Dermatol & Syph 57:141, 1948

2. Katz AD: The frequency and risk of metastases in squamous cell carcinoma of the skin. Cancer 10:1162–1166, 1957

3. Lund HZ: How often does squamous cell carcinoma of the skin metastasize? Arch Dermatol 92:635–637, 1965

4. Pollack SV, Goslen JB, Sherertz EF, et al: The biology of basal cell carcinoma: A review. J Am Acad Dermatol 7:569–577, 1982

5. Safai B, Good RA: Basal cell carcinoma with metastasis: Review of literature. Arch Pathol Lab Med 101:327–331, 1977

6. Strayer DS, Santa Crus DJ: Carcinoma *in situ* of the skin: A review of histopathology. J Cutan Pathol 7:244–259, 1980

CARCINOMA OF THE SKIN (EXCLUDING EYELID, VULVA, AND PENIS)

Data Form for Cancer Staging

Patient identification
Name _____
Address _____
Hospital or clinic number _____
Age _____ Sex _____ Race _____

Institution identification
Hospital or clinic _____
Address _____

Oncology Record

Anatomic site of cancer _____
Histologic type _____
Grade (G) _____
Date of classification _____

Chronology of classification
[ ]   Clinical (use all data prior to first treatment)
[ ]   Pathologic (if definitively resected specimen available)

DEFINITIONS

Clin	Path		

Primary Tumor (T)

Clin	Path		
[ ]	[ ]	TX	Primary tumor cannot be assessed
[ ]	[ ]	T0	No evidence of primary tumor
[ ]	[ ]	Tis	Carcinoma *in situ*
[ ]	[ ]	T1	Tumor 2 cm or less in greatest dimension
[ ]	[ ]	T2	Tumor more than 2 cm but not more than 5 cm in greatest dimension
[ ]	[ ]	T3	Tumor more than 5 cm in greatest dimension
[ ]	[ ]	T4	Tumor invades deep extradermal structures, *i.e.,* cartilage, skeletal muscle or bone

Lymph Node (N)

Clin	Path		
[ ]	[ ]	NX	Regional lymph nodes cannot be assessed
[ ]	[ ]	N0	No regional lymph node metastasis
[ ]	[ ]	N1	Regional lymph node metastasis

Distant Metastasis (M)

Clin	Path		
[ ]	[ ]	MX	Presence of distant metastasis cannot be assessed
[ ]	[ ]	M0	No distant metastasis
[ ]	[ ]	M1	Distant metastasis

Stage Grouping

Clin	Path				
[ ]	[ ]	0	Tis	N0	M0
[ ]	[ ]	I	T1	N0	M0
[ ]	[ ]	II	T2	N0	M0
			T3	N0	M0
[ ]	[ ]	III	T4	N0	M0
			Any T	N1	M0
[ ]	[ ]	IV	Any T	Any N	M1

Histopathologic Grade (G)

[ ] GX   Grade cannot be assessed
[ ] G1   Well differentiated
[ ] G2   Moderately differentiated
[ ] G3   Poorly differentiated
[ ] G4   Undifferentiated

Illustrations

Indicate on diagram primary tumor and regional nodes involved.

Histopathologic Type

The staging system is used primarily for squamous cell and basal cell carcinomas of the skin. It also applies to adenocarcinomas developing from sweat or sebaceous glands and a spindle cell variant of squamous cell carcinoma. Squamous cell tumors may also be described as verrucous.

A form of *in situ* carcinoma or intraepidermal carcinoma is often referred to as Bowen's disease. This lesion should be coded as Tis.

Staged by _____ M.D.
_____ Registrar
Date _____

24

Malignant Melanoma of the Skin (Excluding Eyelid)

C44.0 Skin of lip, NOS
C44.2 External ear
C44.3 Skin of other and unspec-
      ified parts of face
C44.4 Skin of scalp and neck
C44.5 Skin of trunk
C44.6 Skin of upper limb and
      shoulder
C44.7 Skin of lower limb and
      hip
C44.8 Overlapping lesion of
      skin
C44.9 Skin, NOS

C51 Vulva

C60 Penis

C63.2 Scrotum

Malignant melanomas are most common in fair-skinned persons, often with a history of chronic sun exposure. They can occur in any skin area, including the palms, soles, and nail beds. Rarely, melanomas may arise in other sites, such as the mucous membranes of the oral cavity, nasopharynx, vagina, urethra, and anal canal. Melanomas may also arise from the pigmented tissues of the eye and from giant hairy nevi. In some cases of disseminated disease, a primary lesion may not be found. Melanomas can be transmitted from mother to infant during pregnancy. Early detection and treatment of incipient melanomas have resulted in a significant decrease in the mortality from this disease. The staging classification outlined in this chapter applies only to melanomas arising in the skin. These tumors are staged histologically by measuring the depth of penetration into the underlying dermis or subcutis and by a statement on the level of invasion, with the cutaneous anatomic structures used as reference.

ANATOMY

Primary Site. The great majority of melanomas arise from the pigmented melanocytes located in the basal layer of the epidermis. The tumor often develops from a pre-existing pigmented lesion, although some arise from apparently normal skin. Melanomas are found on all skin surfaces. The tumor may grow into the dermis (nodular type) or spread horizontally along the skin (superficial spreading type). Multiple primary tumors may occur.

Regional Lymph Nodes. The regional lymph nodes depend on the location of the primary tumor. Regional nodes are as follows:

Unilateral Tumors

Head and neck	Ipsilateral preauricular, submandibular, cervical, and supraclavicular lymph nodes
Thorax	Ipsilateral axillary lymph nodes
Arm	Ipsilateral epitrochlear and axillary lymph nodes
Abdomen, loins, and buttocks	Ipsilateral inguinal lymph nodes
Leg	Ipsilateral popliteal and inguinal lymph nodes
Anal margin and perianal skin	Ipsilateral inguinal lymph nodes

With tumors in the boundary zones between the above, the lymph nodes pertaining to the regions on both sides of the boundary zone are considered regional lymph nodes. The following 4 cm-wide bands are considered as boundary zones:

Between (Right/left)	*Along* (Midline)
Head and neck/thorax	Claviculo-acromion-upper 　shoulder blade edge
Thorax/arm	Shoulder-axilla-shoulder
Thorax/abdomen, 　loins, and buttocks	Front: Middle between navel 　and costal arch
	Back: Lower border of thoracic 　vertebrae (midtransverse-axis)
Abdomen, loins, 　and buttock/leg	Groin-trochanter-gluteal sulcus

Iliac nodes are considered sites of distant metastasis and should be coded as M1.

Lesions arising in the midtransverse axis of the trunk at a level between the umbilicus and the lower costal margin anteriorly and extending laterally to the posterior level between the tenth thoracic spine (T10) and the first lumbar spine (L1) may spread with equal propensity to either contralateral or ipsilateral (or both) axillary or inguinal nodes.

Metastatic Sites. Melanomas can metastasize widely. No organ or tissue is exempt. In some cases, metastatic deposits may not become apparent for years. Melanomas commonly involve skin, subcutaneous tissues, lymph nodes, liver, bone, lung, brain, and visceral organs.

For staging purposes, two sub-M categories, identified as "a" and "b", are included. Metastasis to the skin, subcutaneous tissue, or lymph nodes beyond the site of the primary lymph node drainage is considered M1a. Metastasis to other distant sites—often referred to as visceral metastasis—is considered M1b. This distinction is based on the more favorable response to therapy by patients with skin or subcutaneous metastases only.

RULES FOR CLASSIFICATION

Clinical Staging. Clinical T classification ordinarily is not possible. Excisional biopsy and pathologic interpretation of the primary lesion are necessary for proper staging. Ulceration of the primary lesion may indicate a bad prognosis and should be recorded, but its presence does not alter staging.

Pathologic Staging. Pathologic staging of the primary melanoma is based on microscopic assessment of the depth of invasion and thickness of the primary tumor. Therefore, evaluation of the entire primary tumor, rather than a wedge or punch biopsy, is always advised. The

SURVIVAL ACCORDING TO AJCC STAGE
MELANOMA

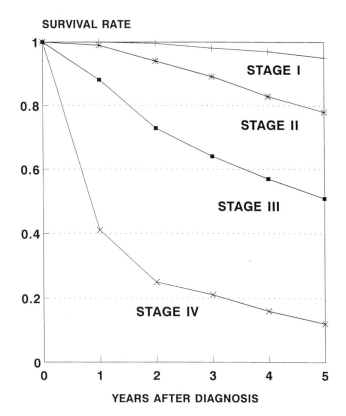

Fig. 24-1. Relative survival rates according to the stage of disease. Data taken from 8,479 patients who were diagnosed between 1977 and 1982. Patients are listed in the Surveillance, Epidemiology, and End Results Program of the National Cancer Institute. Stage I represents 4,286 patients; Stage II, 3,328; Stage III, 649; and Stage IV, 216.

entire thickness of the skin is needed for accurate classification. Regional nodes should be carefully evaluated, if available, and the number of positive nodes should be identified with the total number of lymph nodes removed.

Both the thickness and the level of invasion have prognostic significance, and both parameters should be reported by the pathologist.

Maximal thickness of the tumor is measured with an ocular micrometer at a right angle to the adjacent normal skin. The upper reference point is the top of the granular cell layer of the epidermis of the overlying skin, or the base of the lesion if the tumor is ulcerated. The lower reference point is usually the deepest point of invasion. It may be the invading edge of a single tumor mass or an isolated cell or group of cells deep to the main mass. Actual measurement should be recorded.

If no primary lesion is found, the tumor is coded as TX.

DEFINITION OF TNM

Both the level of invasion and the maximum thickness determine the T classification and should be recorded. In case of discrepancy between tumor thickness and level, the pT category is based on the less favorable finding.

Satellite lesions or subcutaneous nodules more than 2 cm from the primary tumor but not beyond the site of the primary lymph node drainage are considered in-transit metastases and are listed under the N categories.

The extent of tumor is classified after excision.

Primary Tumor (pT)

pTX   Primary tumor cannot be assessed
pT0   No evidence of primary tumor
pTis   Melanoma *in situ* (atypical melanocytic hyperplasia, severe melanocytic dysplasia), not an invasive lesion (Clark's Level I)
pT1   Tumor 0.75 mm or less in thickness and invading the papillary dermis (Clark's Level II)
pT2   Tumor more than 0.75 mm but not more than 1.5 mm in thickness and/or invades to the papillary-reticular dermal interface (Clark's Level III)
pT3   Tumor more than 1.5 mm but not more than 4 mm in thickness and/or invades the reticular dermis (Clark's Level IV)
    pT3a   Tumor more than 1.5 mm but not more than 3mm in thickness
    pT3b   Tumor more than 3 mm but not more than 4 mm in thickness
pT4   Tumor more than 4 mm in thickness and/or invades the subcutaneous tissue (Clark's Level V) and/or satellite(s) within 2 cm of the primary tumor
    pT4a   Tumor more than 4 mm in thickness and/or invades the subcutaneous tissue
    pT4b   Satellite(s) within 2 cm of the primary tumor

Regional Lymph Nodes (N)

NX   Regional lymph nodes cannot be assessed
N0   No regional lymph node metastasis
N1   Metastasis 3 cm or less in greatest dimension in any regional lymph node(s)
N2   Metastasis more than 3 cm in greatest dimension in any regional lymph node(s) and/or in-transit metastasis
    N2a   Metastasis more than 3 cm in greatest dimension in any regional lymph nodes
    N2b   In-transit metastasis
    N2c   Both (N2a and N2b)

Distant Metastasis (M)

MX   Presence of distant metastasis cannot be assessed
M0   No distant metastasis
M1   Distant metastasis
    M1a   Metastasis in skin or subcutaneous tissue or lymph node(s) beyond the regional lymph nodes
    M1b   Visceral metastasis

Note: In-transit metastasis involves skin or subcutaneous tissue more than 2 cm from the primary tumor not beyond the regional lymph nodes.

STAGE GROUPING

Stage	pT	N	M
Stage 0	pTis	N0	M0
Stage I	pT1	N0	M0
	pT2	N0	M0
Stage II	pT3	N0	M0
	pT4	N0	M0
Stage III	Any pT	N1	M0
	Any pT	N2	M0
Stage IV	Any pT	Any N	M1

HISTOPATHOLOGIC TYPE

The types of malignant melanoma are as follows:

Lentigo maligna (Hutchinson's freckle)
Radial spreading (superficial spreading)
Nodular
Acral lentiginous
Unclassified

A rare desmoplastic variant also exists.

Melanomas are identified according to site (e.g., mucosal, ocular, vaginal, anal, urethral). The staging classification described in this chapter applies only to those arising in the skin.

BIBLIOGRAPHY

1. Balch CM, Murad TM, Soong SJ, et al: A multifactorial analysis of melanoma: Prognostic histopathological features comparing Clark's and Breslow's staging lesions. Ann Surg 188:732–742, 1978
2. Breslow A: Thickness, cross-sectional areas and depth of invasion in the prognosis of cutaneous melanoma. Ann Surg 172:902–908, 1970
3. Breslow A: Prognosis in cutaneous melanoma: Tumor thickness as a guide to treatment. Pathol Annu Part 1:1–20, 1980
4. Clark WH Jr: The histogenesis and biological behavior of primary malignant melanoma of the skin. Cancer Res 29:705–717, 1969
5. Kopf AW, Rodriquez-Sains RS, Rigel DS, et al: "Small" melanomas: Relation of prognostic variables to diameter of superficial spreading melanomas. J Dermatol Surg Oncol 8:765–770, 1982

MALIGNANT MELANOMA OF THE SKIN (EXCLUDING EYELID)

Data Form for Cancer Staging

Patient identification
Name _____
Address _____
Hospital or clinic number _____
Age _____ Sex _____ Race _____

Institution identification
Hospital or clinic _____
Address _____

Oncology Record

Anatomic site of cancer _____
Histologic type _____
Grade (G) _____
Date of classification _____

Chronology of classification
[ ] Clinical (use all data prior to first treatment)
[ ] Pathologic (if definitively resected specimen available)

DEFINITIONS

Primary Tumor (pT)

Clin	Path		
[ ]	[ ]	pTX	Primary tumor cannot be assessed
[ ]	[ ]	pT0	No evidence of primary tumor
[ ]	[ ]	pTis	Melanoma *in situ* (atypical melanocytic hyperplasia, severe melanocytic dysplasia, not an invasive lesion (Clark's Level I)
[ ]	[ ]	pT1	Tumor 0.75 mm or less in thickness and invades the papillary dermis (Clark's Level II)
[ ]	[ ]	pT2	Tumor more than 0.75 mm but not more than 1.5 mm in thickness and/or invades to papillary-reticular dermal interface (Clark's Level III)
[ ]	[ ]	pT3	Tumor more than 1.5 mm but not more than 4 mm in thickness and/or invades the reticular dermis (Clark's Level IV)
[ ]	[ ]	pT3a	Tumor more than 1.5 mm but not more than 3 mm in thickness
[ ]	[ ]	pT3b	Tumor more than 3 mm but not more than 4 mm in thickness
[ ]	[ ]	pT4	Tumor more than 4 mm in thickness and/or invades the subcutaneous tissue (Clark's Level V) and/or satellite(s) within 2 cm of the primary tumor
[ ]	[ ]	pT4a	Tumor more than 4 mm in thickness and/or invades the subcutaneous tissue
[ ]	[ ]	pT4b	Satellite(s) within 2 cm of primary tumor

Lymph Node (N)

Clin	Path		
[ ]	[ ]	NX	Regional lymph nodes cannot be assessed
[ ]	[ ]	N0	No regional lymph node metastasis
[ ]	[ ]	N1	Metastasis 3 cm or less in greatest dimension in any regional lymph node(s)
[ ]	[ ]	N2	Metastasis more than 3 cm in greatest dimension in any regional lymph node(s) and/or in-transit metastasis
[ ]	[ ]	N2a	Metastasis more than 3 cm in greatest dimension in any regional lymph node(s)
[ ]	[ ]	N2b	In-transit metastasis
[ ]	[ ]	N2c	Both (N2a and N2b)

Distant Metastasis (M)

Clin	Path		
[ ]	[ ]	MX	Presence of distant metastasis cannot be assessed
[ ]	[ ]	M0	No distant metastasis
[ ]	[ ]	M1	Distant metastasis
[ ]	[ ]	M1a	Metastasis in skin or subcutaneous tissue or lymph node(s) beyond the regional lymph nodes
[ ]	[ ]	M1b	Visceral metastasis

Stage Grouping

Clin	Path				
[ ]	[ ]	0	pTis	N0	M0
[ ]	[ ]	I	pT1	N0	M0
			pT2	N0	M0
[ ]	[ ]	II	pT3	N0	M0
			pT4	N0	M0
[ ]	[ ]	III	Any pT	N1	M0
			Any pT	N2	M0
[ ]	[ ]	IV	Any pT	Any N	M1

Staged by _____ M.D.
_____ Registrar
Date _____

(continued on next page)

American Joint Committee on Cancer—1992

Histopathologic Type

The types of malignant melanoma are as follows:

Lentigo maligna (Hutchinson's freckle)
Radial spreading (superficial spreading)
Nodular
Acral lentiginous
Unclassified

A rare desmoplastic variant also exists.
Melanomas are identified according to site (mucosal, ocular, vaginal, anal, urethral, and so forth). The staging classification described in this chapter applies only to those arising in the skin.

Sites of Distant Metastasis

[ ] Pulmonary   PUL
[ ] Osseous   OSS
[ ] Hepatic   HEP
[ ] Brain   BRA
[ ] Lymph nodes   LYM
[ ] Bone marrow   MAR
[ ] Pleura   PLE
[ ] Peritoneum   PER
[ ] Skin   SKI
[ ] Other   OTH

Depth of Invasion

[ ] Level I (not a melanoma and further characterization is not necessary)
[ ] Level II
[ ] Level III
[ ] Level IV
[ ] Level V
Other description_____
Maximal thickness (mm)_____
Site of primary lesion (check diagram) _____
_____
Extent of primary lesion (include all pigmentation)_____
_____
Size in greatest diameter _____ cm

Illustrations

Indicate on diagrams primary tumor and regional nodes involved.

BREAST

25

Breast

C50.0 Nipple
C50.1 Central portion
C50.2 Upper-inner quadrant
C50.3 Lower-inner quadrant
C50.4 Upper-outer quadrant
C50.5 Lower-outer quadrant
C50.6 Axillary tail
C50.8 Overlapping lesion
C50.9 Breast, NOS

The following TNM definitions and stage groupings for carcinoma of the breast are the same for the AJCC and the UICC/TNM projects. This staging system for carcinoma of the breast applies to infiltrating and *in situ* carcinomas. Microscopic confirmation of the diagnosis is mandatory and the histologic type and grade of carcinoma should be recorded.

ANATOMY

Primary Site. Situated on the anterior chest wall, the mammary gland is composed of glandular tissue within a dense fibroareolar stroma. The glandular tissue consists of approximately 20 lobes, each of which terminates in a separate excretory duct in the nipple.

Regional Lymph Nodes. The breast lymphatics drain by way of three major routes: axillary, transpectoral, and internal mammary. Intramammary lymph nodes are considered with the axillary lymph nodes for staging purposes. Metastases to any other lymph nodes—including supraclavicular, cervical, and contralateral internal mammary nodes—are considered distant (M1). (Please refer to diagram.) The regional lymph nodes are:

(1) Axillary (ipsilateral): interpectoral (Rotter's) nodes and lymph nodes along the axillary vein and its tributaries, which may be divided into the following levels:

(i) Level I (low-axilla): lymph nodes lateral to the lateral border of the pectoralis minor muscle

(ii) Level II (mid-axilla): lymph nodes between the medial and lateral borders of the pectoralis minor muscle and the interpectoral (Rotter's) lymph nodes

(iii) Level III (apical axilla): lymph nodes medial to the medial margin of the pectoralis minor muscle, including those designated as subclavicular, infraclavicular, or apical.

Note: Intramammary lymph nodes are coded as axillary lymph nodes.

(2) Internal mammary (ipsilateral): lymph nodes in the intercostal spaces along the edge of the sternum in the endothoracic fascia.

Any other lymph node metastasis is coded as a distant metastasis (M1), including supraclavicular, cervical, or contralateral internal mammary lymph nodes.

Metastatic Sites. All distant visceral sites are potential sites of metastases. The four major sites of involvement are bone, lung, brain, and liver, but this widely metastasizing disease has been found in almost every remote site.

RULES FOR CLASSIFICATION

Clinical Staging. Clinical staging includes physical examination, with careful inspection and palpation of

REGIONAL LYMPH NODES

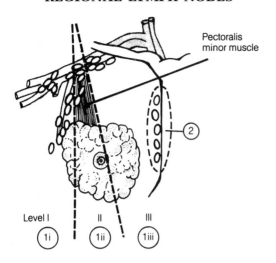

the skin, mammary gland, and lymph nodes (axillary, supraclavicular, and cervical), pathologic examination of the breast or other tissues, and imaging to establish the diagnosis of breast carcinoma. The extent of tissues examined pathologically for clinical staging is less than that required for pathologic staging (see Pathologic Staging). Appropriate operative findings are elements of clinical staging, including the size of the primary tumor and chest wall invasion and the presence or absence of regional or distant metastasis.

Pathologic Staging. Pathologic staging includes all data used for clinical staging and surgical resection as well as pathologic examination of the primary carcinoma, including not less than excision of the primary carcinoma with no tumor in any margin of resection by gross pathologic examination. A case can be included in the pathologic stage if there is only microscopic, but not gross, involvement at the margin. If there is tumor in the margin of resection by gross examination, it is coded as TX, because the extent of primary tumor cannot be assessed. Resection of at least the low axillary lymph nodes (Level I)—that is, those lymph nodes located lateral to the lateral border of the pectoralis minor muscle—should be carried out. Such a resection ordinarily will include six or more lymph nodes. Metastatic nodules in the fat adjacent to the mammary carcinoma, without evidence of residual lymph node tissue, are considered regional lymph node metastases.

TNM CLASSIFICATION

Primary Tumor

The clinical measurement used for classifying the primary tumor (T) should be the one judged most accurate (e.g., physical examination or mammogram). Pathologically, the tumor size for classification (T) is a measure-

ment of the invasive component. For example, if there is a large *in situ* component (4 cm) and a small invasive component (0.5 cm), the tumor is classified as T1a. The size of the primary tumor should be measured before any tissue is removed for special studies, such as for estrogen receptors.

Multiple Simultaneous Ipsilateral Primary Cancers

The following guidelines should be used when classifying multiple simultaneous ipsilateral primary (infiltrating, grossly measurable) carcinomas. These criteria do not apply to one grossly detected tumor associated with multiple separate microscopic foci.

1. Use the largest primary carcinoma to classify T.
2. Enter into the record that this is a case of multiple simultaneous ipsilateral primary carcinomas. Such cases should be analyzed separately.

Simultaneous Bilateral Breast Carcinomas

Each carcinoma is staged separately.

Inflammatory Carcinoma

Inflammatory carcinoma is a clinicopathologic entity characterized by diffuse brawny induration of the skin of the breast with an erysipeloid edge, usually without an underlying palpable mass. Radiologically, there may be a detectable mass and characteristic thickening of the skin over the breast. This clinical presentation is due to tumor embolization of dermal lymphatics. The tumor of inflammatory carcinoma is classified as T4d.

Paget's Disease of the Nipple

Paget's disease of the nipple without an associated tumor mass (clinical) or invasive carcinoma (pathologic) is classified as Tis. Paget's disease with a demonstrable mass (clinical) or an invasive component (pathologic) is classified according to the size of the tumor mass or invasive component.

Skin of the Breast

Dimpling of the skin, nipple retraction, or any other skin change except those described under T4b and T4d may occur in T1, T2, or T3 without changing the classification.

Chest Wall

The chest wall includes the ribs, intercostal muscles, and serratus anterior muscle but not the pectoral muscle.

BREAST CANCER
SURVIVAL ACCORDING TO AJCC STAGE

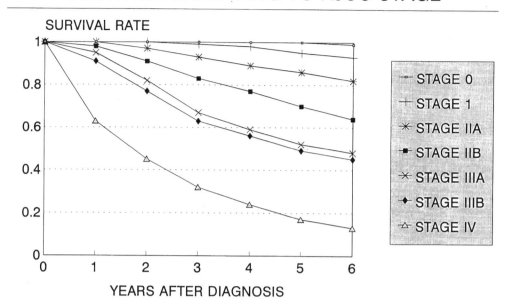

Fig. 25-1. Relative survival rates according to stage of disease. Data taken from 50,834 patients listed in the Surveillance, Epidemiology, and End Results Program of the National Cancer Institute. Patients were diagnosed between 1983 and 1987. Stage 0 represents 4,601 patients; Stage I, 16,519; Stage IIA, 14,692; Stage IIB, 8,283; Stage IIIA, 1,656; Stage IIIB, 1,389; and Stage IV, 3,694.

DEFINITION OF TNM

Primary Tumor (T)

Definitions for classifying the primary tumor (T) are the same for clinical and for pathologic classification. The telescoping method of classification can be applied. If the measurement is made by physical examination, the examiner will use the major headings (T1, T2, or T3). If other measurements, such as mammographic or pathologic, are used, the examiner can use the telescoped subsets of T1.

TX   Primary tumor cannot be assessed
T0   No evidence of primary tumor
Tis   Carcinoma *in situ:* intraductal carcinoma, lobular carcinoma in situ, or Paget's disease of the nipple with no tumor
T1   Tumor 2 cm or less in greatest dimension
    T1a   0.5 cm or less in greatest dimension
    T1b   More than 0.5 cm but not more than 1 cm in greatest dimension
    T1c   More than 1 cm but not more than 2 cm in greatest dimension
T2   Tumor more than 2 cm but not more than 5 cm in greatest dimension
T3   Tumor more than 5 cm in greatest dimension

T4   Tumor of any size with direct extension to chest wall or skin
    T4a   Extension to chest wall
    T4b   Edema (including peau d'orange) or ulceration of the skin of the breast or satellite skin nodules confined to the same breast
    T4c   Both (T4a and T4b)
    T4d   Inflammatory carcinoma (See the definition of inflammatory carcinoma in the introduction.)

Note: Paget's disease associated with a tumor is classified according to the size of the tumor.

Regional Lymph Nodes (N)

NX   Regional lymph nodes cannot be assessed (e.g., previously removed)
N0   No regional lymph node metastasis
N1   Metastasis to movable ipsilateral axillary lymph node(s)
N2   Metastasis to ipsilateral axillary lymph node(s) fixed to one another or to other structures
N3   Metastasis to ipsilateral internal mammary lymph node(s)

Pathologic Classification (pN)

pNX   Regional lymph nodes cannot be assessed (e.g., previously removed, or not removed for pathologic study)

pN0   No regional lymph node metastasis

pN1   Metastasis to movable ipsilateral axillary lymph node(s)

      pN1a   Only micrometastasis (none larger than 0.2 cm)

      pN1b   Metastasis to lymph node(s), any larger than 0.2 cm

         pN1bi   Metastasis in one to three lymph nodes, any more than 0.2 cm and all less than 2 cm in greatest dimension

         pN1bii   Metastasis to four or more lymph nodes, any more than 0.2 cm and all less than 2 cm in greatest dimension

         pN1biii   Extension of tumor beyond the capsule of a lymph node metastasis less than 2 cm in greatest dimension

         pN1biv   Metastasis to a lymph node 2 cm or more in greatest dimension

pN2   Metastasis to ipsilateral axillary lymph nodes that are fixed to one another or to other structures

pN3   Metastasis to ipsilateral internal mammary lymph node(s)

Distant Metastasis (M)

MX   Presence of distant metastasis cannot be assessed

M0   No distant metastasis

M1   Distant metastasis (includes metastasis to ipsilateral supraclavicular lymph node(s))

HISTOPATHOLOGIC TYPE

The histologic types are as follows:

Carcinoma, NOS (not otherwise specified)
Ductal
   Intraductal (*in situ*)
   Invasive with predominant intraductal component
   Invasive, NOS
   Comedo
   Inflammatory
   Medullary with lymphocytic infiltrate
   Mucinous (colloid)
   Papillary
   Scirrhous
   Tubular
   Other

Lobular
   In situ
   Invasive with predominant *in situ* component
   Invasive

Nipple
   Paget's disease, NOS
   Paget's disease with intraductal carcinoma
   Paget's disease with invasive ductal carcinoma
   Other
   Undifferentiated carcinoma

HISTOPATHOLOGIC GRADE (G)

GX   Grade cannot be assessed

G1   Well differentiated

G2   Moderately differentiated

G3   Poorly differentiated

G4   Undifferentiated

STAGE GROUPING

Stage 0	Tis	N0	M0
Stage I	T1	N0	M0
Stage IIA	T0	N1	M0
	T1	N1*	M0
	T2	N0	M0
Stage IIB	T2	N1	M0
	T3	N0	M0
Stage IIIA	T0	N2	M0
	T1	N2	M0
	T2	N2	M0
	T3	N1	M0
	T3	N2	M0
Stage IIIB	T4	Any N	M0
	Any T	N3	M0
Stage IV	Any T	Any N	M1

*Note: The prognosis of patients with N1a is similar to that of patients with pN0.

Data Form for Cancer Staging

Patient identification	Institution identification
Name _____	Hospital or clinic _____
Address _____	Address _____
Hospital or clinic number _____	
Age _____ Sex _____ Race _____	

Oncology Record

Anatomic site of cancer _____

Histologic type _____

Grade (G) _____

Date of classification _____

Chronology of classification

[ ]   Clinical (use all data prior to first treatment)

[ ]   Pathologic (if definitively resected specimen available)

DEFINITIONS

Primary Tumor (T)

Clin	Path		
[ ]	[ ]	TX	Primary tumor cannot be assessed
[ ]	[ ]	T0	No evidence of primary tumor
[ ]	[ ]	Tis	Carcinoma *in situ*: Intraductal carcinoma, lobular carcinoma *in situ*, or Paget's disease of the nipple with no tumor
[ ]	[ ]	T1	Tumor 2 cm or less in greatest dimension
[ ]	[ ]	T1a	0.5 cm or less in greatest dimension
[ ]	[ ]	T1b	More than 0.5 cm but not more than 1 cm in greatest dimension
[ ]	[ ]	T1c	More than 1 cm but not more than 2 cm in greatest dimension
[ ]	[ ]	T2	Tumor more than 2 cm but not more than 5 cm in greatest dimension
[ ]	[ ]	T3	Tumor more than 5 cm in greatest dimension
[ ]	[ ]	T4	Tumor of any size with direct extension to chest wall or skin
[ ]	[ ]	T4a	Extension to chest wall
[ ]	[ ]	T4b	Edema (including peau d'orange) or ulceration of the skin of breast or satellite skin nodules confined to same breast
[ ]	[ ]	T4c	Both T4a and T4b
[ ]	[ ]	T4d	Inflammatory carcinoma

Lymph Node (N)

Clin	Path		
[ ]	[ ]	NX	Regional lymph nodes cannot be assessed (*e.g.* previously removed)
[ ]	[ ]	N0	No regional lymph node metastasis
[ ]	[ ]	N1	Metastasis to movable ipsilateral axillary lymph node(s)
[ ]	[ ]	N2	Metastasis to ipsilateral axillary lymph node(s) fixed to one another or to other structures
[ ]	[ ]	N3	Metastasis to ipsilateral internal mammary lymph node(s)

Pathologic Classification (pN)

Path		
[ ]	pNX	Regional lymph nodes cannot be assessed (*e.g.* previously removed, or not removed for pathologic study)
[ ]	pN0	No regional lymph node metastasis
[ ]	pN1	Metastasis to movable ipsilateral axillary lymph node(s)
[ ]	pN1a	Only micrometastasis (none larger than 0.2 cm)
[ ]	pN1b	Metastasis to lymph nodes, any larger than 0.2 cm
[ ]	pN1bi	Metastasis in 1 to 3 lymph nodes, any more than 0.2 cm and all less than 2 cm in greatest dimension
[ ]	pN1bii	Metastasis to 4 or more lymph nodes, any more than 0.2 cm and all less than 2 cm in greatest dimension
[ ]	pN1biii	Extension of tumor beyond the capsule of a lymph node metastasis less than 2 cm in greatest dimension
[ ]	pN1biv	Metastasis to a lymph node 2 cm or more in greatest dimension
[ ]	pN2	Metastasis to ipsilateral axillary lymph nodes that are fixed to one another or to other structures
[ ]	pN3	Metastasis to ipsilateral internal mammary lymph node(s)

Distant Metastasis (M)

Clin	Path		
[ ]	[ ]	MX	Presence of distant metastasis cannot be assessed
[ ]	[ ]	M0	No distant metastasis
[ ]	[ ]	M1	Distant metastasis (includes metastasis to ipsilateral supraclavicular lymph node(s))

(continued on next page)

American Joint Committee on Cancer—1992

Clin	Path	Stage Grouping			
[ ]	[ ]	0	Tis	N0	M0
[ ]	[ ]	I	T1	N0	M0
[ ]	[ ]	IIA	T0	N1	M0
			T1	N1*	M0
			T2	N0	M0
[ ]	[ ]	IIB	T2	N1	M0
			T3	N0	M0
[ ]	[ ]	IIIA	T0	N2	M0
			T1	N2	M0
			T2	N2	M0
			T3	N1	M0
			T3	N2	M0
[ ]	[ ]	IIIB	T4	Any N	M0
			Any T	N3	M0
[ ]	[ ]	IV	Any T	Any N	M1

Note: The prognosis of patients with pN1a is similar to that of patients with pN0.

Staged by _____ M.D.

_____Registrar

Date _____

Histopathologic Grade (G)

[ ] GX   Grade cannot be assessed
[ ] G1   Well differentiated
[ ] G2   Moderately differentiated
[ ] G3   Poorly differentiated
[ ] G4   Undifferentiated

Histopathologic Type

The histologic types are the following:

Carcinoma, NOS (not otherwise specified)
Ductal
  Intraductal (*in situ*)
  Invasive with predominant intraductal component
  Invasive, NOS (not otherwise specified)
  Comedo
  Inflammatory
  Medullary with lymphocytic infiltrate
  Mucinous (colloid)
  Papillary
  Scirrhous
  Tubular
  Other
Lobular
  In situ
  Invasive with predominant *in situ* component
  Invasive
Nipple
  Paget's disease, NOS (not otherwise specified)
  Paget's disease with intraductal carcinoma
  Paget's disease with invasive ductal carcinoma
Other
  Undifferentiated carcinoma

Illustrations

REGIONAL LYMPH NODES

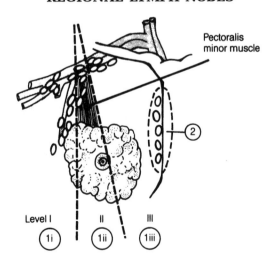

Pectoralis minor muscle

Level I   II   III

Indicate on diagram primary tumor and regional nodes involved.

GYNECOLOGIC TUMORS

The cervix uteri, corpus uteri, ovary, vagina, and vulva are the sites included in this section. The cervix uteri and corpus uteri were among the first sites to be classified by the TNM system. The League of Nations stages for carcinoma of the cervix have been used with minor modifications for nearly 50 years, and, because these are accepted by the International Federation of Gynecology and Obstetrics (FIGO), the TNM categories have been defined to correspond to the FIGO stages. Some amendments have been made in collaboration with FIGO, and the classifications now published have the approval of FIGO, AJCC, and all other national TNM committees of the Union Internationale Contre le Cancer (UICC).

The AJCC has worked closely with FIGO in the classification of cancer at gynecologic sites. Staging of malignant tumors is essentially the same, and stages are comparable in the two systems.

26

Cervix Uteri

C53.0 Endocervix
C53.1 Exocervix
C53.8 Overlapping lesion
C53.9 Cervix uteri

ANATOMY

Primary Site. The cervix is the lower third of the uterus. It is roughly cylindrical in shape, projects through the upper anterior vaginal wall, and communicates with the vagina through an orifice called the external os. Cancer of the cervix may originate on the vaginal surface or in the canal.

Regional Lymph Nodes. The cervix is drained by preureteral, postureteral, and uterosacral routes into the following first station nodes:

Paracervical
Parametrial
Hypogastric (obturator)
Common iliac
Internal and external iliac
Presacral
Sacral

Para-aortic node involvement is considered distant metastasis and is coded as M1.

Metastatic Sites. The most common sites of distant spread are the lungs and skeleton.

RULES FOR CLASSIFICATION

The classification applies only to carcinomas. There should be histologic confirmation of the disease.

Clinical Staging. Careful clinical examination should be performed in all cases, preferably by an experienced examiner and with anesthesia. The clinical staging must not be changed because of subsequent findings. When doubt exists as to the stage to which a particular cancer should be allocated, the earlier stage is mandatory. The following examinations are permitted: palpation, inspection, colposcopy, endocervical curettage, hysteroscopy, cystoscopy, proctoscopy, intravenous urography, and x-ray examination of the lungs and skeleton. Suspected bladder or rectal involvement should be confirmed by biopsy and histologic evidence. Optional examinations include lymphangiography, arteriography, venography, laparoscopy, and other imaging methods. Because these are not yet generally available and because the interpretation of results is variable, the findings of optional studies should not be the basis for changing the clinical staging.

Pathologic Staging. In cases treated by surgical procedures, the pathologist's findings in the removed tissues can be the basis for extremely accurate statements on the extent of disease. These findings should not be allowed to change the clinical staging but should be recorded in the manner described for the pathologic staging of disease. The pTNM nomenclature is appropriate for this purpose. Infrequently, hysterectomy is carried out in the presence of unsuspected extensive invasive cervical carcinoma. Such cases cannot be clinically staged or included in therapeutic statistics, but it is desirable that they be reported separately. Only if the rules for clinical staging are strictly observed will it be possible to compare results among clinics and by different modes of therapy.

Anatomic Subsites

Endocervix
Exocervix

DEFINITION OF TNM

The definitions of the T categories correspond to the several stages accepted by FIGO. Both systems are included for comparison.

Primary Tumor (T)

TNM	FIGO	DEFINITION
TX	—	Primary tumor cannot be assessed
T0	—	No evidence of primary tumor
Tis	—	Carcinoma *in situ*
T1	I	Cervical carcinoma confined to the uterus (extension to the corpus should be disregarded)
T1a	IA	Preclinical invasive carcinoma, diagnosed by microscopy only
T1a1	IA1	Minimal microscopic stromal invasion
T1a2	IA2	Tumor with an invasive component 5 mm or less in depth taken from the base of the epithelium and 7 mm or less in horizontal spread
T1b	IB	Tumor larger than T1a2
T2	II	Cervical carcinoma invades beyond the uterus but not to the pelvic wall or to the lower third of the vagina
T2a	IIA	Tumor without parametrial invasion
T2b	IIB	Tumor with parametrial invasion
T3	III	Cervical carcinoma extends to the pelvic wall and/or involves the lower third of the vagina and/or causes hydronephrosis or nonfunctioning kidney
T3a	IIIA	Tumor involves the lower third of the vagina, with no extension to the pelvic wall
T3b	IIIB	Tumor extends to the pelvic wall and/or causes hydronephrosis or a nonfunctioning kidney
T4*	IVA	Tumor invades the mucosa of the bladder or rectum and/ or extends beyond the true pelvis
M1	IVB	Distant metastasis

Note: Presence of bullous edema is not sufficient evidence to classify a tumor as T4.

Regional Lymph Nodes (N)

NX   Regional lymph nodes cannot be assessed
N0   No regional lymph node metastasis
N1   Regional lymph node metastasis

Distant Metastasis (M)

TNM	FIGO	DEFINITION
MX		Presence of distant metastasis cannot be assessed
M0		No distant metastasis
M1	IVB	Distant metastasis

pTNM Pathologic Classification

The pT, pN, and pM categories correspond to the T, N, and M categories.

STAGE GROUPING

AJCC/UICC				FIGO
Stage 0	Tis	N0	M0	
Stage IA	T1a	N0	M0	Stage IA
Stage IB	T1b	N0	M0	Stage IB
Stage IIA	T2a	N0	M0	Stage IIA
Stage IIB	T2b	N0	M0	Stage IIB
Stage IIIA	T3a	N0	M0	Stage IIIA
Stage IIIB	T1	N1	M0	Stage IIIB
	T2	N1	M0	
	T3a	N1	M0	
	T3b	Any N	M0	
Stage IVA	T4	Any N	M0	Stage IVA
Stage IVB	Any T	Any N	M1	Stage IVB

HISTOPATHOLOGIC TYPE

Cases should be classified as carcinoma of the cervix if the primary growth is in the cervix. All histologic types must be included. Grading is encouraged but is not a basis for modifying the stage groupings. When surgery is the primary treatment, the histologic findings permit the case to have pathologic staging. In this, the pTNM nomenclature is to be used.

The histopathologic types are:

Cervical intraepithelial neoplasia, grade III
Squamous cell carcinoma *in situ*
Squamous cell carcinoma
    Keratinizing
    Nonkeratinizing
    Verrucous
Adenocarcinoma *in situ*
Adenocarcinoma *in situ*, endocervical type
Endometrioid adenocarcinoma
Clear cell adenocarcinoma

Adenosquamous carcinoma
Adenoid cystic carcinoma
Small cell carcinoma
Undifferentiated carcinoma

HISTOPATHOLOGIC GRADE (G)

GX   Grade cannot be assessed
G1   Well differentiated
G2   Moderately differentiated
G3   Poorly differentiated
G4   Undifferentiated

Data Form for Cancer Staging

Patient identification
Name _____
Address _____
Hospital or clinic number _____
Age _____ Sex _____ Race _____

Institution identification
Hospital or clinic _____
Address _____

Oncology Record

Anatomic site of cancer _____
Histologic type _____
Grade (G) _____
Date of classification _____

Chronology of classification
[ ] Clinical (use all data prior to first treatment)
[ ] Pathologic (if definitively resected specimen available)

DEFINITIONS

Primary Tumor (T)

Clin	Path	TNM category	FIGO* stage	
[ ]	[ ]	TX		Primary tumor cannot be assessed
[ ]	[ ]	T0		No evidence of primary tumor
[ ]	[ ]	Tis		Carcinoma *in situ*
[ ]	[ ]	T1	I	Cervical carcinoma confined to uterus (extension to corpus should be disregarded)
[ ]	[ ]	T1a	IA	Preclinical invasive carcinoma, diagnosed by microscopy only
[ ]	[ ]	T1a1	IA1	Minimal microscopic stromal invasion
[ ]	[ ]	T1a2	IA2	Tumor with invasive component 5 mm or less in depth taken from the base of the epithelium and 7 mm or less in horizontal spread
[ ]	[ ]	T1b	IB	Tumor larger than T1a2
[ ]	[ ]	T2	II	Cervical carcinoma invades beyond uterus but not to pelvic wall or to the lower third of vagina
[ ]	[ ]	T2a	IIA	Tumor without parametrial invasion
[ ]	[ ]	T2b	IIB	Tumor with parametrial invasion
[ ]	[ ]	T3	III	Cervical carcinoma extends to pelvic wall and/or involves lower third of vagina and/or causes hydronephrosis or nonfunctioning kidney
[ ]	[ ]	T3a	IIIA	Tumor involves lower third of vagina, no extension to pelvic wall
[ ]	[ ]	T3b	IIIB	Tumor extends to pelvic wall and/or causes hydronephrosis or nonfunctioning kidney
[ ]	[ ]	T4**	IVA	Tumor invades mucosa of bladder or rectum and/or extends beyond the true pelvis

Lymph Node (N)

Clin	Path	TNM category	FIGO stage	
[ ]	[ ]	NX		Regional lymph nodes cannot be assessed
[ ]	[ ]	N0		No regional lymph node metastasis
[ ]	[ ]	N1		Regional lymph node metastasis

Distant Metastasis (M)

Clin	Path	TNM category	FIGO stage	
[ ]	[ ]	MX		Presence of distant metastasis cannot be assessed
[ ]	[ ]	M0		No distant metastasis
[ ]	[ ]	M1	IVB	Distant metastasis

Stage Grouping

Clin	Path	AJCC/UICC				FIGO
[ ]	[ ]	0	Tis	N0	M0	
[ ]	[ ]	IA	T1a	N0	M0	I A
[ ]	[ ]	IB	T1b	N0	M0	I B
[ ]	[ ]	IIA	T2a	N0	M0	II A
[ ]	[ ]	IIB	T2b	N0	M0	II B
[ ]	[ ]	IIIA	T3a	N0	M0	III A
[ ]	[ ]	IIIB	T1	N1	M0	III B
			T2	N1	M0	
			T3a	N1	M0	
			T3b	Any N	M0	
[ ]	[ ]	IVA	T4	Any N	M0	IV A
[ ]	[ ]	IVB	Any T	Any N	M1	IV B

* FIGO: *Federation Internationale de Gynecologie et d'Obstetrique*
** Note: *Presence of bullous edema is not sufficient evidence to classify a tumor T4.*

Staged by _____ M.D.
_____ Registrar
Date _____

(continued on next page)

Histopathologic Grade (G)

[ ] GX   Grade cannot be assessed
[ ] G1   Well differentiated
[ ] G2   Moderately differentiated
[ ] G3   Poorly differentiated
[ ] G4   Undifferentiated

Histopathologic Type

Cases should be classified as carcinoma of the cervix if the primary growth is in the cervix. All histologic types must be included. Grading is encouraged but is not a basis for modifying the stage groupings. When surgery is the primary treatment, the histologic findings permit the case to have pathologic staging. In this, the pTNM nomenclature is to be used.

The histopathologic types are:

Cervical intraepithelial neoplasia, grade III
Squamous cell carcinoma *in situ*
Squamous cell carcinoma
    Keratinizing
    Nonkeratinizing
    Verrucous
Adenocarcinoma *in situ*
Adenocarcinoma *in situ*, endocervical type
Endometroid adenocarcinoma
Clear cell adenocarcinoma
Adenosquamous carcinoma
Adenoid cystic carcinoma
Small cell carcinoma
Undifferentiated carcinoma

Illustrations

Indicate on diagrams primary tumor and regional nodes involved.

27

Corpus Uteri

C54.0 Isthmus uteri
C54.1 Endometrium
C54.2 Myometrium
C54.3 Fundus uteri
C54.8 Overlapping lesion
C54.9 Corpus uteri
C55.9 Uterus, NOS

ANATOMY

Primary Site. The corpus uteri refers to the upper two-thirds of the uterus above the level of the internal cervical os. The fallopian tubes enter at the upper lateral corners of this pear-shaped body. The portion lying above a line joining the tubo-uterine orifices is often referred to as the fundus.

Regional Lymph Nodes. The regional lymph nodes include:

Para-aortic
Parametrial
Presacral
Internal iliac
Paracervical
Obturator
Hypogastric
External iliac
Common iliac
Presacral
Sacral promontory (Gerota's)
Uterosacral

Metastatic Sites. The vagina and lung are the common metastatic sites.

RULES FOR CLASSIFICATION

The classification applies only to carcinoma. There should be histologic verification and grading of the tumor.

Clinical Staging. Careful clinical staging should be performed, preferably by an experienced examiner and with anesthesia, before any definitive therapy begins. The clinical staging must not be changed because of subsequent findings. When doubt exist about the stage to which a particular cancer should be allocated, the earlier stage is mandatory. The following examinations are permitted: palpation, inspection, colposcopy, endocervical curettage, hysteroscopy, cystoscopy, proctoscopy, intravenous urography, and imaging examination of lungs and skeleton. Optional examinations include lymphangiography, arteriography, venography, and laparoscopy. Sounding and determination of uterine cavity depth is an important step. Fractional curettage is essential, with separation of endometrial and endocervical curettings. Careful inspection and palpation of the vagina should be done to assess the entire length of the vaginal tube from the apex to the urethra.

Pathologic Staging. Hysterectomy with or without pelvic node dissection provides the basis for surgical-pathologic staging and should not be substituted for clinical staging.

Anatomic Subsites

Corpus uteri
Isthmus uteri

DEFINITION OF TNM

The definitions of the T categories correspond to the several stages accepted by FIGO. (FIGO stages are further subdivided by histologic grade of tumor.) Both systems are included for comparison.

Primary Tumor (T)

TNM	FIGO	DEFINITION
TX	—	Primary tumor cannot be assessed
T0	—	No evidence of primary tumor
Tis	—	Carcinoma in situ
T1	I	Tumor confined to the corpus uteri
T1a	IA	Tumor limited to the endometrium
T1b	IB	Tumor invades up to or less than one-half of the myometrium
T1c	IC	Tumor invades more than one-half of the myometrium
T2	II	Tumor invades the cervix but not extending beyond the uterus
T2a	IIA	Endocervical glandular involvement only
T2b	IIB	Cervical stromal invasion
T3 and/or N1	III	Local and/or regional spread as specified in T3a, b, N1 and FIGO IIIA, B, and C below
T3a	IIIA	Tumor involves the serosa and/or adnexa (direct extension or metastasis) and/or cancer cells in ascites or peritoneal washings
T3b	IIIB	Vaginal involvement (direct extension or metastasis)
N1	IIIC	Metastasis to the pelvic and/or para-aortic lymph nodes
T4*	IVA	Tumor invades the bladder mucosa or the rectum and/or the bowel mucosa
M1	IVB	Distant metastasis (*excluding* metastasis to the vagina, pelvic serosa, or adnexa; *including* metastasis to intra-abdominal lymph nodes other than paraaortic, and/or inguinal lymph nodes.)

* *Note:* The presence of bullous edema is not sufficient evidence to classify a tumor as T4.

Regional Lymph Nodes (N)

NX Regional lymph nodes cannot be assessed
N0 No regional lymph node metastasis
N1 Regional lymph node metastasis

Distant Metastasis (M)

TNM	FIGO	DEFINITION
MX	—	Presence of distant metastasis cannot be assessed
M0	—	No distant metastasis
M1	IVB	Distant metastasis

pTNM Pathologic Classification

The pT, pN, and pM categories correspond to the T, N, and M categories.

STAGE GROUPING

AJCC/UICC				FIGO
Stage 0	Tis	N0	M0	
Stage IA	T1a	N0	M0	Stage IA
Stage IB	T1b	N0	M0	Stage IB
Stage IC	T1c	N0	M0	Stage IC
Stage IIA	T2a	N0	M0	Stage IIA
Stage IIB	T2b	N0	M0	Stage IIB
Stage IIIA	T3a	N0	M0	Stage IIIA
Stage IIIB	T3b	N0	M0	Stage IIIB
Stage IIIC	T1	N1	M0	Stage IIIC
	T2	N1	M0	
	T3a	N1	M0	
	T3b	N1	M0	
Stage IVA	T4	Any N	M0	Stage IVA
Stage IVB	Any T	Any N	M1	Stage IVB

NOTES ABOUT STAGING

Studies of large series of cases of endometrial carcinoma limited to the corpus have shown that the prognosis is related to some extent to the size of the uterus. However, uterine enlargement may be caused by fibroids, adenomyosis, and other disorders. Therefore, the size of the uterus cannot serve as a basis for subgrouping Stage I cases. The length and the width of the uterine cavity are related to the prognosis. The great majority of cases of corpus cancer belong to Stage I. Extension of the carcinoma to the endocervix is confirmed by fractional curettage, hysterography, or hysteroscopy. Scraping the cervix should be the first step of the curettage; the specimens from the cervix should be examined separately. Occasionally, it may be difficult to decide whether the endocervix is involved by the cancer. In such cases, the simultaneous presence of normal cervical glands and cancer in the same section will give the final diagnosis.

Extension of the carcinoma outside the uterus should refer a case to Stage III or Stage IV.

The presence of metastases in the vagina or in the ovary permits allotment of a case to Stage III.

HISTOPATHOLOGIC TYPE

It is desirable that Stage I cases be subgrouped according to the degree of differentiation described on microscopic examination. The predominant lesion is adenocarcinoma, but all histologic types should be reported. However, choriocarcinomas, sarcomas, mixed mesodermal tumors, and carcinosarcomas should be presented separately.

The histopathologic types are:

Endometrioid carcinoma
  Adenocarcinoma
  Adenocanthoma (adenocarcinoma with squamous metaplasia)
  Adenosquamous carcinoma (mixed adenocarcinoma and squamous cell carcinoma)
Mucinous adenocarcinoma
Serous adenocarcinoma
Clear cell adenocarcinoma
Squamous cell adenocarcinoma
Undifferentiated adenocarcinoma

HISTOPATHOLOGIC GRADE (G)

GX   Grade cannot be assessed
G1   Well differentiated
G2   Moderately differentiated
G3-4 Poorly differentiated or undifferentiated

Note: For details of FIGO histologic grading of endometrial carcinoma, please see the following publications:

FIGO: Annual report on the results of treatment of gynecological cancer. Int J Gynecol Obstet 28:189–193, 1989

FIGO: Changes in gynecologic cancer staging by the International Federation of Gynecology and Obstetrics. Am J Obstet Gynecol 162: 610–611, 1990.

Data Form for Cancer Staging

Patient identification
Name _____
Address _____
Hospital or clinic number _____
Age _____ Sex _____ Race _____

Institution identification
Hospital or clinic _____
Address _____

Oncology Record

Anatomic site of cancer _____
Histologic type _____
Grade (G) _____
Date of classification _____

Chronology of classification
[ ] Clinical (use all data prior to first treatment)
[ ] Pathologic (if definitively resected specimen available)

DEFINITIONS

Primary Tumor (T)

Clin	Path	TNM category	FIGO* stage	
[ ]	[ ]	TX		Primary tumor cannot be assessed
[ ]	[ ]	T0		No evidence of primary tumor
[ ]	[ ]	Tis		Carcinoma in situ
[ ]	[ ]	T1	I	Tumor confined to corpus uteri
[ ]	[ ]	T1a	IA	Tumor limited to endometrium
[ ]	[ ]	T1b	IB	Tumor invades up to or less than one half of the myometrium
[ ]	[ ]	T1c	IC	Tumor invades to more than one half of the myometrium
[ ]	[ ]	T2	II	Tumor invades cervix but does not extend beyond uterus
[ ]	[ ]	T2a	IIA	Endocervical glandular involvement only
[ ]	[ ]	T2b	IIB	Cervical stromal invasion
[ ]	[ ]	T3 &/or N1	III	Local and/or regional spread as specified in T3a, b, N1 and FIGO IIIA, B and C below
[ ]	[ ]	T3a	IIIA	Tumor involves serosa and/or adnexae (direct extension or metastasis) and/or cancer cells in ascites or peritoneal washings
[ ]	[ ]	T3b	IIIB	Vaginal involvement (direct extension or metastasis)
[ ]	[ ]	N1	IIIC	Metastasis to the pelvic and/or paraaortic lymph nodes
[ ]	[ ]	T4**	IVA	Tumor invades bladder mucosa and/or bowel mucosa
[ ]	[ ]	M1	IVB	Distant metastasis. (Excluding metastasis to vagina, pelvic serosa or adnexae. Including metastasis to intraabdominal lymph nodes other than paraaortic, and/or inguinal lymph nodes.)

Lymph Node (N)

Clin	Path		
[ ]	[ ]	NX	Regional lymph nodes cannot be assessed
[ ]	[ ]	N0	No regional lymph node metastasis
[ ]	[ ]	N1	Regional lymph node metastasis

Distant Metastasis (M)

Clin	Path			
[ ]	[ ]	MX		Presence of distant metastasis cannot be assessed
[ ]	[ ]	M0		No distant metastasis
[ ]	[ ]	M1	IVB	Distant metastasis

Stage Grouping

Clin	Path	AJCC/UICC				FIGO
[ ]	[ ]	0	Tis	N0	M0	
[ ]	[ ]	IA	T1a	N0	M0	Stage IA
		IB	T1b	N0	M0	Stage IB
		IC	T1c	N0	M0	Stage IC
[ ]	[ ]	IIA	T2a	N0	M0	Stage IIA
		IIB	T2b	N0	M0	Stage IIB
[ ]	[ ]	IIIA	T3a	N0	M0	Stage IIIA
[ ]	[ ]	IIIB	T3b	N0	M0	Stage IIIB
[ ]	[ ]	IIIC	T1	N1	M0	Stage IIIC
			T2	N1	M0	
			T3a	N1	M0	
			T3b	N1	M0	
[ ]	[ ]	IVA	T4	Any N	M0	Stage IVA
[ ]	[ ]	IVB	Any T	Any N	M1	Stage IVB

Staged by _____ M.D.
_____ Registrar
Date _____

* FIGO: Federation Internationale de Gynecologie et d'Obstetrique

** Note: The presence of bullous edema is not sufficient evidence to classify a tumor T4.

(continued on next page)

Histopathologic Type

It is desirable that Stage I cases be subgrouped according to the degree of differentiation described on microscopic examination. The predominant lesion is adenocarcinoma, but all histologic types should be reported. However, choriocarcinomas, sarcomas, mixed mesodermal tumors, and carcinosarcomas should be presented separately.

The histopathologic types are:

Endometrioid carcinoma
    Adenocarcinoma
    Adenocanthoma (adenocarcinoma with squamous metaplasia)
    Adenosquamous carcinoma (mixed adenocarcinoma and squamous cell carcinoma)
Mucinous adenocarcinoma
Serous adenocarcinoma
Clear cell adenocarcinoma
Squamous cell adenocarcinoma
Undifferentiated adenocarcinoma

Histopathologic Grade (G)

[   ] GX   Grade cannot be assessed
[   ] G1   Well differentiated
[   ] G2   Moderately differentiated
[   ] G3-G4   Poorly differentiated or undifferentiated

Illustrations

Indicate on diagrams primary tumor and regional nodes involved.

28

Ovary

C56.9 Ovary

ANATOMY

Primary Site. Ovaries are a pair of solid, flattened ovoids 2 to 4 cm in diameter connected by a peritoneal fold to the broad ligament and by the infundibulopelvic ligament to the lateral wall of the pelvis.

Regional Lymph Nodes. The lymphatic drainage occurs by the utero-ovarian and round ligament trunks and an external iliac accessory route into the following regional nodes:

External iliac
Common iliac
Hypogastric
Internal iliac
Obturator
Lateral sacral
Aortic nodes
Inguinal nodes
Pelvic, NOS
Retroperitoneal, NOS

Metastatic Sites. The peritoneum, including the omentum and pelvic and abdominal viscera are common sites for seeding. Diaphragmatic involvement and liver metastases are common. Pulmonary and pleural involvement also occur. Liver capsule and peritoneal metastases are T3/Stage III.

RULES FOR CLASSIFICATION

There should be histologic confirmation of the disease to permit division of cases by histopathologic type. In accordance with FIGO,* a simplified version of the WHO** histologic typing (1973 publication No. 9) is recommended. The extent of differentiation (grade) should be recorded.

* FIGO: Federation Internationale de Gynecologie et d'Obstetrique
** World Health Organization

It is desirable to have a clinical stage grouping of ovarian tumors similar to those already existing for other malignant tumors in the female pelvis. Rarely is it possible to come to a final diagnosis by inspection or palpation or by any of the other methods recommended for clinical staging of carcinoma of the uterus and vagina. Therefore, the Cancer Committee of FIGO has recommended that clinical staging of primary carcinoma of the ovary be based on findings by laparoscopy or laparotomy, as well as on the usual clinical examination and roentgen studies.

Clinical Staging. Although clinical studies similar to those for other sites may be used, establishing a diagnosis most often requires a laparotomy, which is most widely accepted in clinical staging. Clinical studies include routine chest radiography. Computed tomography or other imaging studies may be helpful in both initial staging and follow-up of the tumors.

Pathologic Staging. This should include laparotomy and resection of ovarian masses, as well as hysterectomy. Biopsies of suspicious sites, such as the omentum, mesentery, liver, diaphragm, and pelvic and para-aortic nodes, are required.

DEFINITION OF TNM

The definitions of the T categories correspond to the several stages accepted by FIGO. Both systems are included for comparison.

Primary Tumor (T)

TNM	FIGO	DEFINITION
TX	—	Primary tumor cannot be assessed
T0	—	No evidence of primary tumor
T1	I	Tumor limited to ovaries (one or both)

TNM	FIGO	DEFINITION
T1a	IA	Tumor limited to one ovary; capsule intact, no tumor on ovarian surface, no malignant cells in ascites or peritoneal washings
T1b	IB	Tumor limited to both ovaries; capsules intact, no tumor on ovarian surface, no malignant cells in ascites or peritoneal washings
T1c	IC	Tumor limited to one or both ovaries with any of the following: capsule ruptured, tumor on ovarian surface, malignant cells in ascites or peritoneal washings
T2	II	Tumor involves one or both ovaries with pelvic extension
T2a	IIA	Extension and/or implants on the uterus and/or tube(s); no malignant cells in ascites or peritoneal washings
T2b	IIB	Extension to other pelvic tissues; no malignant cells in ascites or peritoneal washings
T2c	IIC	Pelvic extension (2a or 2b) with malignant cells in ascites or peritoneal washings
T3 and/or N1	III	Tumor involves one or both ovaries with microscopically confirmed peritoneal metastasis outside the pelvis and/or regional lymph node metastasis
T3a	IIIA	Microscopic peritoneal metastasis beyond the pelvis
T3b	IIIB	Macroscopic peritoneal metastasis beyond the pelvis 2 cm or less in the greatest dimension
T3c and/or N1	IIIC	Peritoneal metastasis beyond the pelvis more than 2 cm in the greatest dimension and/or regional lymph node metastasis
M1	IV	Distant metastasis (excludes peritoneal metastasis)

Note: Liver capsule and peritoneal metastases are T3/Stage III; liver parenchymal metastasis, M1/Stage IV. Pleural effusion must have positive cytology for M1/Stage IV.

Regional Lymph Nodes (N)

NX Regional lymph nodes cannot be assessed
N0 No regional lymph node metastasis
N1 Regional lymph node metastasis

Distant Metastasis (M)

TNM	FIGO	DEFINITION
MX	—	Presence of distant metastasis cannot be assessed
M0	—	No distant metastasis
M1	IV	Distant metastasis (excludes peritoneal metastasis)

Note: The presence of nonmalignant ascites is not classified. The presence of ascites does not affect staging unless malignant cells are present.

pTNM Pathologic Classification

The pT, pN, and pM categories correspond to the T, N, and M categories.

STAGE GROUPING

AJCC/UICC				FIGO
Stage IA	T1a	N0	M0	Stage IA
Stage IB	T1b	N0	M0	Stage IB
Stage IC	T1c	N0	M0	Stage IC
Stage IIA	T2a	N0	M0	Stage IIA
Stage IIB	T2b	N0	M0	Stage IIB
Stage IIC	T2c	N0	M0	Stage IIC
Stage IIIA	T3a	N0	M0	Stage IIIA
Stage IIIB	T3b	N0	M0	Stage IIIB
Stage IIIC	T3c	N0	M0	Stage IIIC
	Any T	N1	M0	
Stage IV	Any T	Any N	M1	Stage IV

HISTOPATHOLOGIC TYPE

The types currently recommended are serous tumors, mucinous tumors, endometrioid tumors, clear cell (mesonephroid) tumors, undifferentiated tumors, and unclassified tumors. Malignant tumors other than those of the common epithelial types are not to be included with the categories listed below. However, the more common ones—such as granulosa cell tumor, immature teratoma, dysgerminoma, and endodermal sinus tumor—may be collected and reported separately by institutions so desiring, particularly those with a pediatric population among their patients.

The histopathologic types are:

Serous cystomas
   Serous cystadenomas with proliferating activity of the epithelial cells and nuclear abnormalities, but with no infiltrative destructive growth (low potential or borderline malignancy)
   Serous cystadenocarcinomas
Mucinous cystomas
   Mucinous cystadenomas with proliferating activity of the epithelial cells and nuclear abnormalities, but with no infiltrative destructive growth (low potential or borderline malignancy)
   Mucinous cystadenocarcinomas

Endometrioid tumors (similar to adenocarcinomas in the endometrium)

    Endometrioid tumors with proliferating activity of the epithelial cells and nuclear abnormalities, but with no infiltrative destructive growth (low potential or borderline malignancy)

    Endometrioid adenocarcinomas

Clear cell (mesonephroid) tumors

    Clear cell tumors with proliferating activity of the epithelial cells and nuclear abnormalities, but with no infiltrative destructive growth (low potential or borderline malignancy)

    Clear cell cystadenocarcinomas

Unclassified tumors

In some cases of inoperable widespread malignant tumor, it may be impossible for the gynecologist and the pathologist to decide the origin of the growth. In order to evaluate the results obtained in the treatment of carcinoma of the ovary, however, it is necessary that all patients be reported on, including those thought to have a malignant ovarian tumor. If clinical examination cannot exclude the possibility that the lesion is a primary ovarian carcinoma, the case should be reported in the group "special category" and belong to the histologic group of unclassified tumors.

HISTOPATHOLOGIC GRADE (G)

GX   Grade cannot be assessed
GB   Borderline malignancy
G1   Well differentiated
G2   Moderately differentiated
G3-4 Poorly differentiated or undifferentiated

Data Form for Cancer Staging

Patient identification
Name _____
Address _____
Hospital or clinic number _____
Age _____ Sex _____ Race _____

Institution identification
Hospital or clinic _____
Address _____

Oncology Record

Anatomic site of cancer _____
Histologic type _____
Grade (G) _____
Date of classification _____

Chronology of classification
[   ]   Clinical (use all data prior to first treatment)
[   ]   Pathologic (if definitively resected specimen available)

DEFINITIONS

Primary Tumor (T)

Clin	Path	TNM category	FIGO* stage	
[ ]	[ ]	TX		Primary tumor cannot be assessed
[ ]	[ ]	T0		No evidence of primary tumor
[ ]	[ ]	T1	I	Tumor limited to ovaries (one or both)
[ ]	[ ]	T1a	IA	Tumor limited to one ovary; capsule intact, no tumor on ovarian surface. No malignant cells in ascites or peritoneal washings.
[ ]	[ ]	T1b	IB	Tumor limited to both ovaries; capsules intact, no tumor on ovarian surface. No malignant cells in ascites or peritoneal washings.
[ ]	[ ]	T1c	IC	Tumor limited to one or both ovaries with any of the following: capsule ruptured, tumor on ovarian surface, malignant cells in ascites, or peritoneal washings.
[ ]	[ ]	T2	II	Tumor involves one or both ovaries with pelvic extension
[ ]	[ ]	T2a	IIA	Extension and/or implants on uterus and/or tube(s). No malignant cells in ascites or peritoneal washings.
[ ]	[ ]	T2b	IIB	Extension to other pelvic tissues. No malignant cells in ascites or peritoneal washings.
[ ]	[ ]	T2c	IIC	Pelvic extension (2a or 2b) with malignant cells in ascites or peritoneal washings.
[ ]	[ ]	T3 &/or N1	III	Tumor involves one or both ovaries with microscopically confirmed peritoneal metastasis outside the pelvis and/or regional lymph node metastasis
[ ]	[ ]	T3a	IIIA	Microscopic peritoneal metastasis beyond pelvis
[ ]	[ ]	T3b	IIIB	Macroscopic peritoneal metastasis beyond pelvis 2 cm or less in greatest dimension
[ ]	[ ]	T3c &/or N1	IIIC	Peritoneal metastasis beyond pelvis more than 2 cm in greatest dimension and/or regional lymph node metastasis
[ ]	[ ]	M1	IV	Distant metastasis (excludes peritoneal metastasis)

Lymph Node (N)

Clin	Path	TNM category		
[ ]	[ ]	NX		Regional lymph nodes cannot be assessed
[ ]	[ ]	N0		No regional lymph node metastasis
[ ]	[ ]	N1		Regional lymph node metastasis

Distant Metastasis (M)

Clin	Path	TNM category	FIGO	
[ ]	[ ]	MX		Presence of distant metastasis cannot be assessed
[ ]	[ ]	M0		No distant metastasis
[ ]	[ ]	M1	IV	Distant metastasis (excludes peritoneal metastasis)

Stage Grouping

Clin	Path	AJCC/UICC				FIGO*
[ ]	[ ]	IA	T1a	N0	M0	Stage IA
[ ]	[ ]	IB	T1b	N0	M0	Stage IB
[ ]	[ ]	IC	T1c	N0	M0	Stage IC
[ ]	[ ]	IIA	T2a	N0	M0	Stage IIA
[ ]	[ ]	IIB	T2b	N0	M0	Stage IIB
[ ]	[ ]	IIC	T2c	N0	M0	Stage IIC
[ ]	[ ]	IIIA	T3a	N0	M0	Stage IIIA
[ ]	[ ]	IIIB	T3b	N0	M0	Stage IIIB
[ ]	[ ]	IIIC	T3c	N0	M0	Stage IIIC
			Any T	N1	M0	
[ ]	[ ]	IV	Any T	Any N	M1	Stage IV

Staged by _____ M.D.
_____ Registrar
Date _____

* FIGO: *Federation Internationale de Gynecologie et d'Obstetrique*
Note: *Liver capsule metastasis is T3/Stage III, liver parenchymal metastasis M1/Stage IV. Pleural effusion must have positive cytology for M1/Stage IV.*

(continued on next page)
American Joint Committee on Cancer—1992

Histopathologic Grade (G)

[ ] GX Grade cannot be assessed
[ ] GB Borderline malignancy
[ ] G1 Well differentiated
[ ] G2 Moderately differentiated
[ ] G3-G4 Poorly differentiated or undifferentiated

Histopathologic Type

The types currently recommended are serous tumors, mucinous tumors, endometrioid tumors, clear cell (mesonephroid) tumors, undifferentiated tumors, and unclassified tumors. Malignant tumors other than those of the common epithelial types are not to be included with the categories listed below. However, the more common ones—such as granulosa cell tumor, immature teratoma, dysgerminoma, and endodermal sinus tumor—may be collected and reported separately by institutions so desiring, particularly those with a pediatric population among their patients.

The histopathologic types are:

Serous cystomas
> Serous cystadenomas with proliferating activity of the epithelial cells and nuclear abnormalities, but with no infiltrative destructive growth (low potential or borderline malignancy)
> Serous cystadenocarcinomas

Mucinous cystomas
> Mucinous cystadenomas with proliferating activity of the epithelial cells and nuclear abnormalities, but with no infiltrative destructive growth (low potential or borderline malignancy)
> Mucinous cystadenocarcinomas

Endometrioid tumors (similar to adenocarcinomas in the endometrium)
> Endometrioid tumors with proliferating activity of the epithelial cells and nuclear abnormalities, but with no infiltrative destructive growth (low potential or borderline malignancy)
> Endometrioid adenocarcinomas

Clear cell (mesonephroid) tumors
> Clear cell tumors with proliferating activity of the epithelial cells and nuclear abnormalities, but with no infiltrative destructive growth (low potential or borderline malignancy)
> Clear cell cystadenocarcinomas

Unclassified tumors

In some cases of inoperable widespread malignant tumor, it may be impossible for the gynecologist and the pathologist to decide the origin of the growth. In order to evaluate the results obtained in the treatment of carcinoma of the ovary, however, it is necessary that all patients be reported on, including those thought to have a malignant ovarian tumor. If clinical examination cannot exclude the possibility that the lesion is a primary ovarian carcinoma, the case should be reported in the group "special category" and belong to the histologic group of unclassified tumors.

Illustrations

Indicate on diagrams primary tumor and regional nodes involved.

29

Vagina

C52.9 Vagina

ANATOMY

Primary Site. The vagina extends from the vulva upward to the uterine cervix.

Regional Lymph Nodes. They are:

Femoral (lower third only)
Inguinal (lower third only)
Common iliac
Internal iliac (hypogastric)
External iliac
Hypogastric
Pelvic, NOS (upper two-thirds only)

Metastatic Sites. The most common sites of distant spread include the lungs and skeleton.

RULES FOR CLASSIFICATION

The classification applies to primary carcinoma only.

A tumor that has extended to the portio and reached the external os should be classified as carcinoma of the cervix.

A tumor involving the vulva should be classified as carcinoma of the vulva.

There should be histologic confirmation of the disease. Any unconfirmed cases must be reported separately.

Clinical Staging. All data available prior to first definitive treatment should be used.

Pathologic Staging. In addition to data used for clinical staging, additional information available from examination of the resected specimen is to be used.

DEFINITION OF TNM

The definitions of the T categories correspond to the several stages accepted by FIGO. Both systems are included for comparison.

Primary Tumor (T)

TNM	FIGO	DEFINITION
TX	—	Primary tumor cannot be assessed
T0	—	No evidence of primary tumor
Tis	0	Carcinoma *in situ*
T1	I	Tumor confined to the vagina
T2	II	Tumor invades paravaginal tissues but not to the pelvic wall
T3	III	Tumor extends to the pelvic wall
T4*	IVA	Tumor invades the mucosa of the bladder or rectum and/or extends beyond the true pelvis
M1	IVB	Distant metastasis

*Note: The presence of bullous edema is not sufficient evidence to classify a tumor as T4. If the mucosa is not involved, the tumor is Stage III.

Regional Lymph Nodes (N)

NX   Regional lymph nodes cannot be assessed
N0   No regional lymph node metastasis

Upper Two-Thirds of the Vagina:

N1   Pelvic lymph node metastasis

Lower One-Third of the Vagina:

N1   Unilateral inguinal lymph node metastasis
N2   Bilateral inguinal lymph node metastasis

Distant Metastasis (M)

TNM	FIGO	DEFINITION
MX	—	Presence of distant metastasis cannot be assessed
M0	—	No distant metastasis
M1	IVB	Distant metastasis

pTNM Pathological Classification

The pT, pN, and pM categories correspond to the T, N, and M categories.

STAGE GROUPING

AJCC/UICC				FIGO
Stage 0	Tis	N0	M0	Stage 0
Stage I	T1	N0	M0	Stage I
Stage II	T2	N0	M0	Stage II
Stage III	T1	N1	M0	Stage III
	T2	N1	M0	
	T3	N0	M0	
	T3	N1	M0	
Stage IVA	T1	N2	M0	Stage IVA
	T2	N2	M0	
	T3	N2	M0	
	T4	Any N	M0	
Stage IVB	Any T	Any N	M1	Stage IVB

HISTOPATHOLOGIC TYPE

The squamous cell carcinoma is the most common type of cancer occurring in the vagina but infrequently an adenocarcinoma may occur in the upper one third.

HISTOPATHOLOGIC GRADE (G)

GX   Grade cannot be assessed
G1   Well differentiated
G2   Moderately differentiated
G3   Poorly differentiated
G4   Undifferentiated

Data Form for Cancer Staging

Patient identification
Name _____

Address _____

Hospital or clinic number _____

Age _____ Sex _____ Race _____

Institution identification
Hospital or clinic _____

Address _____

Oncology Record

Anatomic site of cancer _____

Histologic type _____

Grade (G) _____

Date of classification _____

Chronology of classification
[ ] Clinical (use all data prior to first treatment)
[ ] Pathologic (if definitively resected specimen available)

Clin	Path	TNM category	FIGO stage	DEFINITIONS

DEFINITIONS

Primary Tumor (T)

Clin	Path	TNM category	FIGO stage	
[ ]	[ ]	TX		Primary tumor cannot be assessed
[ ]	[ ]	T0		No evidence of primary tumor
[ ]	[ ]	Tis	0	Carcinoma in situ
[ ]	[ ]	T1	I	Tumor confined to vagina
[ ]	[ ]	T2	II	Tumor invades paravaginal tissues but not to pelvic wall
[ ]	[ ]	T3	III	Tumor extends to pelvic wall
[ ]	[ ]	T4*	IVA	Tumor invades mucosa of bladder or rectum and/or extends beyond the true pelvis
[ ]	[ ]	M1	IVB	Distant metastasis

Lymph Node (N)

Clin	Path	TNM	FIGO	
[ ]	[ ]	NX		Regional lymph nodes cannot be assessed
[ ]	[ ]	N0		No regional lymph node metastasis

Upper two-thirds of vagina:

Clin	Path	TNM		
[ ]	[ ]	N1		Pelvic lymph node metastasis

Lower one-third of vagina:

Clin	Path	TNM		
[ ]	[ ]	N1		Unilateral inguinal lymph node metastasis
[ ]	[ ]	N2		Bilateral inguinal lymph node metastasis

Distant Metastasis (M)

Clin	Path	TNM	FIGO	
[ ]	[ ]	MX		Presence of distant metastasis cannot be assessed
[ ]	[ ]	M0		No distant metastasis
[ ]	[ ]	M1	IVB	Distant metastasis

Stage Grouping

Clin	Path	AJCC/UICC				FIGO
[ ]	[ ]	0	Tis	N0	M0	Stage 0
[ ]	[ ]	I	T1	N0	M0	Stage I
[ ]	[ ]	II	T2	N0	M0	Stage II
[ ]	[ ]	III	T1	N1	M0	Stage III
			T2	N1	M0	
			T3	N0	M0	
			T3	N1	M0	
[ ]	[ ]	IVA	T1	N2	M0	Stage IVA
			T2	N2	M0	
			T3	N2	M0	
			T4	Any N	M0	
[ ]	[ ]	IVB	Any T	Any N	M1	Stage IVB

Staged by _____ M.D.

_____ Registrar

Date _____

* Note: The presence of bullous edema is not sufficient evidence to classify a tumor T4. If the mucosa is not involved the tumor is stage III.

(continued on next page)

American Joint Committee on Cancer—1992

Histopathologic Type

Squamous cell carcinoma
Adenocarcinoma infrequently
  Upper one third

Histopathologic Grade (G)

[ ] GX Grade cannot be assessed
[ ] G1 Well differentiated
[ ] G2 Moderately differentiated
[ ] G3 Poorly differentiated
[ ] G4 Undifferentiated

Illustrations

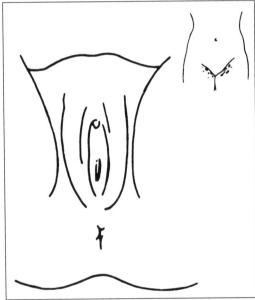

Indicate on diagrams primary tumor and regional nodes involved.

30

Vulva

C51.0 Labium majus
C51.1 Labium minus
C51.2 Clitoris
C51.8 Overlapping lesion
C51.9 Vulva, NOS

The staging classification for carcinomas of the vulva is taken directly from FIGO.

Cases should be classified as carcinoma of the vulva when the primary site of the growth is in the vulva. Tumors present in the vulva as secondary growths from either a genital or extragenital site should be excluded. Malignant melanoma should be reported separately.

ANATOMY

Primary Site. The vulva is the anatomic area immediately external to the vagina.

Regional Lymph Nodes. The femoral and inguinal nodes are the sites of regional spread.

Metastatic Sites. These include any site beyond the area of the regional lymph nodes. Internal iliac, external iliac, and hypogastric lymph nodes are now considered distant metastasis.

RULES FOR CLASSIFICATION

The classification applies only to primary carcinoma of the vulva. There should be histologic confirmation of the cancer. A carcinoma of the vulva that has extended to the vagina should be classified as carcinoma of the vulva. Malignant melanoma should be reported separately.

Clinical Staging. The rules for staging are similar to those for carcinoma of the cervix.

Pathologic Staging. The rules of staging are similar to those for carcinoma of the cervix.

DEFINITION OF TNM

TNM classification of carcinoma of the vulva is based on the FIGO classification.

Primary Tumor (T)

TX   Primary tumor cannot be assessed
T0   No evidence of primary tumor
Tis Carcinoma *in situ* (preinvasive carcinoma)
T1   Tumor confined to the vulva or to the vulva and perineum, 2 cm or less in greatest dimension
T2   Tumor confined to the vulva or to the vulva and perineum, more than 2 cm in greatest dimension
T3   Tumor invades any of the following: lower urethra, vagina, or anus
T4   Tumor invades any of the following: bladder mucosa, upper urethral mucosa, or rectal mucosa, or is fixed to the bone

Regional Lymph Nodes (N)

NX   Regional lymph nodes cannot be assessed
N0   No regional lymph node metastasis
N1   Unilateral regional lymph node metastasis
N2   Bilateral regional lymph node metastasis

Distant Metastasis (M)

MX   Presence of distant metastasis cannot be assessed
M0   No distant metastasis
M1   Distant metastasis (Pelvic lymph node metastasis is M1.)

STAGE GROUPING

(Correlation of the FIGO, UICC, and AJCC nomenclatures)

AJCC/UICC				FIGO
Stage 0	Tis	N0	M0	
Stage I	T1	N0	M0	Stage I
Stage II	T2	N0	M0	Stage II
Stage III	T1	N1	M0	Stage III
	T2	N1	M0	
	T3	N0	M0	
	T3	N1	M0	
Stage IVA	T1	N2	M0	Stage IVA
	T2	N2	M0	
	T3	N2	M0	
	T4	Any N	M0	
Stage IVB	Any T	Any N	M1	Stage IVB

HISTOPATHOLOGIC TYPE

Squamous cell carcinoma is the most common form of cancer of the vulva. Malignant melanoma should be reported separately.

The histopathologic types are:

Vulvar intraepithelial neoplasia, grade III
Squamous cell carcinoma *in situ*
Squamous cell carcinoma
Verrucous carcinoma
Paget's disease of the vulva
Adenocarcinoma, NOS
Basal cell carcinoma, NOS
Bartholin's gland carcinoma

HISTOPATHOLOGIC GRADE (G)

GX   Grade cannot be assessed
G1   Well differentiated
G2   Moderately differentiated
G3   Poorly differentiated
G4   Undifferentiated

Data Form for Cancer Staging

Patient identification
Name _____
Address _____
Hospital or clinic number _____
Age _____ Sex _____ Race _____

Institution identification
Hospital or clinic _____
Address _____

Oncology Record

Anatomic site of cancer _____
Histologic type _____
Grade (G) _____
Date of classification _____

Chronology of classification
[ ]   Clinical (use all data prior to first treatment)
[ ]   Pathologic (if definitively resected specimen available)

Clin	Path		
		DEFINITIONS	
		Primary Tumor (T)	
[ ]	[ ]	TX	Primary tumor cannot be assessed
[ ]	[ ]	T0	No evidence of primary tumor
[ ]	[ ]	Tis	Preinvasive carcinoma (carcinoma *in situ*)
[ ]	[ ]	T1	Tumor confined to the vulva or to the vulva and perineum, 2 cm or less in greatest dimension
[ ]	[ ]	T2	Tumor confined to the vulva or to the vulva and perineum, more than 2 cm in greatest dimension
[ ]	[ ]	T3	Tumor involves any of the following: lower urethra, vagina, or anus
[ ]	[ ]	T4	Tumor invades any of the following: bladder mucosa, upper part of urethral mucosa, rectal mucosa or tumor fixed to the bone

Lymph Node (N)

Regional lymph nodes are the femoral and inguinal nodes

Clin	Path		
[ ]	[ ]	NX	Regional lymph nodes cannot be assessed
[ ]	[ ]	N0	No regional lymph node metastasis
[ ]	[ ]	N1	Unilateral regional lymph node metastasis
[ ]	[ ]	N2	Bilateral regional lymph node metastasis

Distant Metastasis (M)

Clin	Path		
[ ]	[ ]	MX	Presence of distant metastasis cannot be assessed
[ ]	[ ]	M0	No distant metastasis
[ ]	[ ]	M1	Distant metastasis (Pelvic lymph node metastasis is M1)

Stage Grouping

Clin	Path	AJCC/UICC				Figo
[ ]	[ ]	0	Tis	N0	M0	
[ ]	[ ]	I	T1	N0	M0	I
[ ]	[ ]	II	T2	N0	M0	II
[ ]	[ ]	III	T1	N1	M0	III
			T2	N1	M0	
			T3	N0	M0	
			T3	N1	M0	
[ ]	[ ]	IVA	T1	N2	M0	IVA
			T2	N2	M0	
			T3	N2	M0	
			T4	Any N	M0	
[ ]	[ ]	IVB	Any T	Any N	M1	IVB

Staged by _____ **M.D.**
_____**Registrar**
Date _____

(continued on next page)

Histopathologic Grade (G)

[ ] GX   Grade cannot be assessed
[ ] G1   Well differentiated
[ ] G2   Moderately differentiated
[ ] G3   Poorly differentiated
[ ] G4   Undifferentiated

Histopathologic Type

Squamous cell carcinoma is the most frequent form of cancer of the vulva. Malignant melanoma should be reported separately.

The histopathologic types are:

Vulvar intraepithelial neoplasia, grade III
Squamous cell carcinoma *in situ*
Squamous cell carcinoma
Verrucous carcinoma
Paget's disease of the vulva
Adenocarcinoma, NOS
Basal cell carcinoma, NOS
Bartholin's gland carcinoma

Illustrations

Indicate on diagrams primary tumor and regional nodes involved.

GENITOURINARY CANCERS

31

Prostate

C61.9 Prostate gland

Prostatic cancer is the most common cancer in men, with increasing incidence in older age groups. Carcinomas of the prostate are responsive to sex hormones and presumably, therefore, have many analogies with breast cancer. They are stimulated by androgens and inhibited by estrogens. Prostatic cancer has a tendency to metastasize to bone. Early detection may now be possible with a blood test, (prostate specific antigen, PSA) and transrectal ultrasound. This TNM classification for carcinomas of the prostate is new.

ANATOMY

Primary Site. Adenocarcinomas of the prostate usually arise within the peripheral zone and are less commonly seen in the benign hyperplastic enlargement that occurs around the prostatic urethra in older men. Pathologically, cancers of the prostate are often multifocal in origin. They usually start in the peripheral posterior portion of the gland and therefore are amenable to early detection by rectal examination or by transrectal ultrasound.

There is agreement that the incidence of both clinical and latent carcinoma increases with age. However, this cancer is rarely diagnosed in men under 40 years of age. The size or extent of a localized prostatic tumor may be estimated by digital examination or by various imaging techniques, such as ultrasound. Diagnosis of clinically suspicious areas of the prostate is histologically confirmed by needle biopsy.

The grade of the prostatic cancer is also important for prognosis. The histopathologic grading of these tumors can be complex because of the morphologic heterogeneity so often encountered in surgical specimens. Either a histologic or a pattern type of grading method can be used.

Regional Lymph Nodes. The regional lymph nodes are the nodes of the true pelvis, which essentially are the pelvic nodes below the bifurcation of the common iliac arteries. They include the following groups:

Pelvic, NOS
Hypogastric
Obturator
Iliac (internal, external, NOS)
Periprostatic
Sacral (lateral, presacral, promontory [Gerota's], or NOS)

Distant Lymph Nodes. Distant lymph nodes lie outside the confines of the true pelvis. They can be imaged using ultrasound, computed tomography, magnetic resonance imaging, or lymphangiography.

Aortic (para-aortic, lumbar)
Common iliac
Inguinal, deep
Superficial inguinal (femoral)
Supraclavicular
Cervical
Scalene
Retroperitoneal, NOS

The significance of regional lymph node metastasis, pN, in staging prostate cancer lies in the number of nodes involved with tumor and the size of the metastatic foci present within the lymph nodes.

Metastatic Sites. Metastasis to bone is common with primary carcinomas of the prostate. In addition, tumor frequently spreads to distant lymph nodes. Lung metastases are uncommon and may be lymphangitic in pattern of spread. Liver metastases are usually seen late in the course of the disease.

RULES FOR CLASSIFICATION

The TNM classification serves both clinical and pathological staging.

Clinical Staging. Primary tumor assessment includes digital rectal examination of the prostate and histologic or cytologic confirmation of prostatic carcinoma. Clinical examination, acid phosphatase determination, PSA serum level, and imaging techniques (including transrectal ultrasound) are suggested. All information available prior to first definitive treatment may be used for clinical staging.

Pathologic Staging. Histologic examination of the resected specimen is required. Total prostatoseminalvesiculectomy and pelvic lymph node dissection are required for pathologic staging. In some cases, a pT classification may be possible without prostatoseminalvesiculectomy—for example, a positive biopsy from the rectum. Tumor found in one or both lobes by needle biopsy, but not palpable or visible by imaging, is classified as T1c. Laterality does not affect the N classification.

DEFINITION OF TNM

Primary Tumor (T)

TX   Primary tumor cannot be assessed
T0   No evidence of primary tumor
T1   Clinically inapparent tumor not palpable or visible by imaging
     T1a   Tumor incidental histologic finding in 5% or less of tissue resected
     T1b   Tumor incidental histologic finding in more than 5% of tissue resected
     T1c   Tumor identified by needle biopsy (e.g., because of elevated PSA)
T2   Tumor confined within the prostate*
     T2a   Tumor involves half of a lobe or less
     T2b   Tumor involves more than half of a lobe, but not both lobes
     T2c   Tumor involves both lobes
T3   Tumor extends through the prostatic capsule**
     T3a   Unilateral extracapsular extension
     T3b   Bilateral extracapsular extension
     T3c   Tumor invades the seminal vesicle(s)
T4   Tumor is fixed or invades adjacent structures other than the seminal vesicles
     T4a   Tumor invades any of: bladder neck, external sphincter, or rectum
     T4b   Tumor invades levator muscles and/or is fixed to the pelvic wall

*Note: Tumor found in one or both lobes by needle biopsy, but not palpable or visible by imaging, is classified as T1c.

**Note: Invasion into the prostatic apex or into (but not beyond) the prostatic capsule is not classified as T3, but as T2.

Regional Lymph Nodes (N)

NX   Regional lymph nodes cannot be assessed
N0   No regional lymph node metastasis
N1   Metastasis in a single lymph node, 2 cm or less in greatest dimension
N2   Metastasis in a single lymph node, more than 2 cm but not more than 5 cm in greatest dimension; or multiple lymph node metastases, none more than 5 cm in greatest dimension
N3   Metastasis in a lymph node more than 5 cm in greatest dimension

Distant Metastasis* (M)

MX   Presence of distant metastasis cannot be assessed
M0   No distant metastasis
M1   Distant metastasis
     M1a   Nonregional lymph node(s)
     M1b   Bone(s)
     M1c   Other site(s)

*Note: When more than one site of metastasis is present, the most advanced category (pM1c) is used.

STAGE GROUPING

Stage	T	N	M	G
Stage 0	T1a	N0	M0	G1
Stage I	T1a	N0	M0	G2, 3-4
	T1b	N0	M0	Any G
	T1c	N0	M0	Any G
	T1	N0	M0	Any G
Stage II	T2	N0	M0	Any G
Stage III	T3	N0	M0	Any G
Stage IV	T4	N0	M0	Any G
	Any T	N1	M0	Any G
	Any T	N2	M0	Any G
	Any T	N3	M0	Any G
	Any T	Any N	M1	Any G

HISTOPATHOLOGIC TYPE

This classification applies to adenocarcinoma, but not to sarcoma or transitional cell carcinoma of the prostate.

HISTOPATHOLOGIC GRADE (G)

GX   Grade cannot be assessed
G1   Well differentiated (slight anaplasia)
G2   Moderately differentiated (moderate anaplasia)
G3-4   Poorly differentiated or undifferentiated (marked anaplasia)

BIBLIOGRAPHY

1. Babaian RJ, Camps JL, Frangos DN, et al: Monoclonal prostate-specific antigen in untreated prostate cancer: Relationship to clinical stage and grade. Cancer 67:2200–2206, 1991
2. Drago JR, Badalament RA, Nesbitt JA, et al: Localized staging of prostate carcinoma: Comparison of transrectal ultrasound and magnetic resonance imaging. Urology 35:511–512, 1990
3. Epstein JI, Steinberg GD: The significance of low-grade prostate cancer on needle biopsy: A radical prostatectomy study of tumor grade, volume, and stage of the biopsied and multifocal tumor. Cancer 66:1927–1932, 1990
4. Flocks RH, Culp DA, Porto R: Lymphatic spread from prostatic cancer. J Urol 81:194–196, 1959
5. Greskovich FJ 3d, Johnson DE, Tenney DM, et al: Prostate specific antigen in patients with clinical stage C prostate cancer: Relation to lymph node status and grade. J Urol 145:798–801, 1991
6. Hernandez AD, Smith JA Jr: Transrectal ultrasonography for the early detection and staging of prostate cancer. Urol Clin North Am 17:745–757, 1990
7. Huben RP, Murphy GP: Prostate cancer: An update. CA—Cancer J Clin 36:274–292, 1986
8. McDowell GC 2d, Johnson JW, Tenney DM, et al: Pelvic lymphadenectomy for staging clinically localized prostate cancer: Indications, complications, and results in 217 cases. Urology 35:476–482, 1990
9. McNeal JE, Villers AA, Redwine EA, et al: Histologic differentiation, cancer volume, and pelvic lymph node metastasis in adenocarcinoma of the prostate. Cancer 66:1225–1233, 1990.
10. Optenberg SA, Thompson IM: Economics of screening for carcinoma of the prostate. Urol Clin N Amer 17(4):719–737, 1990
11. Partin AW, Carter HB, Chan DW, et al: Prostate specific antigen in the staging of localized prostate cancer: Influence of tumor differentiation, tumor volume, and benign hyperplasia. J Urol 143:747–752, 1990
12. Rifkin MD, Zerhouni EA, Gatsonis CA, et al: Comparison of magnetic resonance imaging and ultrasonography in staging early prostate cancer: Results of a multi-institutional cooperative trial. N Engl J Med 323:621–626, 1990
13. Schnall MD, Imai Y, Tomaszewski J, et al: Prostate cancer: Local staging with endorectal surface coil MR imaging. Radiology 178:797–802, 1991
14. Spirnak JP, Resnick M: Clinical staging of prostatic cancer: New modalities. Urol Clin N Am 11:221–235, 1984
15. Wheeler TM: Anatomic considerations in carcinoma of the prostate. Urol Clin N Amer 16(4):623–634, 1989
16. Winkler HZ, Rainwater LM, Myers RP, et al: Stage D1 prostatic adenocarcinoma: Significance of nuclear DNA ploidy patterns studied by flow cytometry. Mayo Clin Proc, 63:103–112, 1988

Data Form for Cancer Staging

Patient identification
Name _____
Address _____
Hospital or clinic number _____
Age _____ Sex _____ Race _____

Institution identification
Hospital or clinic _____
Address _____

Oncology Record

Anatomic site of cancer _____
Histologic type _____
Grade (G) _____
Date of classification _____

Chronology of classification
[ ] Clinical (use all data prior to first treatment)
[ ] Pathologic (if definitively resected specimen available)

DEFINITIONS

Primary Tumor (T)

Clin	Path		
[ ]	[ ]	TX	Primary tumor cannot be assessed
[ ]	[ ]	T0	No evidence of primary tumor
[ ]	[ ]	T1	Clinically inapparent tumor not palpable or visible by imaging
[ ]	[ ]	T1a	Tumor incidental histologic finding in 5% or less of tissue resected
[ ]	[ ]	T1b	Tumor incidental histologic finding in more than 5% of tissue resected
[ ]	[ ]	T1c	Tumor identified by needle biopsy (e.g. because of elevated PSA)
[ ]	[ ]	T2	Palpable tumor confined within prostate*
[ ]	[ ]	T2a	Tumor involves half of a lobe or less
[ ]	[ ]	T2b	Tumor involves more than half of a lobe, but not both lobes
[ ]	[ ]	T2c	Tumor involves both lobes
[ ]	[ ]	T3	Tumor extends through the prostatic capsule**
[ ]	[ ]	T3a	Unilateral extracapsular extension
[ ]	[ ]	T3b	Bilateral extracapsular extension
[ ]	[ ]	T3c	Tumor invades seminal vesicle(s)
[ ]	[ ]	T4	Tumor is fixed or invades adjacent structures other than seminal vesicles
[ ]	[ ]	T4a	Tumor invades external sphincter and/or bladder neck and/or rectum
[ ]	[ ]	T4b	Tumor invades levator muscles and/or is fixed to pelvic wall

Lymph Node (N)

Clin	Path		
[ ]	[ ]	NX	Regional lymph nodes cannot be assessed
[ ]	[ ]	N0	No regional lymph node metastasis
[ ]	[ ]	N1	Metastasis in a single lymph node, 2 cm or less in greatest dimension
[ ]	[ ]	N2	Metastasis in a single lymph node, more than 2 cm but not more than 5 cm in greatest dimension, or multiple lymph nodes, none more than 5 cm in greatest dimension
[ ]	[ ]	N3	Metastasis in a lymph node more than 5 cm in greatest dimension

Distant Metastasis (M)***

Clin	Path		
[ ]	[ ]	MX	Presence of distant metastasis cannot be assessed
[ ]	[ ]	M0	No distant metastasis
[ ]	[ ]	M1	Distant metastasis
[ ]	[ ]	M1a	Non-regional lymph nodes
[ ]	[ ]	M1b	Bone
[ ]	[ ]	M1c	Other sites

* *Note:* Tumor found in one or both lobes by needle biopsy, but not palpable or visible by imaging, is classified as T1c.

** *Note:* Invasion into the prostatic apex or into (but not beyond) the prostatic capsule is not classified as T3, but as T2.

*** *Note:* When more than one site of metastasis is present, the most advanced category (pM1c) is used.

(continued on next page)

Clin	Path	Stage Grouping				
[ ]	[ ]	0	T1a	N0	M0	G1
[ ]	[ ]	I	T1a	N0	M0	G2
			T1a	N0	M0	G3-4
			T1b	N0	M0	Any G
			T1c	N0	M0	Any G
			T1	N0	M0	Any G
[ ]	[ ]	II	T2	N0	M0	Any G
[ ]	[ ]	III	T3	N0	M0	Any G
[ ]	[ ]	IV	T4	N0	M0	Any G
			Any T	N1	M0	Any G
			Any T	N2	M0	Any G
			Any T	N3	M0	Any G
			Any T	Any N	M1	Any G

Staged by _____ M.D.

_____ Registrar

Date _____

Histopathologic Grade (G)

[ ] GX   Grade cannot be assessed

[ ] G1   Well differentiated (slight anaplasia)

[ ] G2   Moderately well differentiated (moderate anaplasia)

[ ] G3-4   Poorly differentiated or undifferentiated (marked anaplasia)

Histopathologic Type

Almost always adenocarcinoma of variable grades.

Illustrations

This diagram is for use with the prostate diagram. Sketch in extent of tumor.

Indicate on diagram primary tumor and regional nodes involved.

32

Testis

C62.0 Undescended testis
C62.1 Descended testis
C62.9 Testis, NOS

Cancers of the testis are usually found in young adults. Fortunately, they are relatively rare, accounting for less than 1% of all malignancies in males. Cryptorchidism is a predisposing condition. There are two main histologic types: seminomas, which are most common, and teratomas. Most cases of testicular cancer, even when far advanced, can be successfully treated. Circulating tumor markers are found in the serum of patients with cancer of the testis, which enables the clinician to document the course of the disease. These markers are invaluable for the management of testicular malignancies. Staging is based on the extent of disease.

ANATOMY

Primary Site. The testes are composed of convoluted seminiferous tubules with a stroma containing functional endocrine interstitial cells. Both are encased in a dense barrier capsule, the tunica albuginea, with fibrous septa extending into and separating the testes into lobules. The tubules converge and exit at the mediastinum of the testis into the rete testis and efferent ducts, which join a single duct. This duct—the epididymis—coils outside the upper and lower pole of the testicle, then joins the vas deferens, a muscular conduit that accompanies the vessels and lymphatic channels of the spermatic cord. The major route for local extension of cancer is through the lymphatic channels. The tumor emerges from the mediastinum of the testis and courses through the spermatic cord. Occasionally, the epididymis is invaded early, and then the external iliac nodes may become involved. If there has been previous scrotal or inguinal surgery with invasion of the scrotal wall (though this is rare), then the lymphatic spread may be to inguinal nodes.

Regional Lymph Nodes. The regional lymph nodes are:

Aortic
Paraaortic
External iliac
Paracaval
Intrapelvic
Inguinal (after scrotal or inguinal surgery)

Spread of the tumor into contralateral regional or first station nodes of the area occurs in 20% of cases. When there has been previous inguinal or scrotal surgery, inguinal nodes are also considered regional nodes. All nodes outside the regional nodes are distant. As defined, bulky disease has important prognostic significance.

The significance of regional lymph node metastasis in staging testicular cancer lies in the number and size and not in whether metastasis is unilateral or contralateral.

Metastatic Sites. Distant spread of testicular tumors occurs most commonly to the nodes, followed by metastasis to the lung, liver, viscera, and bones. As defined, bulk of disease has important prognostic significance. Serum markers (alphafetoprotein [AFP]) and the beta-subunit of human chorionic gonadotropin (βHCG) should be obtained prior to initial orchiectomy to establish whether the tumor marker is predictive. Markers are helpful in the management of patients with disseminated disease. Stage can be further subdivided by the presence or absence of markers.

RULES FOR CLASSIFICATION

Clinical Staging. Clinical examination and radical orchiectomy are required for clinical staging.

Pathologic Staging. Histologic evaluation of the radical orchiectomy specimen must be used for the pT classification. The specimens from a defined node-bearing area (e.g., retroperitoneal periaortic node dissection) must be used for the pN classification. Histologic verification is required. Laterality does not affect the N classification.

DEFINITION OF TNM

Primary Tumor (T)

The extent of primary tumor is classified after radical orchiectomy.

pTX Primary tumor cannot be assessed (If no radical orchiectomy has been performed, TX is used.)
pT0 No evidence of primary tumor (e.g., histologic scar in testis)
pTis Intratubular tumor: preinvasive cancer
pT1 Tumor limited to the testis, including the rete testis
pT2 Tumor invades beyond the tunica albuginea or into the epididymis
pT3 Tumor invades the spermatic cord
pT4 Tumor invades the scrotum

Regional Lymph Nodes (N)

NX Regional lymph nodes cannot be assessed
N0 No regional lymph node metastasis
N1 Metastasis in a single lymph node, 2 cm or less in greatest dimension
N2 Metastasis in a single lymph node, more than 2 cm but not more than 5 cm in greatest dimension; or multiple lymph nodes, none more than 5 cm in greatest dimension
N3 Metastasis in a lymph node more than 5 cm in greatest dimension

Distant Metastasis (M)

MX Presence of distant metastasis cannot be assessed
M0 No distant metastasis
M1 Distant metastasis

STAGE GROUPING

Stage 0	pTis	N0	M0
Stage I	Any pT	N0	M0
Stage II	Any pT	N1	M0
	Any pT	N2	M0
	Any pT	N3	M0
Stage III	Any pT	Any N	M1

HISTOPATHOLOGIC TYPE

Cell types can be divided into seminomatous and nonseminomatous tumors. The latter can be further divided into teratoma, embryonal carcinoma, yolk sac tumor, and choriocarcinoma. Mixtures of these types should be noted. Lymphomas are excluded. Combinations of embryonal carcinoma and teratoma can be designated as teratocarcinoma.

BIBLIOGRAPHY

1. Hoskin P, Dilly S, Easton D, et al: Prognostic factors in stage I nonseminomatous germ-cell testicular tumors managed by orchiectomy and surveillance: Implications for adjuvanchemotherapy. J Clin Oncol 4:1031–1036, 1986
2. Javadpour N, Canning DA, O'Connell KJ, et al: Predictors of recurrent clinical stage I nonseminomatous testicular cancer: A prospective clinicopathological study. Urology 276:508–511, 1986
3. Mostofi FK, et al: Histological typing of testis tumors. WHO International Classification of Tumors. Geneva, WHO, 1977
4. Pike MC, Chilvers C, Peckham MJ: Effect of age at orchidopexy on risk of testicular cancer. Lancet 1:1246–1248, 1986
5. Rowland RG, Weisman D, Williams SD, et al: Accuracy of preoperative staging in stages A and B nonseminomatous germ cell testis tumors. J Urol 127:718–720, 1982
6. Williams SD, Einhorn LH: Clinical stage I testis tumors: The medical oncologist's view. Cancer Treat Rep 66:15–18, 1981

Data Form for Cancer Staging

Patient identification
Name _____
Address _____
Hospital or clinic number _____
Age _____ Sex _____ Race _____

Institution identification
Hospital or clinic _____
Address _____

Oncology Record

Anatomic site of cancer _____
Histologic type _____
Grade (G) _____
Date of classification _____

Chronology of classification
[ ] Clinical (use all data prior to first treatment)
[ ] Pathologic (if definitively resected specimen available)

DEFINITIONS

Clin	Path		

Primary Tumor (T)

Clin	Path		
[ ]	[ ]	pTX	Primary tumor cannot be assessed. (If no radical orchiectomy has been performed, TX is used)
[ ]	[ ]	pT0	No evidence of primary tumor (*e.g.* histologic scar in testis)
[ ]	[ ]	pTis	Intratubular tumor: preinvasive cancer
[ ]	[ ]	pT1	Tumor limited to testis, including rete testis
[ ]	[ ]	pT2	Tumor invades beyond tunica albuginea or into epididymis
[ ]	[ ]	pT3	Tumor invades spermatic cord
[ ]	[ ]	pT4	Tumor invades scrotum

Lymph Node (N)

Clin	Path		
[ ]	[ ]	NX	Regional lymph nodes cannot be assessed
[ ]	[ ]	N0	No regional lymph node metastasis
[ ]	[ ]	N1	Metastasis in a single lymph node, 2 cm or less in greatest dimension
[ ]	[ ]	N2	Metastasis in a single lymph node, more than 2 cm but not more than 5 cm in greatest dimension, or multiple lymph nodes, none more than 5 cm in greatest dimension
[ ]	[ ]	N3	Metastasis in a lymph node more than 5 cm in greatest dimension

Distant Metastasis (M)

Clin	Path		
[ ]	[ ]	MX	Presence of distant metastasis cannot be assessed
[ ]	[ ]	M0	No distant metastasis
[ ]	[ ]	M1	Distant metastasis

Stage Grouping

Clin	Path				
[ ]	[ ]	0	pTis	N0	M0
[ ]	[ ]	I	Any pT	N0	M0
[ ]	[ ]	II	Any pT	N1	M0
			Any pT	N2	M0
			Any pT	N3	M0
[ ]	[ ]	III	Any pT	Any N	M1

Staged by _____ M.D.
_____ Registrar
Date _____

Histopathologic Type

Cell types can be divided into seminomatous and nonseminomatous tumors. The latter can be further divided into teratoma, embryonal carcinoma, yolk sac tumor, and choriocarcinoma. Mixtures of these types should be noted. Lymphomas are excluded. Combinations of embryonal carcinoma and teratoma can be designated as teratocarcinoma.

Illustrations

Indicate on diagram primary tumor and regional nodes involved.

33

Penis

C60.0 Prepuce
C60.1 Glans penis
C60.2 Body of penis
C60.8 Overlapping lesion
C60.9 Penis, NOS

Cancers of the penis are rare in the United States, and incidence varies in different countries of the world. Most are squamous cell carcinomas arising in the skin or on the glans penis. Prognosis is favorable, provided the lymph nodes are not involved. Melanomas can also occur. The staging classification, however, applies to carcinomas. (Melanomas are staged in Chapter 24.) Some cancers of the penis may be described as verrucous. These are included under this classification. An *in situ* lesion is also included and by definition should be coded as an *in situ* carcinoma of the penis.

ANATOMY

Primary Site. The penis is composed of three cylindrical masses of cavernous tissue bound by fibrous tissue. Two masses are lateral, known as the corpora cavernosa penis. The corpus spongiosum penis, a median mass, contains the greater part of the urethra. The penis is attached to the front and the sides of the pubic arch. The skin covering the penis is thin and loosely connected with the deeper parts of the organ. This skin at the root of the penis is continuous with that over the scrotum and perineum. Distally, the skin folds upon itself to form the prepuce or foreskin. Circumcision has been associated with decreased incidence of cancer of the penis.

Regional Lymph Nodes. The regional lymph nodes are:

Single superficial inguinal (femoral)
Multiple or bilateral superficial inguinal (femoral)
Deep inguinal: Rosenmuller's or Cloquet's node
External iliac
Internal iliac (hypogastric)
Pelvic nodes, NOS

Metastatic Sites. Lung, liver, or bone are most often involved.

RULES FOR CLASSIFICATION

Clinical Staging. Clinical examination, endoscopy (where possible), and histologic confirmation are required. Imaging techniques are indicated for metastatic disease detection.

Pathologic Staging. Complete resection of the primary site with appropriate margins is required. Where regional lymph node involvement is suspected, these should be included.

DEFINITION OF TNM

Primary Tumor (T)

TX   Primary tumor cannot be assessed
T0   No evidence of primary tumor
Tis Carcinoma *in situ*
Ta   Noninvasive verrucous carcinoma
T1   Tumor invades subepithelial connective tissue
T2   Tumor invades the corpus spongiosum or cavernosum
T3   Tumor invades the urethra or prostate
T4   Tumor invades other adjacent structures

Regional Lymph Nodes (N)

NX   Regional lymph nodes cannot be assessed
N0   No regional lymph node metastasis
N1   Metastasis in a single superficial inguinal lymph node

N2   Metastasis in multiple or bilateral superficial inguinal lymph nodes
N3   Metastasis in deep inguinal or pelvic lymph node(s), unilateral or bilateral

Distant Metastasis (M)

MX   Presence of distant metastasis cannot be assessed
M0   No distant metastasis
M1   Distant metastasis

STAGE GROUPING

Stage	T	N	M
Stage 0	Tis	N0	M0
	Ta	N0	M0
Stage I	T1	N0	M0
Stage II	T1	N1	M0
	T2	N0	M0
	T2	N1	M0
Stage III	T1	N2	M0
	T2	N2	M0
	T3	N0	M0
	T3	N1	M0
	T3	N2	M0
Stage IV	T4	Any N	M0
	Any T	N3	M0
	Any T	Any N	M1

HISTOPATHOLOGIC TYPE

Cell types are limited to carcinomas.

HISTOPATHOLOGIC GRADE (G)

GX   Grade cannot be assessed
G1   Well differentiated
G2   Moderately differentiated
G3-4 Poorly differentiated or Undifferentiated

BIBLIOGRAPHY

1. Bassett JW: Carcinoma of the penis. Cancer 5:530–538, 1952
2. Colon JE: Carcinoma of the penis. J Urol 67:702–708, 1952
3. Hanash KA, Furlow WL, Utz DC, et al: Carcinoma of the penis: A clinicopathologic study. J Urol 104:291–297, 1970
4. McDougal WS, Kirchner FK Jr, Edwards RH, et al: Treatment of carcinoma of the penis: The case for primary lymphadenectomy. J Urol 136:38–41, 1986

Data Form for Cancer Staging

Patient identification
Name _____
Address _____
Hospital or clinic number _____
Age _____ Sex _____ Race _____

Institution identification
Hospital or clinic _____
Address _____

Oncology Record

Anatomic site of cancer _____
Histologic type _____
Grade (G) _____
Date of classification _____

Chronology of classification
[ ] Clinical (use all data prior to first treatment)
[ ] Pathologic (if definitively resected specimen available)

Clin	Path	
		DEFINITIONS

DEFINITIONS

Primary Tumor (T)

Clin	Path		
[ ]	[ ]	TX	Primary tumor cannot be assessed
[ ]	[ ]	T0	No evidence of primary tumor
[ ]	[ ]	Tis	Carcinoma *in situ*
[ ]	[ ]	Ta	Noninvasive verrucous carcinoma
[ ]	[ ]	T1	Tumor invades subepithelial connective tissue
[ ]	[ ]	T2	Tumor invades corpus spongiosum or cavernosum
[ ]	[ ]	T3	Tumor invades urethra or prostate
[ ]	[ ]	T4	Tumor invades other adjacent structures

Lymph Node (N)

Clin	Path		
[ ]	[ ]	NX	Regional lymph nodes cannot be assessed
[ ]	[ ]	N0	No regional lymph node metastasis
[ ]	[ ]	N1	Metastasis in a single, superficial inguinal lymph node
[ ]	[ ]	N2	Metastasis in multiple or bilateral superficial inguinal lymph nodes
[ ]	[ ]	N3	Metastasis in deep inguinal or pelvic lymph node(s), unilateral or bilateral

Distant Metastasis

Clin	Path		
[ ]	[ ]	MX	Presence of distant metastasis cannot be assessed
[ ]	[ ]	M0	No distant metastasis
[ ]	[ ]	M1	Distant metastasis

Histopathologic Grade (G)

[ ] GX Grade cannot be assessed
[ ] G1 Well differentiated
[ ] G2 Moderately differentiated
[ ] G3-4 Poorly differentiated or undifferentiated

Histopathologic Type

Cell types are limited to carcinomas.

Stage Grouping

Clin	Path				
[ ]	[ ]	0	Tis	N0	M0
			Ta	N0	M0
[ ]	[ ]	I	T1	N0	M0
[ ]	[ ]	II	T1	N1	M0
			T2	N0	M0
			T2	N1	M0
[ ]	[ ]	III	T1	N2	M0
			T2	N2	M0
			T3	N0	M0
			T3	N1	M0
			T3	N2	M0
[ ]	[ ]	IV	T4	Any N	M0
			Any T	N3	M0
			Any T	Any N	M1

Staged by _____ M.D.
_____ Registrar
Date _____

American Joint Committee on Cancer—1992

34

Urinary Bladder

C67.0 Trigone
C67.1 Dome
C67.2 Lateral wall
C67.3 Anterior wall
C67.4 Posterior wall
C67.5 Bladder neck
C67.6 Ureteric orifice
C67.7 Urachus
C67.8 Overlapping lesion
C67.9 Bladder, NOS

Bladder cancer can present as a low grade papillary lesion, as an indolent *in situ* lesion, which can occupy large areas of the mucosal surface, or as an infiltrative cancer that rapidly extends through the bladder wall. The papillary and *in situ* lesions may be associated with a malignant course, with sudden invasion of the bladder wall. Predisposing factors include exposure to certain chemicals used in the dye industry, and smoking. Bladder cancer is more common in men. Hematuria is the most common presenting sign.

ANATOMY

Primary Site. The urinary bladder consists of three layers: the epithelium and the subepithelial connective tissue, the muscularis, and the perivesical fat (peritoneum covering the superior surface and upper part). In the male, the bladder adjoins the rectum and seminal vesicle posteriorly, the prostate inferiorly, and the pubis and peritoneum anteriorly. In the female, the vagina is located posteriorly and the uterus superiorly. The bladder is located extraperitoneally.

Regional Lymph Nodes. The regional lymph nodes are the nodes of the true pelvis, which essentially are the pelvic nodes below the bifurcation of the common iliac arteries.

The significance of regional lymph node metastasis in staging bladder cancer lies in the number and size and not in whether metastasis is unilateral or contralateral.

Regional nodes include:

Hypogastric
Obturator
Iliac (internal, external, NOS)
Perivesical
Pelvic, NOS
Sacral (lateral, sacral promontory [Gerota's])
Presacral

The common iliac nodes are considered sites of distant metastasis and should be coded as M1.

Metastatic Sites. Distant spread to lymph nodes, lung, bone, and liver is most common.

RULES FOR CLASSIFICATION

Clinical Staging. Primary tumor assessment includes bimanual examination under anesthesia before and after endoscopic surgery (biopsy or transurethral resection) or histologic verification of the presence or absence of tumor when indicated. Add "m" for multiple tumors. Add "is" to any T to indicate associated carcinoma *in situ*. Appropriate imaging techniques for lymph node evaluation should be used. When indicated, evaluation for distant metastases includes imaging of the chest, biochemical studies, and isotopic studies to detect common metastatic sites. Computed tomography or other modalities may subsequently be used to supply information concerning minimal requirements for staging. The primary tumor may be superficial or invasive and can be partially or totally resected with sufficient tissue from the tumor base for evaluation of full depth of tumor invasion. Visually adjacent cystoscopically normal mucosa should be considered for biopsy; urinary cytology and pyelography are important.

Pathologic Staging. Microscopic examination and confirmation of extent is required. Total cystectomy and lymph node dissection generally are required for this staging. Laterality does not affect the N classification.

DEFINITION OF TNM

Primary Tumor (T)

TX   Primary tumor cannot be assessed
T0   No evidence of primary tumor
Ta   Noninvasive papillary carcinoma
Tis Carcinoma *in situ*: "flat tumor"
T1   Tumor invades subepithelial connective tissue
T2   Tumor invades superficial muscle (inner half)
T3   Tumor invades deep muscle or perivesical fat
　　　T3a Tumor invades deep muscle (outer half)
　　　T3b Tumor invades perivesical fat
　　　　　　i.   microscopically
　　　　　　ii. macroscopically (extravesical mass)
T4   Tumor invades any of the following: prostate, uterus, vagina, pelvic wall, or abdominal wall
　　　T4a Tumor invades the prostate, uterus, or vagina
　　　T4b Tumor invades the pelvic wall or abdominal wall

Regional Lymph Nodes (N)

Regional lymph nodes are those within the true pelvis; all others are distant nodes.

NX   Regional lymph nodes cannot be assessed
N0   No regional lymph node metastasis
N1   Metastasis in a single lymph node, 2 cm or less in greatest dimension
N2   Metastasis in a single lymph node, more than 2 cm but not more than 5 cm in greatest dimension; or multiple lymph nodes, none more than 5 cm in greatest dimension
N3   Metastasis in a lymph node more than 5 cm in greatest dimension

Distant Metastasis (M)

MX   Presence of distant metastasis cannot be assessed
M0   No distant metastasis
M1   Distant metastasis

STAGE GROUPING

Stage 0a	Ta	N0	M0
Stage 0is	Tis	N0	M0
Stage I	T1	N0	M0
Stage II	T2	N0	M0
	T3a	N0	M0
Stage III	T3b	N0	M0
	T4a	N0	M0
Stage IV	T4b	N0	M0
	Any T	N1	M0
	Any T	N2	M0
	Any T	N3	M0
	Any T	Any N	M1

HISTOPATHOLOGIC TYPE

The histologic types are:

Transitional cell carcinoma (urothelial)
　　In situ
　　　　Papillary
　　　　Flat
　　With squamous metaplasia
　　With glandular metaplasia
　　With squamous and glandular metaplasia
Squamous cell carcinoma
Adenocarcinoma
Undifferentiated carcinoma

The predominant cancer is a transitional cell carcinoma.

HISTOPATHOLOGIC GRADE (G)

GX   Grade cannot be assessed
G1   Well differentiated
G2   Moderately differentiated
G3-4 Poorly differentiated or undifferentiated

BIBLIOGRAPHY

1. deVere White RW, Olsson CA, Deitch AD: Flow cytometry: Role in monitoring transitional cell carcinoma of bladder. Urology 28:15–20, 1986
2. Jewett HJ, Strong GH: Infiltrating carcinoma of the bladder: Relation of depth of penetration of the bladder wall to incidence of local extension and metastasis. J Urol 55:366–372, 1946
3. Kern WH: The grade and pathologic stage of bladder cancer. Cancer 53:1185–1189, 1984

4. Mostofi FK: Pathological aspects and spread of carcinoma of bladder. JAMA 206:1764–1769, 1968

5. Mostofi FK, et al: Histological typing of urinary bladder tumors. WHO International Histological Classification of Tumors. Geneva, WHO, 1973.

6. Smith JA Jr, Whitmore WF Jr: Regional lymph node metastasis from bladder cancer. J Urol 126:591–593, 1981

7. Whitmore WF Jr: Management of bladder cancer. Curr Probl Cancer 4:3–48, 1979

8. Lipponen PK, Eskelinen MJ, Jauthiainen K, et al. Independent clinical, histological and quantitative prognostic factors in transitional-cell bladder tumours, with special reference to mitotic frequency. Int J Cancer 51(3):396–403, 1992

9. Takashi M, Sakata T, Murase T, et al. Grade 3 bladder cancer with lamina propria invasion (pT1): characteristics of tumor and clinical course. Nagoya J Med Sci 53 (1-4);1–8, 1991

10. Mulder AH, Van Hootegem JC, Sylvester R, et al. Prognostic factors in bladder carcinoma: histologic parameters and expression of a cell cycle-related nuclear antigen (Ki-67). J Pathol 166:37–43, 1992

Data Form for Cancer Staging

Patient identification
Name _____
Address _____
Hospital or clinic number _____
Age _____ Sex _____ Race _____

Institution identification
Hospital or clinic _____
Address _____

Oncology Record

Anatomic site of cancer _____
Histologic type _____
Grade (G) _____
Date of classification _____

Chronology of classification
[ ]   Clinical (use all data prior to first treatment)
[ ]   Pathologic (if definitively resected specimen available)

DEFINITIONS

Primary Tumor (T)

Clin	Path		
[ ]	[ ]	TX	Primary tumor cannot be assessed
[ ]	[ ]	T0	No evidence of primary tumor
[ ]	[ ]	Ta	Non invasive papillary carcinoma
[ ]	[ ]	Tis	Carcinoma *in situ:* "flat tumor"
[ ]	[ ]	T1	Tumor invades subepithelial connective tissue
[ ]	[ ]	T2	Tumor invades superficial muscle (inner half)
[ ]	[ ]	T3	Tumor invades deep muscle or perivesical fat
		T3a	Tumor invades deep muscle (outer half)
[ ]	[ ]	T3b	Tumor invades perivesical fat
			i. microscopically
			ii. macroscopically (extravesical mass)
[ ]	[ ]	T4	Tumor invades prostate, uterus, vagina, pelvic wall or abdominal wall
[ ]	[ ]	T4a	Tumor invades prostate, uterus, vagina
[ ]	[ ]	T4b	Tumor invades pelvic wall or abdominal wall

Lymph Node (N)

Clin	Path		
[ ]	[ ]	NX	Regional lymph nodes cannot be assessed
[ ]	[ ]	N0	No regional lymph node metastasis
[ ]	[ ]	N1	Metastasis in a single lymph node, 2 cm or less in greatest dimension
[ ]	[ ]	N2	Metastasis in a single lymph node, more than 2 cm but not more than 5 cm in greatest dimension, or multiple lymph nodes, none more than 5 cm in greatest dimension
[ ]	[ ]	N3	Metastasis in a lymph node more than 5 cm in greatest dimension

Distant Metastasis (M)

Clin	Path		
[ ]	[ ]	MX	Presence of distant metastasis cannot be assessed
[ ]	[ ]	M0	No distant metastasis
[ ]	[ ]	M1	Distant metastasis

Stage Grouping

Clin	Path				
[ ]	[ ]	0a	Ta	N0	M0
[ ]	[ ]	0is	Tis	N0	M0
[ ]	[ ]	I	T1	N0	M0
[ ]	[ ]	II	T2	N0	M0
			T3a	N0	M0
[ ]	[ ]	III	T3b	N0	M0
			T4a	N0	M0
[ ]	[ ]	IV	T4b	N0	M0
			Any T	N1	M0
			Any T	N2	M0
			Any T	N3	M0
			Any T	Any N	M1

Staged by _____ M.D.
_____ Registrar
Date _____

(continued on next page)

American Joint Committee on Cancer—1992

Histopathologic Grade (G)

[ ] GX   Grade cannot be assessed
[ ] G1   Well differentiated
[ ] G2   Moderately differentiated
[ ] G3-4 Poorly differentiated or undifferentiated

Histopathologic Type

The histologic types are:

Transitional cell carcinoma (urothelial)
   In situ
      Papillary
      Flat
   With squamous metaplasia
   With glandular metaplasia
   With squamous and glandular metaplasia
Squamous cell carcinoma
Adenocarcinoma
Undifferentiated carcinoma

The predominant cancer is a transitional cell cancer.

Illustrations

Male

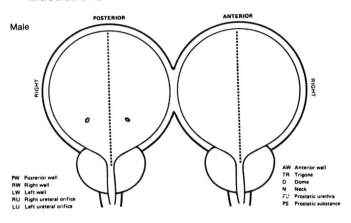

PW Posterior wall
RW Right wall
LW Left wall
RU Right ureteral orifice
LU Left ureteral orifice

AW Anterior wall
TR Trigone
D Dome
N Neck
PU Prostatic urethra
PS Prostatic substance

Female

PW Posterior wall
RW Right wall
LW Left wall
RU Right ureteral orifice
LU Left ureteral orifice

AW Anterior wall
TR Trigone
D Dome
N Neck
U Urethra

Indicate on diagrams primary tumor and regional nodes involved.

35

Kidney

C64.9 Kidney, NOS

Cancers of the kidney are relatively rare, accounting for less than 3% of all malignancies. Nearly all malignant tumors are carcinomas arising from the renal tubular epithelium or, less frequently, from the renal pelvis (see chapter 36). These tumors are more common in males. Pain and hematuria are the common presenting features. Renal carcinomas may be associated with erythrocytosis, secondary to release of erythropoietin from the tumor cells. These carcinomas have a tendency to extend along the renal vein and even into the vena cava. Rarely, they also may regress spontaneously. Staging depends on the size of the primary tumor, invasion of the adjacent structures, and vascular extension.

ANATOMY

Primary Site. Encased by a fibrous capsule and surrounded by perirenal fat, the kidney consists of the cortex (glomeruli, convoluted tubules) and the medulla (Henle's loops, pyramids of converging tubules). Each papilla opens into the minor calices; these in turn unite in the major calices and drain into the renal pelvis. At the hilus are the pelvis, ureter, and renal artery and vein. Gerota's fascia overlies the psoas and quadrants lumborum.

Regional Lymph Nodes. The regional lymph nodes include:

Renal hilar
Paracaval
Aortic (para-aortic, periaortic, lateral aortic)
Retroperitoneal, NOS

Metastatic Sites. Common metastatic sites include bone, liver, lung, brain, and distant nodes.

RULES FOR CLASSIFICATION

The classification applies only to the renal-cell carcinomas. Adenoma is excluded. There should be histologic confirmation of the disease. Refer to Histopathologic Type.

Clinical Staging. Clinical examination, urography, and appropriate imaging techniques are required for assessment of the primary tumor and its extensions, both local and distant. Evaluation for distant metastases should be done by laboratory biochemical studies, chest x-rays, and isotopic studies. Clinical staging may also include laparotomy and biopsy of distant sites.

Pathologic Staging. Histologic examination and confirmation of extent is required. Resection of the primary tumor, kidney, Gerota's fascia, perinephric fat, renal vein, and appropriate lymph nodes is required. Laterality does not affect the N classification.

DEFINITION OF TNM

Primary Tumor (T)

TX Primary tumor cannot be assessed
T0 No evidence of primary tumor
T1 Tumor 2.5 cm or less in greatest dimension limited to the kidney
T2 Tumor more than 2.5 cm in greatest dimension limited to the kidney
T3 Tumor extends into major veins or invades the adrenal gland or perinephric tissues but not beyond Gerota's fascia
    T3a Tumor invades the adrenal gland or perinephric tissues but not beyond Gerota's fascia
    T3b Tumor grossly extends into the renal vein(s) or vena cava below the diaphragm
    T3c Tumor grossly extends into the vena cava above the diaphragm
T4 Tumor invades beyond Gerota's fascia

Regional Lymph Nodes (N)*

NX Regional lymph nodes cannot be assessed
N0 No regional lymph node metastasis

N1   Metastasis in a single lymph node, 2 cm or less in greatest dimension

N2   Metastasis in a single lymph node, more than 2 cm but not more than 5 cm in greatest dimension; or multiple lymph nodes, none more than 5 cm in greatest dimension

N3   Metastasis in a lymph node more than 5 cm in greatest dimension

* *Note:* Laterality does not affect the N classification.

Distant Metastasis (M)

MX   Presence of distant metastasis cannot be assessed
M0   No distant metastasis
M1   Distant metastasis

STAGE GROUPING

Stage I	T1	N0	M0
Stage II	T2	N0	M0
Stage III	T1	N1	M0
	T2	N1	M0
	T3a	N0	M0
	T3a	N1	M0
	T3b	N0	M0
	T3b	N1	M0
	T3c	N0	M0
	T3c	N1	M0
Stage IV	T4	Any N	M0
	Any T	N2	M0
	Any T	N3	M0
	Any T	Any N	M1

HISTOPATHOLOGIC TYPE

The histopathologic types are:

Renal cell carcinoma
Adenocarcinoma
Renal papillary adenocarcinoma
Tubular carcinoma
Granular cell carcinoma
Clear cell carcinoma (hypernephroma)

The predominant cancer is adenocarcinoma; subtypes are clear-cell and granular-cell carcinoma. A grad-

ing system as provided below is recommended when feasible. The staging system does not apply to sarcomas of the kidney; a separate classification is published for nephroblastomas.

HISTOPATHOLOGIC GRADE (G)

GX   Grade cannot be assessed
G1   Well differentiated
G2   Moderately differentiated
G3-4 Poorly differentiated of undifferentiated

BIBLIOGRAPHY

1. Angervall L, Carlstrom E, Wahlquist L, et al: Effects of clinical and morphological variables on spread of renal carcinoma in an operative series. Scand J Urol Nephrol 3:134–140, 1969
2. Bennington JL, Beckwith JB: Tumors of the kidney, renal pelvis, and ureter. Atlas of Tumor Pathology, Second Series, Fascicle 12. Washington DC, Armed Forces Institute of Pathology, 1975
3. Holland JM: Cancer of the kidney—Natural history and staging. Cancer 32:1030–1042, 1973
4. Hermanek P and Schrott KM: Evaluation of the new tumor, nodes, and metastases classification of renal cell carcinoma. J of Urology 144:238–242, 1990.
5. Hulten L, Rosencrantz M, Seeman T, et al: Occurrence and localization of lymph node metastases in renal carcinoma: Lymphographic and histopathologic investigation in connection with nephrectomy. Scand J Urol Nephrol 3:129–133, 1966
6. Katz SA, Davis JE: Renal adenocarcinoma: Prognostics and treatment reflected by survival. Urology 10:10–11, 1977
7. McDonald JR, Priestley JT: Malignant tumors of the kidney: Surgical and prognostic significance of tumor thrombosis of the renal vein. Surg Gynecol Obstet 77:295, 1983
8. Mostofi FK, et al: Histological typing of kidney tumors. WHO International Histological Classification of Tumors. Geneva, WHO, 1981
9. Ramchandani P, Soulen RL, Schnall RI, et al: Impact of magnetic resonance on staging of renal carcinoma. Urology 27:564–568, 1986
10. Weyman PJ, McClennan BL, Stanley RJ, et al: Comparison of computer tomography and angiography in the evaluation of renal carcinoma. Radiology 137:417–424, 1980

Data Form for Cancer Staging

Patient identification
Name _____
Address _____
Hospital or clinic number _____
Age _____ Sex _____ Race _____

Institution identification
Hospital or clinic _____
Address _____

Oncology Record

Anatomic site of cancer _____
Histologic type _____
Grade (G) _____
Date of classification _____

Chronology of classification
[ ] Clinical (use all data prior to first treatment)
[ ] Pathologic (if definitively resected specimen available)

Clin	Path		
		DEFINITIONS	
		Primary Tumor (T)	
[ ]	[ ]	TX	Primary tumor cannot be assessed
[ ]	[ ]	T0	No evidence of primary tumor
[ ]	[ ]	T1	Tumor 2.5 cm or less in greatest dimension limited to the kidney
[ ]	[ ]	T2	Tumor more than 2.5 cm in greatest dimension limited to the kidney
[ ]	[ ]	T3	Tumor extends into major veins or invades adrenal gland or perinephric tissues but not beyond Gerota's fascia
[ ]	[ ]	T3a	Tumor invades adrenal gland or perinephric tissues but not beyond Gerota's fascia
[ ]	[ ]	T3b	Tumor grossly extends into renal vein(s) or vena cava below diaphragm
[ ]	[ ]	T3c	Tumor grossly extends into vena cava above diaphragm
[ ]	[ ]	T4	Tumor invades beyond Gerota's fascia
		Lymph Node (N)	
[ ]	[ ]	NX	Regional lymph nodes cannot be assessed
[ ]	[ ]	N0	No regional lymph node metastasis
[ ]	[ ]	N1	Metastasis in a single lymph node, 2 cm or less in greatest dimension
[ ]	[ ]	N2	Metastasis in a single lymph node, more than 2 cm but not more than 5 cm in greatest dimension, or multiple lymph nodes, none more than 5 cm in greatest dimension
[ ]	[ ]	N3	Metastasis in a lymph node more than 5 cm in greatest dimension
		Distant Metastasis (M)	
[ ]	[ ]	MX	Presence of distant metastasis cannot be assessed
[ ]	[ ]	M0	No distant metastasis
[ ]	[ ]	M1	Distant metastasis

Clin	Path				
		Stage Grouping			
[ ]	[ ]	I	T1	N0	M0
[ ]	[ ]	II	T2	N0	M0
[ ]	[ ]	III	T1	N1	M0
			T2	N1	M0
			T3a	N0	M0
			T3a	N1	M0
			T3b	N0	M0
			T3b	N1	M0
			T3c	N0	M0
			T3c	N1	M0
[ ]	[ ]	IV	T4	Any N	M0
			Any T	N2	M0
			Any T	N3	M0
			Any T	Any N	M1

Staged by _____ M.D.
_____ Registrar
Date _____

(continued on next page)

Histopathologic Grade (G)

[ ] GX Grade cannot be assessed
[ ] G1 Well differentiated
[ ] G2 Moderately differentiated
[ ] G3-4 Poorly differentiated or undifferentiated

Histopathologic Type

The histopathologic types are:

Renal cell carcinoma
Adenocarcinoma
Renal papillary adenocarcinoma
Tubular carcinoma
Granular cell carcinoma
Clear cell carcinoma—Hypernephroma

The predominant cancer is adenocarcinoma; subtypes are clear-cell and granular-cell carcinoma. A grading system is recommended when feasible. The staging system does not apply to sarcomas of the kidney. A separate classification is published for nephroblastomas.

Illustrations

This drawing is to be used with the checklist. Sketch in the urographic, angiographic, ultrasound, or CT extent of tumor.

This drawing is to be used with the checklist and the upper drawing. Sketch in the pathologic extent of tumor.

36

Renal Pelvis and Ureter

C65.9 Renal pelvis
C66.9 Ureter

Tumors of the renal pelvis and ureter are not common. Tumors of the renal pelvis comprise only 5% to 10% of all renal cancers. Most cases are found in adults. Commonly, malignant tumors in the renal pelvis or ureter are multiple and associated with cancers located in other parts of the urinary tract. For instance, carcinomas of the ureter are often associated with tumors in the urinary bladder. Most tumors are transitional cell carcinomas, although other types can occur. Tumors in the renal pelvis may be associated with calculi. Staging depends on the extent of disease. T3 differs between the renal pelvis and the ureter, but all other definitions are the same.

ANATOMY

Primary Site. The renal pelvis and ureter form a single unit that cephalad is continuous with the collecting ducts of the renal pyrimides and comprises the minor and major calyces, which are continuous with the renal pelvis. The ureteropelvic junction is variable in position and location, but serves as a "landmark" that separates the renal pelvis and the ureter, which continues caudad and traverses the wall of the urinary bladder as the intramural ureter opening on the trigone of the bladder at the ureteral orifice. The renal pelvis and ureter are composed of the following layers: epithelium, subepithelial connective tissue, and muscularis, which is continuous with a connective tissue adventitial layer. It is in this outer layer that the major blood supply and lymphatics are found.

The intrarenal portion of the renal pelvis is surrounded by renal parenchyma; the extrarenal pelvis, by perihilar fat. The ureter courses through the retroperitoneum adjacent to the parietal peritoneum and rests on the retroperitoneal musculature above the pelvic vessels. As it crosses the vessels and enters the deep pelvis, the ureter is surrounded by pelvic fat until it traverses the bladder wall.

Regional Lymph Nodes. The regional lymph nodes include:

Renal pelvis:
Renal hilar
Paracaval
Aortic
Retroperitoneal, NOS

Ureter:
Renal hilar
Iliac (common, internal hypogastric, external)
Paracaval
Periureteral
Pelvic, NOS

The significance of regional lymph node metastasis in staging renal cancer lies in the number and size and not in whether metastasis is unilateral or contralateral.

Metastatic Sites. Distant spread to lung, bone, and liver is most common.

RULES FOR CLASSIFICATION

Clinical Staging. Primary tumor assessment includes radiographic imaging, endoscopic evaluation, and ureteroscopy when applicable. Material in cytoscopic study should be obtained. The possible concurrent presence of bladder tumors is not a prognostic factor in this staging system. These tumors should be staged separately. Evaluation of distant metastatic sites includes radiographic, radioisotopic, and appropriate blood studies.

Pathologic Staging. Histologic confirmation of extent of disease is required. Resection of primary tumor, kidney, ureter, appropriate regional lymph nodes, and bladder cuff is usually required. Special circumstances may limit the magnitude of resection, but, at a minimum, the tumor with appropriate margins and regional lymph nodes must be available for pathologic evaluation. Laterality does not affect N classification.

DEFINITION OF TNM

Primary Tumor (T)

TX   Primary tumor cannot be assessed
T0   No evidence of primary tumor
Ta   Papillary noninvasive carcinoma
Tis Carcinoma *in situ*
T1   Tumor invades subepithelial connective tissue
T2   Tumor invades the muscularis
T3   (For renal pelvis only) Tumor invades beyond the muscularis into peripelvic fat or the renal parenchyma
T3   (For ureter only) Tumor invades beyond the muscularis into periureteric fat
T4   Tumor invades adjacent organs, or through the kidney into the perinephric fat.

Regional Lymph Nodes (N)*

NX   Regional lymph nodes cannot be assessed
N0   No regional lymph node metastasis
N1   Metastasis in a single lymph node, 2 cm or less in greatest dimension
N2   Metastasis in a single lymph node, more than 2 cm but not more than 5 cm in greatest dimension; or multiple lymph nodes, none more than 5 cm in greatest dimension
N3   Metastasis in a lymph node more than 5 cm in greatest dimension

* *Note:* Laterality does not affect N classification.

Distant Metastasis (M)

MX   Presence of distant metastasis cannot be assessed
M0   No distant metastasis
M1   Distant metastasis

HISTOPATHOLOGIC TYPE

The histologic types are:

Transitional cell carcinoma
Papillary carcinoma
Squamous cell carcinoma
Epidermoid carcinoma
Adenocarcinoma
Urothelial carcinoma

HISTOPATHOLOGIC GRADE

GX   Grade cannot be assessed
G1   Well differentiated
G2   Moderately differentiated
G3-4 Poorly differentiated or undifferentiated

BIBLIOGRAPHY

1. Batata MA, Whitmore WF, Hilaris BS, et al: Primary carcinoma of the ureter: A prognostic study. Cancer 35:1626–1632, 1975
2. Bloom NA, Vidone RA, Lytton B: Primary carcinoma of the ureter. A report of 102 new cases. J Urol 103:590–598, 1970
3. Claymen RV, Williams RD, Fraley EE: The pursuit of the renal mass. N Engl J Med 300:72–74, 1979
4. Johansson S, Angervall L, Bengtsson U, et al: A clinico-pathologic and prognostic study of epithelial tumors of the renal pelvis. Cancer 37:1376–1383, 1976
5. Wagle DG, Moore RH, Murphy GP: Primary carcinoma of the renal pelvis. Cancer 33:1642–1648, 1974
6. Kidney Cancer, Results in Treating Cancer. Report No. 12, CIER Committee, American Cancer Society, Illinois Division, 1989
7. Huben RP, Mounzer AM, Murphy GP: Tumor grade and stage as prognostic variables in upper tract urothelial tumors. Cancer 62:2016–2020, 1988

STAGE GROUPING

Stage	T	N	M
Stage 0a	Ta	N0	M0
Stage 0is	Tis	N0	M0
Stage I	T1	N0	M0
Stage II	T2	N0	M0
Stage III	T3	N0	M0
Stage IV	T4	N0	M0
	Any T	N1	M0
	Any T	N2	M0
	Any T	N3	M0
	Any T	Any N	M1

Data Form for Cancer Staging

Patient identification
Name _____
Address _____
Hospital or clinic number _____
Age _____ Sex _____ Race _____

Institution identification
Hospital or clinic _____
Address _____

Oncology Record

Anatomic site of cancer _____
Histologic type _____
Grade (G) _____
Date of classification _____

Chronology of classification
[ ]   Clinical (use all data prior to first treatment)
[ ]   Pathologic (if definitively resected specimen available)

Clin	Path		
[ ]	[ ]	TX	Primary tumor cannot be assessed
[ ]	[ ]	T0	No evidence of primary tumor
[ ]	[ ]	Ta	Papillary noninvasive carcinoma
[ ]	[ ]	Tis	Carcinoma *in situ*
[ ]	[ ]	T1	Tumor invades subepithelial connective tissue
[ ]	[ ]	T2	Tumor invades muscularis
[ ]	[ ]	T3	Tumor invades beyond muscularis into peripelvic fat or renal parenchyma (For renal pelvis only)
[ ]	[ ]	T3	Tumor invades beyond muscularis into periureteric fat (For ureter only)
[ ]	[ ]	T4	Tumor invades adjacent organs or through the kidney into perinephric fat

DEFINITIONS
Primary Tumor (T)

Lymph Node (N)

Clin	Path		
[ ]	[ ]	NX	Regional lymph nodes cannot be assessed
[ ]	[ ]	N0	No regional lymph node metastasis
[ ]	[ ]	N1	Metastasis in a single lymph node, 2 cm or less in greatest dimension
[ ]	[ ]	N2	Metastasis in a single lymph node, more than 2 cm but not more than 5 cm in greatest dimension, or multiple lymph nodes, none more than 5 cm in greatest dimension
[ ]	[ ]	N3	Metastasis in a lymph node more than 5 cm in greatest dimension

Distant Metastasis (M)

Clin	Path		
[ ]	[ ]	MX	Presence of distant metastasis cannot be assessed
[ ]	[ ]	M0	No distant metastasis
[ ]	[ ]	M1	Distant metastasis

Stage Grouping

Clin	Path				
[ ]	[ ]	0a	Ta	N0	M0
[ ]	[ ]	0is	Tis	N0	M0
[ ]	[ ]	I	T1	N0	M0
[ ]	[ ]	II	T2	N0	M0
[ ]	[ ]	III	T3	N0	M0
[ ]	[ ]	IV	T4	N0	M0
			Any T	N1	M0
			Any T	N2	M0
			Any T	N3	M0
			Any T	Any N	M1

Histopathologic Grade (G)
[ ]   GX   Grade cannot be assessed
[ ]   G1   Well differentiated
[ ]   G2   Moderately differentiated
[ ]   G3-4 Poorly differentiated or undifferentiated

Histopathologic Type
The histopathologic types are:

Transitional cell carcinoma
Papillary carcinoma
Squamous cell carcinoma
Epidermoid carcinoma
Adenocarcinoma
Urothelial carcinoma

Staged by _____ M.D.
_____ Registrar
Date _____

37

Urethra

C68.0 Urethra
C68.1 Paraurethral gland
C68.8 Overlapping lesion
C68.9 Urinary system, NOS

In both sexes, cancers of the urethra are exceedingly rare. Most carcinomas of the female urethra occur at the junction of the transitional and stratified squamous epithelium at the meatus. In males, the cancer may be associated with a venereal disease, such as gonorrhea; the most common location is the bulbomembranous portion. In females and males, most tumors are squamous cell carcinomas. In males, transitional cell carcinomas are found in the prostatic portion. Staging depends on the depth of penetration and local extension.

ANATOMY

Primary Site. In the *male*, the urethra is divided into anterior, penile (pendulous), and posterior (bulbomembranous and prostate). The urethra consists of mucosa, submucosal stroma, and the surrounding corpus spongiosum. Histologically, the meatal and parameatal urethra are lined with squamous epithelium; the penile and bulbomembranous urethra, with pseudostratified or stratified columnar epithelium; and the prostatic urethra, with transitional cell epithelium. The corpora cavernosum is contiguous to the bulbous and penile urethra.

The *female* urethra is divided into proximal and distal sections. The epithelium is supported on subepithelial connective tissue. The periurethral glands of Skene are concentrated near the meatus but extend along the entire urethra. The urethra is surrounded by a longitudinal layer of smooth muscle continuous with the bladder. The distal third of the urethra is contiguous to the vaginal wall. The distal two-thirds of the urethra is lined with squamous epithelium; the proximal one third, with transitional epithelium. The periurethral glands are lined with pseudostratified and stratified columnar epithelium.

Regional Lymph Nodes. The regional lymph nodes include:

Iliac (common, internal [hypogastric] obturator, external)
Inguinal (superficial or deep)
Presacral
Sacral, NOS
Pelvic, NOS

The significance of regional lymph node metastasis in staging urethral cancer lies in the number and size and not in whether metastasis is unilateral or bilateral.

Metastatic Sites. Distant spread to lung, liver, and bone is most common.

RULES FOR CLASSIFICATION

Clinical Staging. Radiographic imaging, cystourethroscopy, palpation, and biopsy or cytology of the tumor prior to definitive treatment are desirable. The site of origin should be confirmed to exclude metastatic disease.

Pathologic Staging. Histologic examination and confirmation of extent and location of disease are required. The extent of resection, including removal of regional lymph nodes, will depend on tumor location, depth of penetration, and sex of patient. Laterality does not affect the N classification.

DEFINITION OF TNM

Primary Tumor (T) (male and female)

TX   Primary tumor cannot be assessed
T0   No evidence of primary tumor
Ta   Noninvasive papillary, polypoid, or verrucous carcinoma

Tis   Carcinoma *in situ*
T1   Tumor invades subepithelial connective tissue
T2   Tumor invades the corpus spongiosum or the pros-
      tate, or the periurethral muscle
T3   Tumor invades the corpus cavernosum or beyond
      the prostatic capsule, or the anterior vagina or
      bladder neck
T4   Tumor invades other adjacent organs

Regional Lymph Nodes (N)

NX   Regional lymph nodes cannot be assessed
N0   No regional lymph node metastasis
N1   Metastasis in a single lymph node, 2 cm or less in
      greatest dimension
N2   Metastasis in a single lymph node, more than 2 cm
      but not more than 5 cm in greatest dimension;
      or multiple lymph nodes, none more than 5 cm
      in greatest dimension
N3   Metastasis in a lymph node more than 5 cm in
      greatest dimension

Distant Metastasis (M)

MX   Presence of distant metastasis cannot be assessed
M0   No distant metastasis
M1   Distant metastasis

STAGE GROUPING

Stage 0a	Ta	N0	M0
Stage 0is	Tis	N0	M0
Stage I	T1	N0	M0
Stage II	T2	N0	M0
Stage III	T1	N1	M0
	T2	N1	M0
	T3	N0	M0
	T3	N1	M0
Stage IV	T4	N0	M0
	T4	N1	M0
	Any T	N2	M0
	Any T	N3	M0
	Any T	Any N	M1

HISTOPATHOLOGIC TYPE

Cell types can be divided into transitional, squamous,
and glandular.

HISTOPATHOLOGIC GRADE (G)

GX   Grade cannot be assessed
G1   Well differentiated
G2   Moderately differentiated
G3-4 Poorly differentiated or undifferentiated

BIBLIOGRAPHY

1. Levine RL: Urethral cancer. Cancer 45:1965–1972,
   1980
2. Rogers RE, Burns B: Carcinoma of the female urethra.
   Obstet Gynecol 33:54–57, 1969
3. Vernon HK, Wilkins RD: Primary carcinoma of the
   male urethra. Br J Urol 21:232–235, 1950

Data Form for Cancer Staging

Patient identification
Name _____
Address _____
Hospital or clinic number _____
Age _____ Sex _____ Race _____

Institution identification
Hospital or clinic _____
Address _____

Oncology Record

Anatomic site of cancer _____
Histologic type _____
Grade (G) _____
Date of classification _____

Chronology of classification
[ ] Clinical (use all data prior to first treatment)
[ ] Pathologic (if definitively resected specimen available)

DEFINITIONS

Primary Tumor (T)

Clin	Path		
[ ]	[ ]	TX	Primary tumor cannot be assessed
[ ]	[ ]	T0	No evidence of primary tumor
[ ]	[ ]	Ta	Noninvasive papillary, polypoid, or verrucous carcinoma
[ ]	[ ]	Tis	Carcinoma *in situ*
[ ]	[ ]	T1	Tumor invades subepithelial connective tissue
[ ]	[ ]	T2	Tumor invades corpus spongiosum or prostate or periurethral muscle
[ ]	[ ]	T3	Tumor invades corpus cavernosum or beyond prostatic capsule or the anterior vagina or bladder neck
[ ]	[ ]	T4	Tumor invades other adjacent organs

Lymph Node (N)

Clin	Path		
[ ]	[ ]	NX	Regional lymph nodes cannot be assessed
[ ]	[ ]	N0	No regional lymph node metastasis
[ ]	[ ]	N1	Metastasis in a single lymph node, 2 cm or less in greatest dimension
[ ]	[ ]	N2	Metastasis in a single lymph node, more than 2 cm but not more than 5 cm in greatest dimension, or multiple lymph nodes, none more than 5 cm in greatest dimension
[ ]	[ ]	N3	Metastasis in a lymph node more than 5 cm in greatest dimension

Distant Metastasis (M)

Clin	Path		
[ ]	[ ]	MX	Presence of distant metastasis cannot be assessed
[ ]	[ ]	M0	No distant metastasis
[ ]	[ ]	M1	Distant metastasis

Histopathologic Type

Cell types can be divided into transitional, squamous, and glandular.

Histopathologic Grade (G)

[ ] GX   Grade cannot be assessed
[ ] G1   Well differentiated
[ ] G2   Moderately differentiated
[ ] G3-4 Poorly differentiated or undifferentiated

Stage Grouping

Clin	Path				
[ ]	[ ]	0a	Ta	N0	M0
[ ]	[ ]	0is	Tis	N0	M0
[ ]	[ ]	I	T1	N0	M0
[ ]	[ ]	II	T2	N0	M0
[ ]	[ ]	III	T1	N1	M0
			T2	N1	M0
			T3	N0	M0
			T3	N1	M0
[ ]	[ ]	IV	T4	N0	M0
			T4	N1	M0
			Any T	N2	M0
			Any T	N3	M0
			Any T	Any N	M1

Staged by _____ M.D.
_____ Registrar
Date _____

American Joint Committee on Cancer—1992

OPHTHALMIC CANCERS

The orbit and its contents—primarily the eye—contain many types of tissues. Consequently, a wide variety of malignant tumors occur in this anatomic area. This section includes recommendations for staging these cancers based on data available in the literature and on knowledge of the experts serving on the American Joint Committee on Cancer's Task Force for Staging of Cancer of the Eye.

The following sites are included:

Eyelid
Conjunctiva
Uvea
Retina
Orbit
Lacrimal gland

38

Carcinoma of the Eyelid

C44.1 Eyelid

ANATOMY

Primary Site. The eyelid is covered externally by epidermis and internally by conjunctiva, which becomes continuous with the conjunctiva covering the eyeball. Basal cell carcinomas and squamous cell carcinomas arise from the epidermal surface. Sebaceous cell carcinomas arise from the meibomian glands in the tarsus, the glands of Zeis at the lid margin, and the sebaceous glands of the caruncle. Other adnexal carcinomas arise from the sweat glands of Moll and the hair follicles.

Regional Lymph Nodes. The eyelids are supplied with lymphatics that drain into the preauricular, infra-auricular, facial, submandibular, and cervical lymph nodes.

Metastatic Sites. Tumors of the eyelids not only metastasize to distant sites by way of the regional lymphatics and bloodstream but also spread directly into the orbit, including the lacrimal gland, and into the eyeball.

RULES FOR CLASSIFICATION

The classification applies only to carcinoma. There should be histologic verification of the cancer. This verification permits a division of cases by histologic type (i.e., basal cell, squamous cell, and sebaceous carcinoma). Any unconfirmed case must be reported separately.

Clinical Staging. The assessment of the cancer is based on inspection, slit-lamp examination, palpation of the regional lymph nodes, and, when indicated, radiologic (including computed tomography) and ultrasonographic examination of the orbit, paranasal sinuses, and chest.

Pathologic Staging. Complete resection of the primary site is indicated. Histologic study of the margins and the deep aspect of resected tissues is necessary. Resection or needle biopsy of enlarged regional lymph nodes or orbital masses is desirable.

DEFINITION OF TNM

The following definitions apply to both clinical and pathologic staging.

Primary Tumor (T)

TX   Primary tumor cannot be assessed
T0   No evidence of primary tumor

Tis   Carcinoma *in situ*
T1   Tumor of any size, not invading the tarsal plate or,
      at the eyelid margin, 5 mm or less in greatest
      dimension
T2   Tumor invades tarsal plate or, at the eyelid margin,
      more than 5 mm but not more than 10 mm in
      greatest dimension
T3   Tumor involves full eyelid thickness or, at the eye-
      lid margin, more than 10 mm in greatest dimen-
      sion
T4   Tumor invades adjacent structures

Regional Lymph Nodes (N)

NX   Regional lymph nodes cannot be assessed
N0   No regional lymph node metastasis
N1   Regional lymph node metastasis

Distant Metastasis (M)

MX   Presence of distant metastasis cannot be assessed
M0   No distant metastasis
M1   Distant metastasis

STAGE GROUPING

No stage grouping is presently recommended.

HISTOPATHOLOGIC TYPE

Basal cell carcinoma
Squamous cell carcinoma
Sebaceous cell carcinoma

HISTOPATHOLOGIC GRADE (G)

GX   Grade cannot be assessed
G1   Well differentiated
G2   Moderately differentiated
G3   Poorly differentiated
G4   Undifferentiated

BIBLIOGRAPHY

1. Zimmerman LE, et al: Histological typing of tumors of
   the eye and its adnexa. WHO International Histological Classification of Tumors. Geneva, WHO, 1980

Data Form for Cancer Staging

Patient identification
Name _____
Address _____
Hospital or clinic number _____
Age _____ Sex _____ Race _____

Institution identification
Hospital or clinic _____
Address _____

Oncology Record

Anatomic site of cancer _____
Histologic type _____
Grade (G) _____
Date of classification _____

Chronology of classification
[ ]   Clinical (use all data prior to first treatment)
[ ]   Pathologic (if definitively resected specimen available)

DEFINITIONS

Primary Tumor (T)

Clin	Path		
[ ]	[ ]	TX	Primary tumor cannot be assessed
[ ]	[ ]	T0	No evidence of primary tumor
[ ]	[ ]	Tis	Carcinoma *in situ*
[ ]	[ ]	T1	Tumor of any size, not invading the tarsal plate or, at the eyelid margin, 5 mm or less in greatest dimension
[ ]	[ ]	T2	Tumor invades tarsal plate or, at the eyelid margin, more than 5 mm but not more than 10 mm in greatest dimension
[ ]	[ ]	T3	Tumor involves full eyelid thickness or, at the eyelid margin, more than 10 mm in greatest dimension
[ ]	[ ]	T4	Tumor invades adjacent structures

Lymph Node (N)

Clin	Path		
[ ]	[ ]	NX	Regional lymph nodes cannot be assessed
[ ]	[ ]	N0	No regional lymph node metastasis
[ ]	[ ]	N1	Regional lymph node metastasis

Distant Metastasis (M)

Clin	Path		
[ ]	[ ]	MX	Presence of distant metastasis cannot be assessed
[ ]	[ ]	M0	No distant metastasis
[ ]	[ ]	M1	Distant metastasis

Histopathologic Grade (G)

[ ]   GX   Grade cannot be assessed
[ ]   G1   Well differentiated
[ ]   G2   Moderately differentiated
[ ]   G3   Poorly differentiated
[ ]   G4   Undifferentiated

Illustration

Indicate on diagram and describe exact location and characteristics of tumor.

Stage Grouping

No stage grouping is presently recommended.

Staged by _____ M.D.
_____ Registrar
Date _____

Histopathologic Type

Basal cell carcinoma
Squamous cell carcinoma
Sebaceous carcinoma

39

Malignant Melanoma of the Eyelid

C44.1 Eyelid

This chapter has been adapted from the discussion for melanoma of the skin, because that discussion is considered applicable to melanoma of the skin of the eyelid.

No cT categories are presently recommended.

The pT categories correspond to those in the third edition of the AJCC manual and are based on Clark's "levels" and Breslow's "thickness of invasion." Thickness of invasion into the skin is recorded as an actual measurement by an ocular micrometer.

Maximal thickness of the tumor is measured with an ocular micrometer at a right angle to the adjacent normal skin. The upper reference point is the top of the granular cell layer of the epidermis of the overlying skin, or the base of the lesion if the tumor is ulcerated. The lower reference point is usually the deepest point of invasion. It may be the invading edge of a single tumor mass or an isolated cell or group of cells deep to the main mass.

The N and M categories correspond to those of melanoma of the skin.

ANATOMY

Primary Site. The eyelid is covered externally by epidermis and internally by conjunctiva, which becomes continuous with the conjunctiva covering the eyeball.

Regional Lymph Nodes. The eyelids are supplied with lymphatics that drain into the preauricular, infra-auricular, facial, submandibular, and cervical lymph nodes.

Metastatic Sites. Tumors of the eyelid not only metastasize to distant sites by way of the regional lymphatics and bloodstream but also spread directly into the orbit, including the lacrimal gland, and into the eyeball.

RULES FOR CLASSIFICATION

Clinical Staging. Assessment of the cancer is based on inspection, slit-lamp examination, palpation of the regional lymph nodes, and, when indicated, radiologic (including computed tomography) and ultrasonographic examination of the orbit, paranasal sinuses, and chest.

Pathologic Staging. Complete resection of the primary site is indicated. Histologic study of the margins and the deep aspect of resected tissues is necessary. Resection or needle biopsy of enlarged regional lymph nodes or orbital masses is desirable.

DEFINITION OF TNM

Clinical Classification (cTNM)

Primary Tumor (T)

No classification is recommended at present.

Regional Lymph Nodes (N)

NX Regional lymph nodes cannot be assessed
N0 No regional lymph node metastasis
N1 Metastasis 3 cm or less in greatest dimension in any regional lymph node(s)
N2 Metastasis more than 3 cm in greatest dimension in any regional lymph node(s) and/or in-transit metastasis
   N2a Metastasis more than 3 cm in greatest dimension in any regional node(s)
   N2b In-transit metastasis
   N2c Both (N2a and N2b)

Distant Metastasis (M)

MX Presence of distant metastasis cannot be assessed
M0 No distant metastasis
M1 Distant metastasis

DEFINITION OF TNM

Pathologic Classification (pTNM)

Primary Tumor (pT)

pTX   Primary tumor cannot be assessed

pT0   No evidence of primary tumor

pTis   Melanoma *in situ* (atypical melanocytic hyperplasia, severe melanocytic dysplasia), not an invasive malignant lesion (Clark's Level I)

pT1   Tumor 0.75 mm or less in thickness and invades the papillary dermis (Clark's Level II)

pT2   Tumor more than 0.75 mm but not more than 1.5 mm in thickness and/or invades to the papillary-reticular dermal interface (Clark's Level III)

pT3   Tumor more than 1.5 mm but not more than 4 mm in thickness and/or invades the reticular dermis (Clark's Level IV)

    pT3a   Tumor more than 1.5 mm but not more than 3 mm in thickness

    pT3b   Tumor more than 3 mm but not more than 4 mm in thickness

pT4   Tumor more than 4 mm in thickness and/or invades the subcutaneous tissue and/or satellite(s) within 2 cm of the primary tumor (Clark's Level V)

    pT4a   Tumor more than 4 mm in thickness and/or invades the subcutaneous tissue

    pT4b   Satellite(s) within 2 cm of the primary tumor

Regional Lymph Nodes (pN)

pNX   Regional lymph nodes cannot be assessed

pN0   No regional lymph node metastasis

pN1   Metastasis 3 cm or less in greatest dimension in any regional lymph node(s)

pN2   Metastasis more than 3 cm in greatest dimension in any regional lymph node(s) and/or in-transit metastasis

    pN2a   Metastasis more than 3 cm in greatest dimension

    pN2b   In-transit metastasis

    pN2c   Both (pN2a and pN2b)

Distant Metastasis (pM)

pMX   Presence of distant metastasis cannot be assessed

pM0   No distant metastasis

pM1   Distant metastasis

    pM1a   Metastasis in skin or subcutaneous tissue or lymph node(s) beyond the regional lymph nodes

    pM1b   Visceral metastasis

Note: In-transit metastasis involves skin or subcutaneous tissue more than 2 cm from the primary tumor not beyond the regional lymph nodes.

STAGE GROUPING

Stage			
Stage I	pT1	N0	M0
	pT2	N0	M0
Stage II	pT3	N0	M0
Stage III	pT4	N0	M0
	Any pT	N1	M0
	Any pT	N2	M0
Stage IV	Any pT	Any N	M1

HISTOPATHOLOGIC TYPE

This classification is only for melanoma of the eyelid.

BIBLIOGRAPHY

1. Breslow A: Tumor thickness, level of invasion, and node dissection in Stage 1 cutaneous melanoma. Ann Surg 182:572–575, 1975
2. Breslow A: Thickness, cross-sectional areas, and depth of invasion in the prognosis of cutaneous melanoma. Ann Surg 172:902–908, 1970
3. Clark WH Jr, Ainsworth AM, Bernardina EA, et al: The developmental biology of primary human malignant melanomas. Semin Oncol 2:83–103, 1975
4. Elder DE, Jucovy PM, Tuthill RJ, Clark WH Jr: The classification of malignant melanoma. Am J Dermatopathol 2:315–319, 1980

Data Form for Cancer Staging

Patient identification
Name _____
Address _____
Hospital or clinic number _____
Age _____ Sex _____ Race _____

Institution identification
Hospital or clinic _____
Address _____

Oncology Record

Anatomic site of cancer _____
Histologic type _____
Grade (G) _____
Date of classification _____

Chronology of classification
[ ] Clinical (use all data prior to first treatment)
[ ] Pathologic (if definitively resected specimen available)

DEFINITIONS

Primary Tumor (T)

No classification is recommended at present.

Lymph Node (N)

Clin	Path		
[ ]		NX	Regional lymph nodes cannot be assessed
[ ]		N0	No regional lymph node metastasis
[ ]		N1	Metastasis 3 cm or less in greatest dimension in any regional lymph node(s)
[ ]		N2	Metastasis more than 3 cm in greatest dimension in any regional lymph node(s) and/or in-transit metastasis
[ ]		N2a	Metastasis more than 3 cm in greatest dimension in any regional node(s)
[ ]		N2b	In-transit metastasis
[ ]		N2c	Both

Primary Tumor (pT)

Clin	Path		
	[ ]	pTX	Primary tumor cannot be assessed
	[ ]	pT0	No evidence of primary tumor
	[ ]	pTis	Melanoma *in situ* (atypical melanocytic hyperplasia, severe melanocytic dysplasia), not an invasive malignant lesion (Clark's Level I)
	[ ]	pT1	Tumor 0.75 mm or less in thickness and invades the papillary dermis (Clark's Level II)
	[ ]	pT2	Tumor more than 0.75 mm but not more than 1.5 mm in thickness and/or invades to the papillary-reticular dermal interface (Clark's Level III)
	[ ]	pT3	Tumor more than 1.5 mm but not more than 4 mm in thickness and/or invades the reticular dermis (Clark's Level IV)
	[ ]	pT3a	Tumor more than 1.5 mm but not more than 3 mm in thickness
	[ ]	pT3b	Tumor more than 3 mm but not more than 4 mm in thickness
	[ ]	pT4	Tumor more than 4 mm in thickness and/or invades the subcutaneous tissue and/or satellite(s) within 2 cm of the primary tumor (Clark's Level V)
	[ ]	pT4a	Tumor more than 4 mm in thickness and/or invades the subcutaneous tissue
	[ ]	pT4b	Satellite(s) within 2 cm of the primary tumor

Lymph Node (pN)

Clin	Path		
	[ ]	pNX	Regional lymph nodes cannot be assessed
	[ ]	pN0	No regional lymph node metastasis
	[ ]	pN1	Metastasis 3 cm or less in greatest dimension in any regional lymph node(s)
	[ ]	pN2	Metastasis more than 3 cm in greatest dimension in any regional lymph node(s) and/or in-transit metastasis
	[ ]	pN2a	Metastasis more than 3 cm in greatest dimension
	[ ]	pN2b	In-transit metastasis
	[ ]	pN2c	Both (pN2a and pN2b)

Distant Metastasis (pM)

Clin	Path		
	[ ]	pMX	Presence of distant metastasis cannot be assessed
	[ ]	pM0	No distant metastasis
	[ ]	pM1	Distant metastasis
	[ ]	pM1a	Metastasis in skin or subcutaneous tissue or lymph node(s) beyond the regional lymph nodes
	[ ]	pM1b	Visceral metastasis

(continued on next page)

Clin	Path	Stage Grouping			
[ ]	[ ]	I	pT1	N0	M0
			pT2	N0	M0
[ ]	[ ]	II	pT3	N0	M0
[ ]	[ ]	III	pT4	N0	M0
			Any pT	N1	M0
[ ]	[ ]	IV	Any pT	Any N	M1

Staged by _____ M.D.

_____Registrar

Date _____

Histopathologic Type

This classification is only for melanoma of the eyelid.

Note: In-transit metastasis involves skin or subcutaneous tissue more than 2 cm from the primary tumor not beyond the regional lymph nodes.

40

Carcinoma of the Conjunctiva

C69.0 Conjunctiva

ANATOMY

Primary Site. The conjunctiva consists of stratified epithelium that contains mucus-secreting goblet cells; these cells are most numerous in the fornices. Palpebral conjunctiva lines the eyelid; bulbar conjunctiva covers the eyeball. Conjunctival epithelium merges with that of the cornea at the limbus. It is at this site, particularly at the temporal limbus, that carcinoma is most likely to arise. Conjunctival intraepithelial neoplasia (CIN) embraces all forms of intraepithelial dysplasia, including *in situ* carcinoma. Mucinous adenocarcinoma is a rare form of adenocarcinoma of the conjunctival goblet cells.

Regional Lymph Nodes. The regional lymph nodes are:

Preauricular (parotid)
Submandibular
Cervical

Metastatic Sites. Tumors of the conjunctiva, in addition to spread by way of regional lymphatics, may also involve the eyelid proper, the orbit, lacrimal glands, and the brain.

RULES FOR CLASSIFICATION

Clinical Staging. Assessment of the cancer is based on inspection, slit-lamp examination, palpation of the regional lymph nodes, and, when indicated, radiologic examination (including computed tomography) and ultrasonographic examination of the orbit, paranasal sinuses, and chest.

Pathologic Staging. Complete resection of the primary site is indicated. Extensive local involvement of orbital spread requires exenteration. Histologic study of the margins of the deep aspect of resected tissues is necessary.

DEFINITION OF TNM

These definitions apply to both clinical and pathologic staging.

Primary Tumor (T)

TX   Primary tumor cannot be assessed
T0   No evidence of primary tumor
Tis Carcinoma *in situ*
T1   Tumor 5 mm or less in greatest dimension
T2   Tumor more than 5 mm in greatest dimension, without invasion of adjacent structures
T3   Tumor invades adjacent structures, excluding the orbit
T4   Tumor invades the orbit

Regional Lymph Nodes (N)

NX   Regional lymph nodes cannot be assessed
N0   No regional lymph node metastasis
N1   Regional lymph node metastasis

Distant Metastasis (M)

MX   Presence of distant metastasis cannot be assessed
M0   No distant metastasis
M1   Distant metastasis

STAGE GROUPING

No stage grouping is presently recommended.

HISTOPATHOLOGIC TYPE

This classification applies only to carcinoma of the conjunctiva.

HISTOPATHOLOGIC GRADE (G)

GX   Grade cannot be assessed
G1   Well differentiated
G2   Moderately differentiated
G3   Poorly differentiated
G4   Undifferentiated

CARCINOMA OF THE CONJUNCTIVA

Data Form for Cancer Staging

Patient identification
Name _____
Address _____
Hospital or clinic number _____
Age _____ Sex _____ Race _____

Institution identification
Hospital or clinic _____
Address _____

Oncology Record

Anatomic site of cancer _____
Histologic type _____
Grade (G) _____
Date of classification _____

Chronology of classification
[ ] Clinical (use all data prior to first treatment)
[ ] Pathologic (if definitively resected specimen available)

DEFINITIONS

Clin	Path		

Primary Tumor (T)

Clin	Path		
[ ]	[ ]	TX	Primary tumor cannot be assessed
[ ]	[ ]	T0	No evidence of primary tumor
[ ]	[ ]	Tis	Tumor *in situ*
[ ]	[ ]	T1	Tumor 5 mm or less in greatest dimension
[ ]	[ ]	T2	Tumor more than 5 mm in greatest dimension, without invasion of adjacent structures
[ ]	[ ]	T3	Tumor invades adjacent structures, excluding the orbit
[ ]	[ ]	T4	Tumor invades the orbit

Lymph Node (N)

Clin	Path		
[ ]	[ ]	NX	Regional lymph nodes cannot be assessed
[ ]	[ ]	N0	No regional lymph node metastasis
[ ]	[ ]	N1	Regional lymph node metastasis

Distant Metastasis (M)

Clin	Path		
[ ]	[ ]	MX	Presence of distant metastasis cannot be assessed
[ ]	[ ]	M0	No distant metastasis
[ ]	[ ]	M1	Distant metastasis

Illustration

Indicate on diagram and describe exact location and characteristics of tumor.

Stage Grouping

No stage grouping is presently recommended.

Staged by _____ M.D.
_____Registrar
Date _____

Histopathologic Type

This classification applies only to carcinoma of conjunctiva.

Histopathologic Grade (G)

[ ] GX Grade cannot be assessed
[ ] G1 Well differentiated
[ ] G2 Moderately differentiated
[ ] G3 Poorly differentiated
[ ] G4 Undifferentiated

American Joint Committee on Cancer—1992

41

Malignant Melanoma of the Conjunctiva

C69.0 Conjunctiva

ANATOMY

Primary Site. In addition to mucus-secreting goblet cells within the stratified epithelium, melanocytic cells exist in the basal layer. These are of neuroectodermal origin, and melanocytic tumors may arise from these cells. Melanomas may arise from junctional and compound nevi, from primary acquired melanosis, or de novo. Tumors must be distinguished from nontumorous pigmentation.

Regional Lymph Nodes. The regional lymph nodes are:

Parotid
Preauricular
Submandibular
Cervical

Metastatic Sites. In addition to spread by lymphatics and the bloodstream, direct extension to the eyeball and orbit occurs.

RULES FOR CLASSIFICATION

The classification applies only to melanoma. There should be histologic verification of the melanocytic lesion.

Clinical Staging. The assessment of the cancer is based on inspection, slit-lamp examination, palpation of the regional lymph nodes, and, when indicated, radiologic (including computed tomography) and ultrasonographic examination of the orbit, paranasal sinuses, and chest.

Pathologic Staging. Complete resection of the primary site is indicated. Histologic study of the margins and the deep aspect of resected tissues is necessary. Resection or needle biopsy of enlarged regional lymph nodes or orbital masses is desirable.

DEFINITION OF TNM

Clinical Classification

Primary Tumor (T)

TX   Primary tumor cannot be assessed
T0   No evidence of primary tumor
T1   Tumor(s) of the bulbar conjunctiva occupying one quadrant or less
T2   Tumor(s) of the bulbar conjunctiva occupying more than one quadrant
T3   Tumor(s) of the conjunctival fornix and/or palpebral conjunctiva and/or caruncle
T4   Tumor invades the eyelid, cornea, and/or orbit

Regional Lymph Nodes (N)

NX   Regional lymph nodes cannot be assessed
N0   No regional lymph node metastasis
N1   Regional lymph node metastasis

Distant Metastasis (M)

MX   Presence of distant metastasis cannot be assessed
M0   No distant metastasis
M1   Distant metastasis

Pathologic Classification (pTNM)

Primary Tumor (pT)

pTX   Primary tumor cannot be assessed
pT0   No evidence of primary tumor
pT1   Tumor(s) of the bulbar conjunctiva occupying one quadrant or less and 2 mm or less in thickness

pT2   Tumor(s) of the bulbar conjunctiva occupying more than one quadrant and 2 mm or less in thickness

pT3   Tumor(s) of the conjunctival fornix and/or palpebral conjunctiva and/or caruncle or tumor(s) of the bulbar conjunctiva, more than 2 mm in thickness

pT4   Tumor invades the eyelid, cornea, and/or orbit

Regional Lymph Nodes (pN)

pNX   Regional lymph nodes cannot be assessed
pN0   No regional lymph node metastasis
pN1   Regional lymph node metastasis

Distant Metastasis (pM)

pMX   Presence of distant metastasis cannot be assessed
pM0   No distant metastasis
pM1   Distant metastasis

STAGE GROUPING

No stage grouping is presently recommended.

HISTOPATHOLOGIC TYPE

This categorization applies only to melanoma of the conjunctiva.

HISTOPATHOLOGIC GRADE (G)

Histopathologic grade represents the origin of the primary tumor.

GX   Origin cannot be assessed
G0   Primary acquired melanosis
G1   Malignant melanoma arises from a nevus
G2   Malignant melanoma arises from primary acquired melanosis
G3   Malignant melanoma arises de novo

BIBLIOGRAPHY

1. Liesegang TJ, Campbell RJ: Mayo Clinic experience with conjunctival melanomas. Arch Ophthalmol 98: 1385–1389, 1980

2. Silvers DN, Jakobiec FA, Freeman TR, et al: Melanoma of the conjunctiva: A clinicopathologic study. In Jakobiec FA (Ed.), Ocular and Adnexal Tumors. Birmingham, Aesculapius, 1978

3. Zimmerman LE: The histogenesis of conjunctival melanomas: The first Algernon B. Reese lecture. In Jakobiec FA (Ed.), Ocular and Adnexal Tumors. Birmingham, Aesculapius, 1978

Data Form for Cancer Staging

Patient identification
Name _____
Address _____
Hospital or clinic number _____
Age _____ Sex _____ Race _____

Institution identification
Hospital or clinic _____
Address _____

Oncology Record

Anatomic site of cancer _____
Histologic type _____
Grade (G) _____
Date of classification _____

Chronology of classification
[ ]   Clinical (use all data prior to first treatment)
[ ]   Pathologic (if definitively resected specimen available)

Clin	Path		
		DEFINITIONS	
		Primary Tumor (T)	
[ ]		TX	Primary tumor cannot be assessed
[ ]		T0	No evidence of primary tumor
[ ]		T1	Tumor(s) of bulbar conjunctiva occupying one quadrant or less
[ ]		T2	Tumor(s) of bulbar conjunctiva occupying more than one quadrant
[ ]		T3	Tumor(s) of conjunctival fornix and/or palpebral conjunctiva and/or caruncle
[ ]		T4	Tumor invades eyelid, cornea, and/or orbit
		Lymph Node (N)	
[ ]		NX	Regional lymph nodes cannot be assessed
[ ]		N0	No regional lymph node metastasis
[ ]		N1	Regional lymph node metastasis
		Distant Metastasis (M)	
[ ]		MX	Presence of distant metastasis cannot be assessed
[ ]		M0	No distant metastasis
[ ]		M1	Distant metastasis
		Primary Tumor (pT)	
	[ ]	pTX	Primary tumor cannot be assessed
	[ ]	pT0	No evidence of primary tumor
	[ ]	pT1	Tumor(s) of bulbar conjunctiva occupying one quadrant or less and 2 mm or less in thickness
	[ ]	pT2	Tumor(s) of bulbar conjunctiva occupying more than one quadrant and 2 mm or less in thickness
	[ ]	pT3	Tumor(s) of conjunctival fornix and/or palpebral conjunctiva and/or caruncle and/or tumor of the bulbar conjunctiva, more than 2 mm in thickness
	[ ]	pT4	Tumor invades eyelid, cornea, and/or orbit
		Lymph Node (pN)	
	[ ]	pNX	Regional lymph nodes cannot be assessed
	[ ]	pN0	No regional lymph node metastasis
	[ ]	pN1	Regional lymph node metastasis
		Distant Metastasis (pM)	
	[ ]	pMX	Presence of distant metastasis cannot be assessed
	[ ]	pM0	No distant metastasis
	[ ]	pM1	Distant metastasis

Stage Grouping

No stage grouping is presently recommended.

Staged by _____ M.D.
_____ Registrar
Date _____

(continued on next page)

Histopathologic Type

The categorization applies only to malignant melanoma of the conjunctiva.

Histopathologic Grade (G)

[ ] GX   Grade cannot be assessed
[ ] G0   Primary acquired melanosis
[ ] G1   Malignant melanoma arising from a nevus
[ ] G2   Malignant melanoma arising from primary acquired melanosis
[ ] G3   Malignant melanoma arising de novo

Illustration

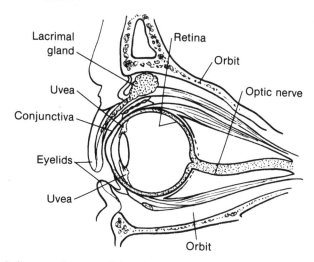

Indicate on diagram and describe exact location and characteristics of tumor.

42

Malignant Melanoma of the Uvea

C69.3 Choroid
C69.4 Ciliary body and iris

The classification applies only to melanoma.

ANATOMY

Primary Site. The middle layer of the eyeball, the uvea (uveal tract) lies between the cornea and sclera externally and the retina and its analogues internally. The uveal tract is divided into three regions: iris, ciliary body, and choroid. It is a highly vascular structure, with the choroid in particular composed of large blood vessels with little intervening connective tissue. There are no lymphatic channels in the uvea. Systemic metastasis from uveal melanomas occurs by hematogenous routes. Uveal melanomas are believed to arise from uveal melanocytes and are, therefore, of neural crest origin. Melanomas may spread by local extension through Bruch's membrane to involve the retina and vitreous, or by extension through the sclera or optic nerve into the orbit.

Most uveal melanomas occur in the choroid. The ciliary body is less commonly the site of origin, and the iris is least commonly involved. Iris melanomas are relatively benign and slow growing, and they rarely metastasize. Melanomas of the ciliary body and choroid are cytologically more malignant and metastasize more frequently.

It may be clinically impossible to distinguish a large nevus from a small melanoma.

Regional Lymph Nodes. Because there are no intraocular lymphatics, this category applies only to extrascleral extension anteriorly. The regional lymph nodes are:

Parotid
Preauricular
Submandibular
Cervical

Nodal involvement implies subconjunctival extension of the primary tumor.

Metastatic Sites. Uveal melanomas can metastasize through hematogenous routes to various organs. The liver is most commonly involved and usually is the first site of clinically detectable metastasis. Less commonly, the lung, pleura, subcutaneous tissues, bone, and other sites may be involved.

RULES FOR CLASSIFICATION

There should be histologic verification of the disease. Any unconfirmed case must be reported separately.

Clinical Staging. The assessment of the tumor is based on clinical examination, including slit-lamp examination and direct and indirect ophthalmoscopy. Additional methods such as ultrasonography, computerized stereometry, fluorescein angiography, and isotope examination may enhance the accuracy of appraisal.

Pathologic Staging. Complete resection of the primary site is indicated. Histologic study of the margins and the deep aspect of resected tissues is necessary. Resection or needle biopsy of enlarged regional lymph nodes or orbital masses is desirable.

DEFINITION OF TNM

These definitions apply to both clinical and pathologic staging.

ANATOMIC SITES

Iris
Ciliary body
Choroid

Iris

Primary Tumor (T)

TX   Primary tumor cannot be assessed
T0   No evidence of primary tumor
T1   Tumor limited to the iris
T2   Tumor involves one quadrant or less, with invasion into the anterior chamber angle
T3   Tumor involves more than one quadrant, with invasion into the anterior chamber angle
T4   Tumor with extraocular extension

Regional Lymph Nodes (N)

NX   Regional lymph nodes cannot be assessed
N0   No regional lymph node metastasis
N1   Regional lymph node metastasis

Distant Metastasis (M)

MX   Presence of distant metastasis cannot be assessed
M0   No distant metastasis
M1   Distant metastasis

Ciliary Body

Primary Tumor (T)

TX   Primary tumor cannot be assessed
T0   No evidence of primary tumor
T1   Tumor limited to the ciliary body
T2   Tumor invades into the anterior chamber and/or iris
T3   Tumor invades the choroid
T4   Tumor with extraocular extension

Regional Lymph Nodes (N)

NX   Regional lymph nodes cannot be assessed
N0   No regional lymph node metastasis
N1   Regional lymph node metastasis

Distant Metastasis (M)

MX   Presence of distant metastasis cannot be assessed
M0   No distant metastasis
M1   Distant metastasis

Choroid

Primary Tumor (T)

TX   Primary tumor cannot be assessed
T0   No evidence of primary tumor
T1*   Tumor 10 mm or less in greatest dimension, with an elevation of 3 mm or less
     T1a   Tumor 7 mm or less in greatest dimension, with an elevation of 2 mm or less

T1b   Tumor more than 7 mm but not more than 10 mm in greatest dimension, with an elevation of more than 2 mm but not more than 3 mm
T2*   Tumor more than 10 mm but not more than 15 mm in greatest dimension, with an elevation of more than 3 mm but not more than 5 mm
T3*   Tumor more than 15 mm in greatest dimension or with an elevation of more than 5 mm
T4   Tumor with extraocular extension

Note: When dimension and elevation show a difference in classification, the highest category should be used for classification.

* *Note:* In clinical practice, the tumor base may be estimated in optic disc diameters (dd) (average: 1 dd = 1.5 mm). The elevation may be estimated in diopters (average: 3 diopters = 1 mm). Other techniques, such as ultrasonography and computerized stereometry, may provide a more accurate measurement.

Regional Lymph Nodes (N)

NX   Regional lymph nodes cannot be assessed
N0   No regional lymph node metastasis
N1   Regional lymph node metastasis

Distant Metastasis (M)

MX   Presence of distant metastasis cannot be assessed
M0   No distant metastasis
M1   Distant metastasis

STAGE GROUPING

The classification of the structure most affected is used when more than one of the uveal structures is involved by tumor.

Iris and Ciliary Body

Stage	T	N	M
Stage I	T1	N0	M0
Stage II	T2	N0	M0
Stage III	T3	N0	M0
Stage IVA	T4	N0	M0
Stage IVB	Any T	N1	M0
	Any T	Any N	M1

Choroid

Stage	T	N	M
Stage IA	T1a	N0	M0
Stage IB	T1b	N0	M0
Stage II	T2	N0	M0
Stage III	T3	N0	M0
Stage IVA	T4	N0	M0
Stage IVB	Any T	N1	M0
	Any T	Any N	M1

HISTOPATHOLOGIC TYPE

The histopathologic types are:

Spindle cell melanoma
Mixed cell melanoma
Epithelioid cell melanoma

HISTOPATHOLOGIC GRADE (G)

GX   Grade cannot be assessed
G1   Spindle cell melanoma
G2   Mixed cell melanoma
G3   Epithelioid cell melanoma

Venous Invasion (V)

VX   Venous invasion cannot be assessed
V0   Veins do not contain tumor
V1   Veins in melanoma contain tumor
V2   Vortex veins contain tumor

Scleral Invasion (S)

SX   Scleral invasion cannot be assessed
S0   Sclera does not contain tumor
S1   Intrascleral* invasion of tumor
S2   Extrascleral extension of tumor

Note: Includes perineural and perivascular invasion of scleral canals.

Data Form for Cancer Staging

Patient identification
Name _____
Address _____
Hospital or clinic number _____
Age _____ Sex _____ Race _____

Institution identification
Hospital or clinic _____
Address _____

Oncology Record

Anatomic site of cancer _____
Histologic type _____
Grade (G) _____
Date of classification _____

Chronology of classification
[ ] Clinical (use all data prior to first treatment)
[ ] Pathologic (if definitively resected specimen available)

Clin	Path		
		DEFINITIONS	
		Iris	
		Primary Tumor (T)	
[ ]	[ ]	TX	Primary tumor cannot be assessed
[ ]	[ ]	T0	No evidence of primary tumor
[ ]	[ ]	T1	Tumor limited to the iris
[ ]	[ ]	T2	Tumor involves one quadrant or less, with invasion into the anterior chamber angle
[ ]	[ ]	T3	Tumor involves more than one quadrant, with invasion into the anterior chamber angle
[ ]	[ ]	T4	Tumor with extraocular extension
		Lymph Node (N)	
[ ]	[ ]	NX	Regional lymph nodes cannot be assessed
[ ]	[ ]	N0	No regional lymph node metastasis
[ ]	[ ]	N1	Regional lymph node metastasis
		Distant Metastasis (M)	
[ ]	[ ]	MX	Presence of distant metastasis cannot be assessed
[ ]	[ ]	M0	No distant metastasis
[ ]	[ ]	M1	Distant metastasis
		Ciliary Body	
		Primary Tumor (T)	
[ ]	[ ]	TX	Primary tumor cannot be assessed
[ ]	[ ]	T0	No evidence of primary tumor
[ ]	[ ]	T1	Tumor limited to ciliary body
[ ]	[ ]	T2	Tumor invades into anterior chamber and/or iris
[ ]	[ ]	T3	Tumor invades choroid
[ ]	[ ]	T4	Tumor with extraocular extension
		Lymph Node (N)	
[ ]	[ ]	NX	Regional lymph nodes cannot be assessed
[ ]	[ ]	N0	No regional lymph node metastasis
[ ]	[ ]	N1	Regional lymph node metastasis
		Distant Metastasis (M)	
[ ]	[ ]	MX	Presence of distant metastasis cannot be assessed
[ ]	[ ]	M0	No distant metastasis
[ ]	[ ]	M1	Distant metastasis
		Choroid	
		Primary Tumor (T)	
[ ]	[ ]	TX	Primary tumor cannot be assessed
[ ]	[ ]	T0	No evidence of primary tumor
[ ]	[ ]	T1	Tumor 10 mm or less in greatest dimension with an elevation 3 mm or less
[ ]	[ ]	T1a	Tumor 7 mm or less in greatest dimension with an elevation 2 mm or less
[ ]	[ ]	T1b	Tumor more than 7 mm but not more than 10 mm in greatest dimension with an elevation more than 2 mm but not more than 3 mm
[ ]	[ ]	T2	Tumor more than 10 mm but not more than 15 mm in greatest dimension with an elevation of more than 3 mm but not more than 5 mm
[ ]	[ ]	T3	Tumor more than 15 mm in greatest dimension or with an elevation more than 5 mm
[ ]	[ ]	T4	Tumor with extraocular extension

(continued on next page)

233

American Joint Committee on Cancer—1992

Clin	Path

Lymph Node (N)

Clin	Path		
[ ]	[ ]	NX	Regional lymph nodes cannot be assessed
[ ]	[ ]	N0	No regional lymph node metastasis
[ ]	[ ]	N1	Regional lymph node metastasis

Distant Metastasis (M)

Clin	Path		
[ ]	[ ]	MX	Presence of distant metastasis cannot be assessed
[ ]	[ ]	M0	No distant metastasis
[ ]	[ ]	M1	Distant metastasis

Stage Grouping

Iris and Ciliary Body

Clin	Path				
[ ]	[ ]	I	T1	N0	M0
[ ]	[ ]	II	T2	N0	M0
[ ]	[ ]	III	T3	N0	M0
[ ]	[ ]	IVA	T4	N0	M0
[ ]	[ ]	IVB	Any T	N1	M0
			Any T	Any N	M1

Choroid

Clin	Path				
[ ]	[ ]	IA	T1a	N0	M0
[ ]	[ ]	IB	T1b	N0	M0
[ ]	[ ]	II	T2	N0	M0
[ ]	[ ]	III	T3	N0	M0
[ ]	[ ]	IVA	T4	N0	M0
[ ]	[ ]	IVB	Any T	N1	M0
			Any T	Any N	M1

Staged by _____ M.D.

_____ Registrar

Date _____

Histopathologic Type

Spindle cell melanoma
Mixed cell melanoma
Epithelioid cell melanoma

Histopathologic Grade (G)

[ ] GX Grade cannot be assessed
[ ] G1 Spindle cell melanoma
[ ] G2 Mixed cell melanoma
[ ] G3 Epithelioid cell melanoma

Venous Invasion (V)

[ ] VX Venous invasion cannot be assessed
[ ] V0 Veins do not contain tumor
[ ] V1 Veins in melanoma contain tumor
[ ] V2 Vortex veins contain tumor

Scleral Invasion (S)

[ ] SX Scleral invasion cannot be assessed
[ ] S0 Sclera does not contain tumor
[ ] S1 Intrascleral invasion of tumor
[ ] S2 Extrascleral invasion of tumor*

*Note: Includes perineural and perivascular invasion of scleral canals.

Illustrations

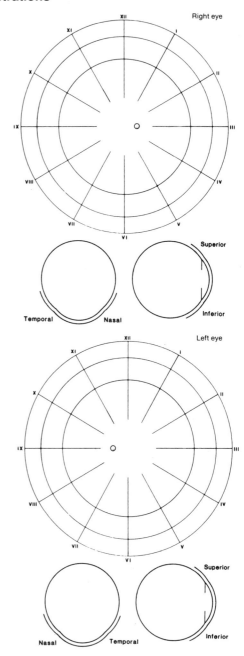

Indicate on diagrams and describe exact location and characteristics of tumor.

43

Retinoblastoma

C69.2 Retina

ANATOMY

Primary Site. The retina comprises neurons and glial cells. The neurons give rise to retinoblastoma, whereas the glial cells give rise to astrocytomas, which in the retina are benign and extremely rare. The retina is limited internally by a membrane separating it from the vitreous cavity. Externally, it is limited by the retinal pigment epithelium and Bruch's membrane, which separate it from the choroid and act as natural barriers to extension of retinal tumors into the choroid. The continuation of the retina with the optic nerve allows direct extension of retinoblastomas into the optic nerve and then to the subarachnoid space. Because the retina has no lymphatics, spread of retinal tumors occurs either by direct extension into adjacent structures or by distant metastasis through hematogenous routes.

Regional Lymph Nodes. Because there are no intraocular lymphatics, the category applies only to anterior extrascleral extension. The regional lymph nodes are:

Parotid
Preauricular
Submandibular
Cervical

Involvement implies subconjunctival extension of the tumor.

Metastatic Sites. Retinoblastoma can metastasize through hematogenous routes to various sites, most notably the skull, long bones, brain, lymph nodes, and viscera.

RULES FOR CLASSIFICATION

Clinical Staging. In bilateral cases, each eye must be classified separately. The classification does not apply to complete spontaneous regression of the tumor. There should be histologic verification of the disease in an enucleated eye. Any unconfirmed case must be reported separately. The extent of retinal involvement is indicated as a percentage.

Pathologic Staging. All clinical and pathologic data from the resected specimen are to be used.

DEFINITION OF TNM

Clinical Classification (cTNM)

Primary Tumor (T)

TX Primary tumor cannot be assessed
T0 No evidence of primary tumor
T1 Tumor(s) limited to 25% or less of the retina
T2 Tumor(s) involve(s) more than 25% but not more than 50% of the retina
T3 Tumor(s) involve(s) more than 50% of the retina and/or invade(s) beyond the retina but remain(s) intraocular

    T3a Tumor(s) involve(s) more than 50% of the retina and/ or tumor cells in the vitreous
    T3b Tumor(s) involve(s) the optic disc
    T3c Tumor(s) involve(s) the anterior chamber and/or uvea

T4 Tumor with extraocular invasion
T4a Tumor invades the retrobulbar optic nerve
T4b Extraocular extension other than invasion of the optic nerve

Note: The following suffixes may be added to the appropriate T categories: "m" indicates multiple tumors (e.g., T2 [m2]); "f" indicates cases with a known family history; and "d" indicates diffuse retinal involvement without the formation of discrete masses.

Regional Lymph Nodes (N)

NX Regional lymph nodes cannot be assessed
N0 No regional lymph node metastasis
N1 Regional lymph node metastasis

Distant Metastasis (M)

MX   Presence of distant metastasis cannot be assessed
M0   No distant metastasis
M1   Distant metastasis

Pathologic Classification (pTNM)

Primary Tumor (pT)

pTX   Primary tumor cannot be assessed
pT0   No evidence of primary tumor
pT1   Tumor(s) limited to 25% or less of the retina
pT2   Tumor(s) involve(s) more than 25% but not more than 50% of the retina
pT3   Tumor(s) involve(s) more than 50% of the retina and/or invade(s) beyond the retina but remain(s) intraocular

    pT3a   Tumor(s) involve(s) more than 50% of the retina and/ or tumor cells in the vitreous

    pT3b   Tumor invades the optic nerve as far as the lamina cribrosa

    pT3c   Tumor in the anterior chamber and/or invasion with thickening of the uvea and/or intrascleral invasion

pT4   Tumor with extraocular invasion

    pT4a   Intraneural tumor beyond the lamina cribrosa but not at the line of resection

    pT4b   Tumor at the line of resection or other extraocular extension

Regional Lymph Nodes (pN)

pNX   Regional lymph nodes cannot be assessed
pN0   No regional lymph node metastasis
pN1   Regional lymph node metastasis

Distant Metastasis (pM)

pMX   Presence of distant metastasis cannot be assessed
pM0   No distant metastasis
pM1   Distant metastasis

STAGE GROUPING

In cases of bilateral disease, the more affected eye is used for the stage grouping.

Stage IA	T1	N0	M0
Stage IB	T2	N0	M0
Stage IIA	T3a	N0	M0
Stage IIB	T3b	N0	M0
Stage IIC	T3c	N0	M0
Stage IIIA	T4a	N0	M0
Stage IIIB	T4b	N0	M0
Stage IV	Any T	N1	M0
	Any T	Any N	M1

Note: Pathologic stage grouping corresponds to the clinical stage grouping.

HISTOPATHOLOGIC TYPE

This classification applies only to retinoblastoma.

Data Form for Cancer Staging

Patient identification
Name _____
Address _____
Hospital or clinic number _____
Age _____ Sex _____ Race _____

Institution identification
Hospital or clinic _____
Address _____

Oncology Record

Anatomic site of cancer _____
Histologic type _____
Grade (G) _____
Date of classification _____

Chronology of classification
[   ] Clinical (use all data prior to first treatment)
[   ] Pathologic (if definitively resected specimen available)

DEFINITIONS

Primary Tumor (T)

Clin	Path		
[ ]	[ ]	TX	Primary tumor cannot be assessed
[ ]	[ ]	T0	No evidence of primary tumor
[ ]	[ ]	T1	Tumor(s) limited to 25% or less of the retina
[ ]	[ ]	T2	Tumor(s) involve(s) more than 25% but not more than 50% of the retina
[ ]	[ ]	T3	Tumor(s) involve(s) more than 50% of the retina and/or invade(s) beyond the retina but remain(s) intraocular
[ ]	[ ]	T3a	Tumor(s) involve(s) more than 50% of the retina and/or tumor cells in the vitreous
[ ]	[ ]	T3b	Tumor(s) involve(s) optic disc
[ ]	[ ]	T3c	Tumor(s) involve(s) anterior chamber and/or uvea
[ ]	[ ]	T4	Tumor with extraocular invasion
[ ]	[ ]	T4a	Tumor invades retrobulbar optic nerve
[ ]	[ ]	T4b	Extraocular extension other than invasion of optic nerve

Lymph Node (N)

Clin	Path		
[ ]	[ ]	NX	Regional lymph nodes cannot be assessed
[ ]	[ ]	N0	No regional lymph node metastasis
[ ]	[ ]	N1	Regional lymph node metastasis

Distant Metastasis (M)

Clin	Path		
[ ]	[ ]	MX	Presence of distant metastasis cannot be assessed
[ ]	[ ]	M0	No distant metastasis
[ ]	[ ]	M1	Distant metastasis

Primary Tumor (pT)

Clin	Path		
[ ]	[ ]	pTX	Primary tumor cannot be assessed
[ ]	[ ]	pT0	No evidence of primary tumor
[ ]	[ ]	pT1	Tumor(s) limited to 25% or less of the retina
[ ]	[ ]	pT2	Tumor(s) involve(s) more than 25% but not more than 50% of the retina
[ ]	[ ]	pT3	Tumor(s) involve(s) more than 50% of the retina and/or invade(s) beyond the retina but remain(s) intraocular
[ ]	[ ]	pT3a	Tumor(s) involve(s) more than 50% of the retina and/or tumor cells in the vitreous
[ ]	[ ]	pT3b	Tumor invades optic nerve as far as the lamina cribrosa
[ ]	[ ]	pT3c	Tumor in anterior chamber and/or invasion with thickening of the uvea and/or intrascleral invasion
[ ]	[ ]	pT4	Tumor with extraocular invasion
[ ]	[ ]	pT4a	Intraneural tumor beyond the lamina cribrosa but not at the line of resection
[ ]	[ ]	pT4b	Tumor at the line of resection or other extraocular extension

Lymph Node (pN)

Clin	Path		
[ ]	[ ]	pNX	Regional lymph nodes cannot be assessed
[ ]	[ ]	pN0	No regional lymph node metastasis
[ ]	[ ]	pN1	Regional lymph node metastasis

Distant Metastasis (pM)

Clin	Path		
[ ]	[ ]	pMX	Presence of distant metastasis cannot be assessed
[ ]	[ ]	pM0	No distant metastasis
[ ]	[ ]	pM1	Distant metastasis

(continued on next page)

Clin	Path	Stage Grouping			
[ ]	[ ]	IA	T1	N0	M0
[ ]	[ ]	IB	T2	N0	M0
[ ]	[ ]	IIA	T3a	N0	M0
[ ]	[ ]	IIB	T3b	N0	M0
[ ]	[ ]	IIC	T3c	N0	M0
[ ]	[ ]	IIIA	T4a	N0	M0
[ ]	[ ]	IIIB	T4b	N0	M0
[ ]	[ ]	IV	Any T	N1	M0
			Any T	Any N	M1

Staged by _____ M.D.

_____ Registrar

Date _____

Histopathologic Type

This classification applies only to retinoblastoma.

Illustrations

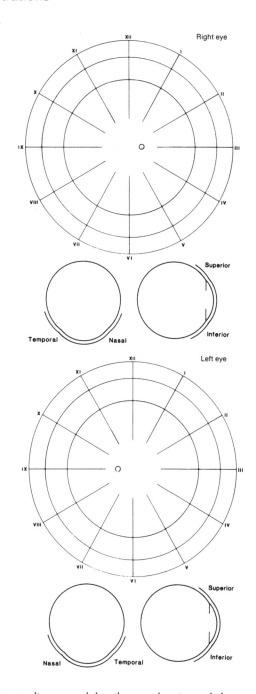

Indicate on diagrams and describe exact location and characteristics of tumor.

_____
_____
_____
_____

44

Sarcoma of the Orbit

C69.6 Orbit, NOS
C69.8 Overlapping lesion

Sarcomas of the orbit include a broad spectrum of soft-tissue tumors and sarcomas of bone.

ANATOMY

Primary Site. Sarcoma of the orbit occurs in the soft tissues and bone of the orbital fossa.

Regional Lymph Nodes. The regional lymph nodes are:

Submandibular
Parotid (preauricular)
Cervical

Metastatic Sites. Metastatic spread occurs by way of the bloodstream to distant sites.

RULES FOR CLASSIFICATION

Clinical Staging. Clinical classification is based on symptoms and signs relating to visual loss, degree of proptosis or displacement, papilledema, and optic atrophy. Diagnostic tests include radiographs of the orbit, computed tomography, and angiography.

Pathologic Staging. Pathologic classification is based on the histopathology of the tumor, its grade, and the extent of removal.

DEFINITION OF TNM

Primary Tumor (T)

TX Primary tumor cannot be assessed
T0 No evidence of primary tumor
T1 Tumor 15 mm or less in greatest dimension
T2 Tumor more than 15 mm in greatest dimension
T3 Tumor of any size with diffuse invasion of orbital tissues and/or bony walls
T4 Tumor invades beyond the orbit to adjacent sinuses and/ or to the cranium

Regional Lymph Nodes (N)

NX Regional lymph nodes cannot be assessed
N0 No regional lymph node metastasis
N1 Regional lymph node metastasis

Distant Metastasis (M)

MX Presence of distant metastasis cannot be assessed
M0 No distant metastasis
M1 Distant metastasis

STAGE GROUPING

No stage grouping is presently recommended.

HISTOPATHOLOGIC TYPE

Sarcomas of the orbit include a broad spectrum of soft-tissue tumors and sarcomas of bone.

HISTOPATHOLOGIC GRADE (G)

GX Grade cannot be assessed
G1 Well differentiated
G2 Moderately differentiated
G3 Poorly differentiated
G4 Undifferentiated

BIBLIOGRAPHY

1. Backwinkel KD, Diddams JA: Hemangiopericytoma: Report of a case and comprehensive review of the literature. Cancer 25:896, 1970
2. Croxatto JO, Font RL: Hemangiopericytoma of the orbit: A clinicopathologic study of 30 cases. Hum Pathol 13:210–218, 1982

3. Ellsworth RM: Rhabdomyosarcoma of the orbit. New Orleans Academy of Ophthalmology Symposium on Surgery of the Orbit and Adnexa. St. Louis, CV Mosby, 1974

4. Enzinger FM, Lattes R, Torioni H: Histologic typing of soft tissue tumors. WHO International Histological Classification of Tumours, No. 3. Geneva, WHO, 1969

5. Font RL, Hidayat A: Fibrous histiocytoma of the orbit: A clinicopathologic study of 150 cases. Hum Pathol 13:199–209, 1982

6. Foos R: Fibrosarcoma of the orbit. Am J Ophthalmol 57:244, 1969

7. Guccion JG, Font RL, Enzinger FM, et al: Extraskeletal-mesenchymal chondrosarcoma. Arch Pathol 95:336–340, 1973

8. Henderson JW, Farrow GM: Primary orbital hemangiopericytoma: An aggressive and potentially malignant neoplasm. Arch Ophthalmol 96:666–673, 1978

9. Jaffe N, Filler RM, Farber S, et al: Rhabdomyosarcoma in children: Improved outlook with a multi-disciplinary approach. Am J Surg 125:482, 1973

10. Jones IS, Reese AB, Krout J: Orbital rhabdomyosarcoma: An analysis of sixty-two cases. Trans Am Ophthalmol Soc 63:223–255, 1965

11. Knowles DM, Jakobiec FA, Potter GD, et al: Ophthalmic striated muscle neoplasms. Surv Ophthalmol 21:219–261, 1976

12. Porterfield JF, Zimmerman LE: Rhabdomyosarcoma of the orbit: A clinicopathologic study of 55 cases. Virchows Arch (Path Anat) 335:329–344, 1962

13. Russell WO, Cohen J, Enzinger F, et al: A clinical and pathological staging system for soft tissue sarcomas. Cancer 40:1562–1570, 1977

14. Suit HD, Russell WO, Martin RG: Sarcoma of soft tissue: Clinical and histopathologic parameters and response to treatment. Cancer 35:1478–1483, 1975

15. Zimmerman LE, Sobin LH: Histological typing of tumors of the eye and its adnexa. WHO International Histological Classification of Tumors, No. 24. Geneva, WHO, 1981

Data Form for Cancer Staging

Patient identification
Name _____
Address _____
Hospital or clinic number _____
Age _____ Sex _____ Race _____

Institution identification
Hospital or clinic _____
Address _____

Oncology Record

Anatomic site of cancer _____
Histologic type _____
Grade (G) _____
Date of classification _____

Chronology of classification
[ ] Clinical (use all data prior to first treatment)
[ ] Pathologic (if definitively resected specimen available)

DEFINITIONS

Primary Tumor (T)

Clin	Path		
[ ]	[ ]	TX	Primary tumor cannot be assessed
[ ]	[ ]	T0	No evidence of primary tumor
[ ]	[ ]	T1	Tumor 15 mm or less in greatest dimension
[ ]	[ ]	T2	Tumor more than 15 mm in greatest dimension
[ ]	[ ]	T3	Tumor of any size with diffuse invasion of orbital tissues and/or bony walls
[ ]	[ ]	T4	Tumor invades beyond the orbit to adjacent sinuses and/or to cranium

Lymph Node (N)

Clin	Path		
[ ]	[ ]	NX	Regional lymph nodes cannot be assessed
[ ]	[ ]	N0	No regional lymph node metastasis
[ ]	[ ]	N1	Regional lymph node metastasis

Distant Metastasis (M)

Clin	Path		
[ ]	[ ]	MX	Presence of distant metastasis cannot be assessed
[ ]	[ ]	M0	No distant metastasis
[ ]	[ ]	M1	Distant metastasis

Stage Grouping

No stage grouping is presently recommended.

Staged by _____ _____ M.D.
_____ Registrar
Date _____

Histopathologic Type

Sarcomas of the orbit include a broad spectrum of soft-tissue tumors and sarcomas of bone.

Histopathologic Grade (G)

[ ] GX Grade cannot be assessed
[ ] G1 Well differentiated
[ ] G2 Moderately differentiated
[ ] G3 Poorly differentiated
[ ] G4 Undifferentiated

Illustration

Indicate on diagrams and describe exact location and characteristics of tumor.

_____
_____
_____
_____

45

Carcinoma of the Lacrimal Gland

C69.5 Lacrimal gland

A retrospective study of 265 epithelial tumors of the lacrimal gland has been completed from material on file in the Registry of Ophthalmic Pathology at the Armed Forces Institute of Pathology. The histologic classification used is a modification of the WHO classification of salivary gland tumors. The lacrimal gland includes both lobules: the superficial (palpebral lobe) portion and the deep intraorbital portion.

ANATOMY

Primary Site. The lacrimal gland lies in a bony excavation covered by periosteum, located in the lateral orbital wall (the fossa of the lacrimal gland). The smaller palpebral portion projects into the lateral portion of the upper lid between the palpebral fascia and the conjunctiva.

Regional Lymph Nodes. The regional lymph nodes include:

Parotid (preauricular)
Submandibular
Cervical

Metastatic Sites. The lung is the most common metastatic site, followed by bone and remote viscera.

RULES FOR CLASSIFICATION

Clinical Staging. A complete physical examination, imaging of the orbit (including computed tomography, ultrasonography, and plane films), and tomography of the adjacent paranasal sinuses should be done. Chest x-ray films, radionuclide bone scans, and blood chemistries should also be available.

Pathologic Staging. After complete resection of the mass, the entire specimen should be evaluated to determine the type of tumor and the grade of malignancy.

DEFINITION OF TNM

This classification applies to both clinical and pathologic staging.

Primary Tumor (T)

TX Primary tumor cannot be assessed
T0 No evidence of primary tumor
T1 Tumor 2.5 cm or less in greatest dimension limited to the lacrimal gland
T2 Tumor 2.5 cm or less in greatest dimension invading the periosteum of the fossa of the lacrimal gland
T3 Tumor more than 2.5 cm but not more than 5 cm in greatest dimension
    T3a Tumor limited to the lacrimal gland
    T3b Tumor invades the periosteum of the fossa of the lacrimal gland
T4 Tumor more than 5 cm in greatest dimension
    T4a Tumor invades the orbital soft tissues, optic nerve, or globe without bone invasion
    T4b Tumor invades the orbital soft tissues, optic nerve, or globe with bone invasion

Regional Lymph Nodes (N)

NX Regional lymph nodes cannot be assessed
N0 No regional lymph node metastasis
N1 Regional lymph node metastasis

Distant Metastasis (M)

MX Presence of distant metastasis cannot be assessed
M0 No distant metastasis
M1 Distant metastasis

<table>
<tr><td>

STAGE GROUPING

No stage grouping is presently recommended.
</td></tr>
</table>

HISTOPATHOLOGIC TYPE

The major malignant primary epithelial tumors include the following:

Carcinoma in pleomorphic adenoma (malignant mixed tumor), which includes adenocarcinoma and adenoid cystic carcinoma arising in benign mixed tumor (BMT)

Adenoid cystic carcinoma (cylindroma), arising de novo

Adenocarcinoma, arising de novo

Mucoepidermoid carcinoma

Squamous cell carcinoma

HISTOPATHOLOGIC GRADE (G)

GX Grade cannot be assessed
G1 Well differentiated
G2 Moderately differentiated: includes adenoid cystic carcinoma without baseloid (solid) pattern
G3 Poorly differentiated: includes adenoid cystic carcinoma with baseloid (solid) pattern
G4 Undifferentiated

BIBLIOGRAPHY

1. Font RL, Gamel JW: Epithelial tumors of the lacrimal gland: An analysis of 265 cases. In Jakobiec FA (Ed.), Ocular and Adnexal Tumors, pp 787–805. Birmingham, Aesculapius, 1978
2. Font RL, Gamel JW: Adenoid cystic carcinoma of the lacrimal gland: A clinicopathologic study of 79 cases. In Nicholson D (Ed.), Ocular Pathology Update, pp 277–283. New York, Masson, 1980
3. Foote FW Jr, Frazell EL: Tumors of the major salivary glands. Atlas of Tumor Pathology, Section IV, Fascicle 11. Washington DC, Armed Forces Institute of Pathology, 1954
4. Forrest A: Pathologic criteria for effective management of epithelial lacrimal gland tumors. Am J Ophthalmol (Suppl) 71:178, 1971
5. Forrest AW: Epithelial lacrimal gland tumors: Pathology as a guide to prognosis. Trans Am Acad Ophthalmol Otolaryngol 58:848, 1954
6. Zimmerman LE, Sanders TE, Ackerman LV: Epithelial tumors of the lacrimal gland: Prognostic and therapeutic significance of histologic types. In Zimmerman LE (Ed.), Tumors of the Eye and Adnexa, Vol. 2, No. 2, p 337. International Ophthalmology Clinics. Boston, Little, Brown & Co, 1962

Data Form for Cancer Staging

Patient identification
Name _____
Address _____
Hospital or clinic number _____
Age _____ Sex _____ Race _____

Institution identification
Hospital or clinic _____
Address _____

Oncology Record

Anatomic site of cancer _____
Histologic type _____
Grade (G) _____
Date of classification _____

Chronology of classification
[ ] Clinical (use all data prior to first treatment)
[ ] Pathologic (if definitively resected specimen available)

DEFINITIONS

Primary Tumor (T)

Clin	Path		
[ ]	[ ]	TX	Primary tumor cannot be assessed
[ ]	[ ]	T0	No evidence of primary tumor
[ ]	[ ]	T1	Tumor 2.5 cm or less in greatest dimension limited to the lacrimal gland and mobile within the lacrimal fossa
[ ]	[ ]	T2	Tumor 2.5 cm or less in greatest dimension invading the periosteum of the fossa of the lacrimal gland
[ ]	[ ]	T3	Tumor more than 2.5 cm but not more than 5 cm in greatest dimension
[ ]	[ ]	T3a	Tumor limited to the lacrimal gland
[ ]	[ ]	T3b	Tumor invades the periosteum of the fossa of the lacrimal gland
[ ]	[ ]	T4	Tumor more than 5 cm in greatest dimension
[ ]	[ ]	T4a	With invasion of orbital soft tissues, optic nerve, or globe, *without* bone invasion
[ ]	[ ]	T4b	With invasion of orbital soft tissues, optic nerve, or globe, *with* bone invasion

Lymph Node (N)

Clin	Path		
[ ]	[ ]	NX	Regional lymph nodes cannot be assessed
[ ]	[ ]	N0	No regional lymph node metastasis
[ ]	[ ]	N1	Regional lymph node metastasis

Distant Metastasis (M)

Clin	Path		
[ ]	[ ]	MX	Presence of distant metastasis cannot be assessed
[ ]	[ ]	M0	No distant metastasis
[ ]	[ ]	M1	Distant metastasis

Stage Grouping

No stage grouping is presently recommended.

Staged by _____ M.D.
_____ Registrar
Date _____

Histopathologic Type

The major malignant primary epithelial tumors include the following:

Carcinoma in pleomorphic adenoma (malignant mixed tumor), which includes adenocarcinoma and adenoid cystic carcinoma arising in benign mixed tumor (BMT)
Adenoid cystic carcinoma (cylindroma) arising de novo
Adenocarcinoma (arising de novo)
Mucoepidermoid carcinoma
Squamous cell carcinoma

Histopathologic Grade (G)

[ ] GX Grade cannot be assessed
[ ] G1 Well differentiated
[ ] G2 Moderately differentiated: includes adenoid cystic carcinoma without baseloid (solid) pattern
[ ] G3 Poorly differentiated: includes adenoid cystic carcinoma with baseloid (solid) pattern
[ ] G4 Undifferentiated

Illustration

Indicate on diagram and describe exact location and characteristics of tumor.

_____
_____

CENTRAL NERVOUS SYSTEMS

46

Brain

C70.0 Cerebral meninges

C71.0 Cerebrum
C71.1 Frontal lobe
C71.2 Temporal lobe
C71.3 Parietal lobe
C71.4 Occipital lobe
C71.5 Ventricle, NOS
C71.6 Cerebellum, NOS
C71.7 Brain stem
C71.8 Overlapping lesion
C71.9 Brain, NOS

The most critical feature in the classification of brain tumors is histopathology. Accurate pathologic criteria and classification are essential to an understanding of the clinical and biologic behavior of the gliomas in particular, and of most other tumors as well. The anatomic location and extent of tumors within the brain are also of clinical and prognostic significance. Neuroradiologic-diagnostic procedures have become increasingly more accurate and reliable in providing topographic and morphologic information on tumors of the brain and are useful at various points in diagnosis and management. The recommendations in this chapter refer to primary tumors of the brain. A system for staging metastatic tumors of the brain is under development and is currently being tested.

ANATOMY

Primary Site. Various tissues within the brain can give rise to neoplasms, including astrocytes and other glial cells, meninges, blood vessels, pituitary and pineal cells, and neural elements proper. The major structural sites involved include the various lobes of the cerebral hemispheres; the midline structures, including the midbrain, pons, and medulla; and the posterior fossa.

Regional Lymph Nodes. There are no lymphatic structures draining the brain.

Metastatic Sites. Certain brain tumors can seed into the subarachnoid space. Hematogenous spread is very uncommon but on rare occasions has occurred in bone and other sites.

RULES FOR CLASSIFICATION

Clinical Staging. This staging is based on neurologic signs and symptoms and on neurologic diagnostic tests, including skull radiography, electroencephalography, isotopic brain scans, cerebral angiography, pneumoencephalography, computed tomography, and magnetic resonant imaging. All diagnostic information available prior to first definitive treatment may be used.

Pathologic Staging. This staging is based on histopathology, grade, and microscopic evidence of completeness of resected tumor removal.

DEFINITION OF TNM

Primary Tumor (T)

TX   Primary tumor cannot be assessed
T0   No evidence of primary tumor

Supratentorial Tumor

T1   Tumor 5 cm or less in greatest dimension; limited to one side

T2   Tumor more than 5 cm in greatest dimension; limited to one side
T3   Tumor invades or encroaches on the ventricular system
T4   Tumor crosses the midline, invades the opposite hemisphere, or invades infratentorially

Infratentorial Tumor

T1   Tumor 3 cm or less in greatest dimension; limited to one side
T2   Tumor more than 3 cm in greatest dimension; limited to one side
T3   Tumor invades or encroaches on the ventricular system
T4   Tumor crosses the midline, invades the opposite hemisphere, or invades supratentorially

Regional Lymph Nodes (N)

This category does not apply to this site.

Distant Metastasis (M)

MX   Presence of distant metastasis cannot be assessed
M0   No distant metastasis
M1   Distant metastasis

HISTOPATHOLOGIC GRADE (G)

GX   Grade cannot be assessed
G1   Well differentiated
G2   Moderately differentiated
G3   Poorly differentiated
G4   Undifferentiated

STAGE GROUPING

Stage IA	G1	T1	M0
Stage IB	G1	T2	M0
	G1	T3	M0
Stage IIA	G2	T1	M0
Stage IIB	G2	T2	M0
	G2	T3	M0
Stage IIIA	G3	T1	M0
Stage IIIB	G3	T2	M0
	G3	T3	M0
Stage IV	G1	T4	M0
	G2	T4	M0
	G3	T4	M0
	G4	Any T	M0
	Any G	Any T	M1

HISTOPATHOLOGIC TYPE

Tumors included in analysis and evaluation are:

Astrocytomas
Oligodendrogliomas
Ependymal and choroid plexus tumors
Glioblastomas
Medulloblastomas
Meningiomas, malignant
Neurilemmomas (neurinomas, schwannomas), malignant
Hemangioblastomas
Neurosarcomas
Other sarcomas

Histologic grade usually correlates with biologic activity of the tumor. This is particularly the case with malignant astrocytomas, the most common form of glioma. The age of the patient at the time of diagnosis is also of major importance for prognosis.

APPENDIX

Histologic Grading of Tumors of the Central Nervous System

Criteria for the Diagnosis of Malignancy in Tumors of the Central Nervous System and Allied Structures

For tumors of the central nervous system and allied structures, the uncritical application of criteria for histologic and biologic malignancy that generally pertain to other neoplasms is inadequate for the following reasons:

1. Irrespective of the histologic malignancy of the tumor, its unimpeded growth within the confines of the skull as a space-occupying and expanding lesion inevitably leads to a fatal termination, which by definition is equated with clinical malignancy.
2. Similarly, the local pressure caused by an intracranial tumor on vital neural structures may result in the clinical effects of malignancy, irrespective of the histologic type of tumor.
3. The obstructive effect of a growing tumor leads to the production of secondary occlusive hydrocephalus.
4. Certain criteria of malignancy of neoplasms that in other body systems pertain to their growth and spread (especially the characteristic of infiltrative growth and the capacity to metastasize, either within or outside the central nervous system) do not necessarily pertain to, or have to be modified to, the evaluation of the malignant behavior of central nervous system tumors.

Thus, tumors of the central nervous system and allied structures, in addition to their intrinsic benign or malignant histologic character that to a considerable extent determines their biologic behavior, may by their specific localization acquire certain characteristics that collectively will add up to a picture regarded as benign, semi-benign, relatively malignant, or highly malignant.

The numerical grading used in this classification is based on histologic criteria of malignancy and should be considered an estimate of the usual behavior of each type of tumor. Numerical grade 1 is considered the least malignant; grades 2, 3, and 4 indicate increasing degrees of malignancy.

In this general evaluation, the pathologist confronted with the problem of malignancy and prognosis is faced with two sets of data. In the first analysis, the evaluation of malignancy must clearly be based on retrospective assessment of the postoperative prognosis and survival rates of other known similar examples, leading to a final and reasonably accurate clinicopathologic correlation that both reinforces the purely histopathologic evaluation of malignancy and is reinforced by it.

Second, the pathologist deduces malignancy from a number of purely histologic and cytologic data. These include increase of cellularity, presence and rate of mitotic figures, presence of atypical mitotic figures, pleomorphism of tumor cells, pleomorphism of tissue architecture (particularly necroses, abnormally prominent stromal reaction, disorderly stromal reaction, and overgrowth), and the formation of pathologic blood vessels (corresponding to the angiographic appearance of arteriovenous fistulas).

On the other hand, other features usually regarded as indicative of or synonymous with malignancy need not necessarily be recognized in the case of tumors of the central nervous system, especially those of neuroectodermal origin. For instance, lack of circumscription and focal parenchymatous invasion is not a necessary accompaniment of cellular anaplasia or ultimate clinical malignancy. Also, the actual presence of mitotic figures (as in oligodendroglioma) does not necessarily imply a particularly malignant behavior; the overall number of mitoses and the presence of abnormal mitotic figures are more important in evaluation. Similarly, local invasion of the leptomeninges is often clearly dissociated from either of the two features just quoted. This is the case, for example, in the pilocytic astrocytoma that involves the wall of the third ventricle, the optic nerve, the cerebellum, and so on.

Although distant meningeal and ventricular metastases are often characteristic of highly malignant tumors such as medulloblastoma, this phenomenon again is not always to be correlated with the highest degrees of cytologic malignancy, as seen in some oligodendrogliomas.

The Question of Grading

Following Broder's classification of epithelial tumors elsewhere in the body, an attempt has been made by Kerno-han and his school to apply a system of grading by ascending degrees of malignancy, numbered 1 to 4, to certain tumors of neuroectodermal origin—namely astrocytoma, oligodendroglioma, ependymoma, and neuro-astrocytoma. This attempt stemmed both from a desire to simplify the then current classification of tumors of the central nervous system and from a need to offer to the neurosurgeon a prognostic evaluation of the tumor removed at surgery, based on certain definite histologic and cytologic criteria. Attractive though this attempt at simplification might be, however, it has to meet with a number of objections:

1. The sample of tissue so analyzed may from surgical necessity not be representative of the tumor as a whole.
2. The specific evolution of the particular tumor in terms of its anaplastic potentialities is not fully expressed by such a scheme of grading. For example, a cerebellar pilocytic astrocytoma graded 1 does not have the same anaplastic potential as a cerebral astrocytoma or some other tumors also graded 1.
3. The pleomorphism of cell and tissue structures so frequently inherent in primary neuroectodermal tumors poses additional difficulties to the application of a simplified system of grading.
4. This cytologic grading makes it extremely difficult to place tumors with mixed cell populations into an already predetermined tumor category.

Nevertheless, the above remarks should not be regarded as basically antagonistic to some attempts at expressing the degree of malignancy of a particular tumor of the central nervous system. Indeed, from the clinical and therapeutic points of view, no classification based on purely histologic entities is satisfactory unless adequate cognizance is taken of, and information provided on, the degree of malignancy of a particular tumor submitted for examination. Thus, it is the duty and prerogative of the pathologist to provide his clinical colleagues with an informed opinion on the likely evolution of a particular tumor, and to some extent this prognostic opinion is embodied in the recognition of specific clinicopathologic neuro-oncologic entities. As an illustration, it might be pointed out that two tumors of similar cellularity, isomorphous appearance, and mitotic rate—such as the medulloblastomas and some oligodendrogliomas—usually do not exhibit the same biologic behavior. This acquired body of knowledge is clearly the result of previous collaboration among clinicians and pathologists in the field of neuro-oncology.

BIBLIOGRAPHY

1. Jelsma R, Bucy PC: Glioblastoma multiforme: Its treatment 161and some factors affecting survival. Arch Neurol 20:161–171, 1969

2. Salcman M: Survival in glioblastoma: Historical perspective. Neurosurgery 7:435–439, 1980

3. Scanlon PW, Taylor WF: Radiotherapy of intracranial astrocytomas: Analysis of 417 cases treated from 1960 through 1969. Neurosurgery 5:301–308, 1979

4. Walker MD, Alexander E Jr, Hunt WE, et al: Evaluation of BCNU and/or radiotherapy in the treatment of anaplastic gliomas: A cooperative clinical trial. J Neurosurg 49:333–343, 1978

5. Wilson CB, Gutin P, Boldrey EB, et al: Single-agent chemotherapy of brain tumors: A five-year review. Arch Neurol 33:739–744, 1976

6. Zulch KJ: Histologic typing of tumors of the central nervous system. WHO International Histological Classification of Tumors, No. 21. Geneva, WHO, 1979

Data Form for Cancer Staging

Patient identification
Name _____
Address _____
Hospital or clinic number _____
Age _____ Sex _____ Race _____

Institution identification
Hospital or clinic _____
Address _____

Oncology Record

Anatomic site of cancer _____
Histologic type _____
Grade (G) _____
Date of classification _____

Chronology of classification
[ ]   Clinical (use all data prior to first treatment)
[ ]   Pathologic (if definitively resected specimen available)

Clin	Path	
		DEFINITIONS
		Primary Tumor (T)
[ ]	[ ]	TX Primary tumor cannot be assessed
[ ]	[ ]	T0 No evidence of primary tumor
		Supratentorial tumor
[ ]	[ ]	T1 Tumor 5 cm or less in greatest dimension; limited to one side
[ ]	[ ]	T2 Tumor more than 5 cm in greatest dimension; limited to one side
[ ]	[ ]	T3 Tumor invades or encroaches upon the ventricular system
[ ]	[ ]	T4 Tumor crosses the midline, invades the opposite hemisphere, or extends infratentorially
		Infratentorial tumor
[ ]	[ ]	T1 Tumor 3 cm or less in greatest dimension; limited to one side
[ ]	[ ]	T2 Tumor more than 3 cm in greatest dimension; limited to one side
[ ]	[ ]	T3 Tumor invades or encroaches upon the ventricular system
[ ]	[ ]	T4 Tumor crosses the midline, invades the opposite hemisphere, or invades supratentorially
		Lymph Node (N)
		This category does not apply to this site.
		Distant Metastasis (M)
[ ]	[ ]	MX Presence of distant metastasis cannot be assessed
[ ]	[ ]	M0 No distant metastasis
[ ]	[ ]	M1 Distant metastasis
		Histopathologic Grade (G)
[ ]	[ ]	GX Grade cannot be assessed
[ ]	[ ]	G1 Well differentiated
[ ]	[ ]	G2 Moderately differentiated
[ ]	[ ]	G3 Poorly differentiated
[ ]	[ ]	G4 Undifferentiated

Stage Grouping

Clin	Path				
[ ]	[ ]	IA	G1	T1	M0
[ ]	[ ]	IB	G1	T2	M0
			G1	T3	M0
[ ]	[ ]	IIA	G2	T1	M0
[ ]	[ ]	IIB	G2	T2	M0
			G2	T3	M0
[ ]	[ ]	IIIA	G3	T1	M0
[ ]	[ ]	IIIB	G3	T2	M0
			G3	T3	M0
[ ]	[ ]	IV	G1	T4	M0
			G2	T4	M0
			G3	T4	M0
			G4	Any T	M0
			Any G	Any T	M1

Staged by _____ M.D.
_____ Registrar
Date _____

(continued on next page)

American Joint Committee on Cancer—1992

Histopathologic Type

Tumors that are included in the analysis and evaluation are as follows:

Astrocytoma
Oligodendroglioma
Ependymal and choroid plexus tumors
Glioblastoma
Medulloblastoma
Meningiomas, malignant
Neurilemmomas (neurinomas, schwannomas), malignant
Hemangioblastoma
Neurosarcomas
Other sarcomas

Illustrations

Size: _____cm

Weight: _____ g

Indicate on diagrams the exact location and characteristics of tumor.

LYMPHOMAS

47

Hodgkin's Disease

A distinctive form of lymphoma, Hodgkin's disease has served as a model for treatment trials, for great strides have been made in therapy for this disease. Staging of Hodgkin's lymphoma is not based on the local extent of disease but rather on its distribution and symptomatology. The classic TNM system is not useful for staging Hodgkin's disease. It is usually not possible to determine the primary tumor site. When the patient presents, the disease is often widely disseminated. Important for staging is the evaluation of many organs and groups of lymph nodes for tumor involvement. The disease is often associated with unusual immunologic abnormalities and a diversity of histologic changes. Staging is considered critical for patient management.

ANATOMY

The major lymphatic structures include groups and chains of lymph nodes, the spleen, and the thymus gland. The digestive system is also an important lymphoid organ that has collections of lymphoid tissue known as Waldeyer's ring in the oropharynx, Peyer's patches in the ileum, and lymphoid nodules in the appendix. Hodgkin's disease can involve almost any organ or tissue, especially the liver, bone marrow, and spleen, in addition to the lymph nodes.

RULES FOR CLASSIFICATION

Clinical Staging. The clinical stage is determined by obtaining an adequate initial biopsy, history, physical examination, laboratory tests, and imaging studies. Such studies usually establish the diagnosis and histologic type of Hodgkin's disease. Histologic confirmation is essential. All symptoms should be recorded, especially fever and weight loss.

Pathologic Staging. Pathologic staging depends on one or more lymph node biopsies, bone marrow biopsy, and, if the result will influence therapy, a laparotomy, which would include liver biopsy, splenectomy, and multiple nodal biopsies to assess distribution of the abdominal disease. Involved organs and sites should be listed.

STAGE GROUPING

Stage I   Involvement of single lymph node region (I) or localized involvement of a single extralymphatic organ or site (I_E).

Stage II   Involvement of two or more lymph node regions on the same side of the diaphragm (II) or localized involvement of a single associated extralymphatic organ or site and its regional lymph node(s) with or without involvement of other lymph node regions on the same side of the diaphragm (II_E).

Note: The number of lymph node regions involved may be indicated by a subscript (e.g., II_3).

Stage III   Involvement of lymph node regions on both sides of the diaphragm (III), which may also be accompanied by localized involvement of an associated extralymphatic organ or site (III_E), by involvement of the spleen (III_S), or both $III_{(E+S)}$.

Stage IV   Disseminated (multifocal) involvement of one or more extralymphatic organs, with or without associated lymph node involvement, or isolated extralymphatic organ involvement with distant (nonregional) nodal involvement.

SYSTEMIC SYMPTOMS

Each stage is subdivided into "A" and "B" categories, "B" for those with defined systemic symptoms and "A" for those without. The B designation is given to those patients with (1) unexplained loss of more than 10% of body weight in the 6 months before diagnosis; (2) unexplained fever with temperatures above 38 C; and (3) drenching night sweats. Pruritus alone does not qualify for B classification, nor does a short febrile illness associated with an infection.*

* *Note:* Pruritus as a systemic symptom remains controversial. This symptom is hard to define quantitatively and uniformly, but when it is recurrent, generalized, and otherwise unexplained, and when it ebbs and flows parallel to disease activity, it may be the equivalent of a B symptom.

HISTOPATHOLOGIC TYPE

Hodgkin's disease is divided into four major histologic types and "unclassified." These types should be recorded because they have prognostic significance. They are:

Nodular sclerosis
Lymphocyte predominance
Mixed cellularity

Lymphocyte depletion
Unclassified

Histologic classification should be based on paraffin-embedded hematoxylin and eosin-stained sections.

BIBLIOGRAPHY

1. Boyd NF, Feinstein AR: Symptoms as an index of growth rates and prognosis in Hodgkin's disease. Clin Invest Med 1:25–31, 1978
2. Carbonne PP, Kaplan HS, Musshoff K, et al: Report of the committee on Hodgkin's disease staging classification. Cancer Res 31:1860–1861, 1971
3. Kaplan HS: Hodgkin's Disease, 2nd ed. Cambridge MA, Harvard University Press, 1980
4. Symposium: "Staging of Hodgkin's Disease." Ann Arbor, MI. Cancer Res 31:1971
5. Hoppe RT, Castellino RA: The staging of Hodgkin's disease. Prin and Pract Oncol 4(7):1–11, July 1990

Data Form for Cancer Staging

Patient identification
Name _____
Address _____
Hospital or clinic number _____
Age _____ Sex _____ Race _____

Institution identification
Hospital or clinic _____
Address _____

Oncology Record

Anatomic site of cancer _____
Histologic type _____
Grade (G) _____
Date of classification _____

Chronology of classification
[ ] Clinical (use all data prior to first treatment)
[ ] Pathologic (if definitively resected specimen available)

Clin	Path	DEFINITIONS
		Stage Grouping
[ ]	[ ]	Stage I Involvement of single lymph node region (I) or localized involvement of a single extralymphatic organ or site (I_E).
[ ]	[ ]	Stage II Involvement of two or more lymph node regions on the same side of the diaphragm (II) or localized involvement of a single associated extralymphatic organ or site and its regional lymph node(s) with or without involvement of other lymph node regions on the same side of the diaphragm (II_E). NOTE: The number of lymph node regions involved may be indicated by a subscript (*e.g.*, II_3).
[ ]	[ ]	Stage III Involvement of lymph node regions on both sides of the diaphragm (III), which may also be accompanied by localized involvement of an associated extralymphatic organ or site (III_E), by involvement of the spleen (III_S), or both (III_{E+S}).
[ ]	[ ]	Stage IV Disseminated (multifocal) involvement of one or more extralymphatic organs, with or without associated lymph node involvement, or isolated extralymphatic organ involvement with distant (non-regional) nodal involvement.

Staged by _____ M.D.
_____ Registrar
Date _____

Histopathologic Type

Hodgkin's disease is divided into four major histologic types and "unclassified." These types should be recorded because they have prognostic significance. They are:

Nodular sclerosis
Lymphocyte predominance
Mixed cellularity
Lymphocyte depletion
Unclassified

Histologic classification should be based on paraffin-embedded hematoxylin and eosin-stained sections.

48

Non-Hodgkin's Lymphoma

The histologic classification of the non-Hodgkin's lymphomas has been an area of considerable controversy. Currently, various competing classifications are in use, including those of Rappaport, Lukes and Collins, WHO, Dorfman, Kiel, and the British National Lymphoma Investigation Group. In an effort to bring some uniformity to the classification of these disorders, an international panel of expert pathologists has generated a Working Formulation, which attempts to provide a means of interpretation of these somewhat divergent classification schemes. This formulation provides a useful format in which to discuss the staging and workup of these lymphomas.

The anatomic staging system currently used was developed for Hodgkin's disease and has been extended to the non-Hodgkin's lymphomas, although it is more directly applicable to Hodgkin's disease. As a result, some difficulties arise in some instances when attempting to apply traditional staging systems to non-Hodgkin's lymphomas. However, in the main it has proved to be a workable system and has the advantage of being similar to that used in Hodgkin's disease and thus familiar.

The TNM classification is not a workable system for staging the malignant lymphomas, however. The site of origin of these diseases is often unclear, and there is no way to differentiate among T, N, and M. In non-Hodgkin's lymphomas, the pattern of node involvement (follicular versus diffuse) and the bulk of disease at individual sites is often more important than anatomic considerations.

ANATOMY

The major lymphatic structures include groups and chains of lymph nodes, the spleen, thymus, Waldeyer's ring, appendix, and Peyer's patches. Minor lymphoid collections are widely dispersed in other viscera and tissues, such as the bone marrow, liver, skin, bone, lung, pleura, and gonads. Involvement of extranodal sites is more commonly seen in the non-Hodgkin's lymphomas than in Hodgkin's disease.

RULES FOR CLASSIFICATION

The diagnosis of malignant lymphoma requires the biopsy of lymph nodes or of an extranodal lymphoid tumor. Frozen sections are never to be used as a definitive diagnostic source, and confirmation rests on the review of the fixed specimen.

Clinical Staging. Staging generally involves a combination of clinical, radiologic, and surgical procedures, progressing sequentially from less invasive to more invasive, necessary to define the final stage and to provide a sound basis for planning and monitoring therapy. Clinical staging includes a carefully recorded medical history, physical examination, urinalysis, chest roentgenography, blood chemistry studies, complete blood examination, and bilateral biopsies of the bone marrow. In addition, most investigators use abdominal computed tomography (CT) scan to fulfill the mandatory staging requirements. Other procedures often useful in full staging of patients include bone roentgenography, technetium 99m-labeled polyphosphate bone scans, or CT scans of the thorax (if the initial chest x-ray is abnormal). Additional procedures helpful under certain circumstances include upper GI series (if Waldeyer's ring is involved or if the patient has GI symptoms), lumbar puncture (for patients with diffuse histologies and bone marrow involvement), ultrasonography, gallium scans, and radioisotopic scans of the spleen and liver. Increasingly, surface marker studies and studies of immunoglobulin gene rearrangement have been used to characterize these lymphomas, although these presently must be thought of as research tools.

Pathologic Staging. Initial diagnosis is almost always made by surgical biopsy. In addition, biopsy of accessible extranodal primary tumors is desirable. Extranodal sites of disease at presentation are seen in about 30% of patients. About 25% of patients with non-Hodgkin's lymphomas present with evidence of abdominal disease requiring laparotomy for diagnosis. However, staging laparotomy is not routinely used in this disease and should only be used when treatment changes would be indicated from the results of the surgery. If liver involvement is suspected, it may be biopsied by a percutaneous needle procedure, or multiple directed biopsies of both lobes may be obtained using peritoneoscopy. Although a staging laparotomy is used selectively and only after careful consideration of its impact on both staging and subsequent therapy, when used it should include splenectomy, wedge liver biopsy, and biopsies of the perisplenic, mesenteric, portahepatic, para-aortic, and bilateral iliac nodes, unless underlying medical problems prohibit such biopsies.

Retreatment Evaluation. Suspected recurrence or relapses require biopsy confirmation, particularly if a complete remission of greater than 1 year has occurred. Patients may be reevaluated for extent of disease at this juncture, using the procedures previously outlined for staging.

STAGE GROUPING

Stage I   Involvement of a single lymph node region (I) or localized involvement of a single extralymphatic organ or site (I_E).

Stage II   Involvement of two or more lymph node regions on the same side of the diaphragm (II), or localized involvement of a single associated extralymphatic organ or site and its regional nodes with or without other lymph node regions on the same side of the diaphragm (II_E).

Note: The number of lymph node regions involved may be indicated by a subscript (e.g., II_3).

Stage III Involvement of lymph node regions on both sides of the diaphragm (III) that may also be accompanied by localized involvement of an extralymphatic organ or site (III_E), by involvement of the spleen (III_S), or both (III_{E+S}).

Stage IV   Disseminated (multifocal) involvement of one or more extralymphatic organs with or without associated lymph node involvement, or isolated extralymphatic organ involvement with distant (nonregional) nodal involvement.

SYSTEMIC SYMPTOMS

Systemic symptoms are not as commonly associated with the non-Hodgkin's lymphomas as with Hodgkin's disease, and patients with non-Hodgkin's lymphomas often have remarkably few symptoms, even though many node

areas and/or extranodal sites are involved. However, when systemic symptoms are seen, they do have prognostic significance.

Each stage is subdivided into "A" and "B" categories: "B" for those with defined systematic symptoms and "A" for those without. The B designation is given to those patients with (1) unexplained loss of more than 10% of body weight in the 6 months before diagnosis; (2) unexplained fever with temperatures above 38 C; and (3) drenching night sweats. Pruritus alone does not qualify for B classification, nor does a short febrile illness associated with an infection.* In addition, an accurate assessment of the performance status (ECOG or Karnofsky) with allowances for unrelated diseases is most important.

Note: Pruritus as a systemic symptom remains controversial. This symptom is hard to define quantitatively and uniformly, but when it is recurrent, generalized, and otherwise unexplained, and when it ebbs and flows parallel to disease activity, it may be the equivalent of a B symptom.

GENERAL CONSIDERATIONS

The anatomic extent of disease in the non-Hodgkin's lymphomas is defined by the appropriate sequence of diagnostic procedures selected for a given histologic subset and a particular individual. The exact sequence of staging procedures and the magnitude of invasive staging will rest on the patient's histology, the therapeutic approach contemplated, and the stage of disease. No invasive staging procedure should be used merely to change the patient's stage, if that change of stage will not alter the therapy selected or the outcome of treatment. There is always some variation—often with good reason—in the degree of completeness and adequacy of the data used for final staging.

In general, the yield from particular staging procedures depends on the histology of the patient's lymphoma. For instance, in the low-grade or indolent follicular lymphomas (see Histopathology), some 80% to 90% of patients will have positive lymphangiograms, 40% will have liver involvement, and more than 40% will have bone marrow involvement as well. When comprehensive staging is done on these patients, over 90% have Stage III–IV disease. This high frequency of advanced disease makes staging laparotomy rarely, if ever, required in the workup of follicular lymphoma, because treatment decisions are rarely influenced by the findings in the majority of patients.

In contrast, in the intermediate- or high-grade lymphomas, a much lower incidence of visceral disease is generally found at initial staging. As an example, some 30% to 40% of patients have positive lymphangiograms, the frequency of positive bone marrows is about 15% to 20%, and about 15% to 20% of liver biopsies are positive. After final comprehensive staging, about 25% to 30% of patients with diffuse aggressive lymphoma appear to have localized (Stage I and II) disease. Again, the importance of the extent of staging rests on the subsequent therapeutic approaches taken and the success of that therapy. Comprehensive staging is required if a localized form of therapy (i.e., involved field irradiation) is being considered.

CT scans are a useful addition to the staging procedures. They should be done before lymphangiography, because after lymphangiography the increase in size of nodes may lead to a false CT. Moreover, foci of lymphoreticular disease in the para-aortic region above the level of the second lumbar vertebra, in the portahepatic, splenic hilus, mesentery, gut wall, and retrocrural nodes, and in other sites in the abdomen cannot be demonstrated by lymphangiography. On the other hand, CT scanning is unable to detect small defects in otherwise normal-sized nodes. Thus, a complementary role of CT scanning and lymphangiography is seen in the non-Hodgkin's lymphomas.

HISTOPATHOLOGIC TYPE

Although individual institutions and particular pathologists may use one of the many classifications of these lymphomas mentioned earlier (see Introduction), the corresponding Working Formulation equivalent should be identified so that interinstitutional comparisons can be made and accurate staging approaches selected. The Working Formulation is listed below. It should be noted that the term non-Hodgkin's lymphoma is not used, follicular is used rather than nodular, and surface markers are not required.

HISTOPATHOLOGIC GRADE (G)

Working Formulation

I. Low-grade malignant lymphoma
 A. Small lymphocytic
 B. Follicular, predominantly small cleaved cell
 C. Follicular mixed, small and large cell
II. Intermediate-grade malignant lymphoma
 D. Follicular, predominantly large cell
 E. Diffuse small cleaved cell
 F. Diffuse mixed, small and large cell
 G. Diffuse large cell, cleaved or noncleaved
III. High-grade malignant lymphoma
 H. Diffuse large cell immunoblastic
 I. Lymphoblastic (convoluted or nonconvoluted)
 J. Small noncleaved cell (Burkitt's or non-Burkitt's)
IV. Miscellaneous
 Composite
 Mycosis fungoides
 Other

BIBLIOGRAPHY

1. Bunn PA Jr, Lamberg SI: Report of the committee on staging and classification of cutaneous T-cell lymphomas. Cancer Treat Rep 63:725–728, 1979
2. Chabner BA, Johnson RE, Young RC, et al: Sequential nonsurgical and surgical staging of non-Hodgkin's lymphoma. Cancer 42:922–925, 1978
3. Nathwani BN: A critical analysis of the classifications of non-Hodgkin's lymphoma. Cancer 44:347–384, 1979
4. Rosenberg SA: National Cancer Institute-sponsored study of classifications of non-Hodgkin's lymphomas: Summary and description of a working formulation for clinical usage. Cancer 49:2112–2135, 1982

Data Form for Cancer Staging

Patient identification
Name _____

Address _____

Hospital or clinic number _____

Age _____ Sex _____ Race _____

Institution identification
Hospital or clinic _____

Address _____

Oncology Record

Anatomic site of cancer _____

Histologic type _____

Grade (G) _____

Date of classification _____

Chronology of classification
[   ]   Clinical (use all data prior to first treatment)
[   ]   Pathologic (if definitively resected specimen available)

Clin	Path	DEFINITIONS
		Stage Grouping
[ ]	[ ]	Stage I Involvement of single lymph node region (I) or localized involvement of a single extralymphatic organ or site (I_E).
[ ]	[ ]	Stage II Involvement of two or more lymph node regions on the same side of the diaphragm (II), or localized involvement of a single associated extralymphatic organ or site and its regional nodes with or without other lymph node regions on the same side of the diaphragm (II_E). NOTE: The number of lymph node regions involved may be indicated by a subscript (e.g., II_3).
[ ]	[ ]	Stage III Involvement of lymph node regions on both sides of the diaphragm (III), which may also be accompanied by localized involvement of an extralymphatic organ or site (III_E), by involvement of the spleen (III_S), or both (III_{E+S}).
[ ]	[ ]	Stage IV Disseminated (multifocal) involvement of one or more extralymphatic organs, with or without associated lymph node involvement, or isolated extralymphatic organ involvement with distant (nonregional) nodal involvement.

Staged by _____ M.D.

_____ Registrar

Date _____

Histopathologic Type

While individual institutions and particular pathologists may use one of the many classifications of these lymphomas mentioned earlier (see Introduction), the corresponding Working Formulation equivalent should be identified so that interinstitutional comparisons can be made and accurate staging approaches selected. The modified Working Formulation is listed below. It should be noted that the term *non-Hodgkin's lymphoma* is not used, *follicular* is employed rather than *nodular*, and surface markers are not required.

Histopathologic Grade (G)
Working Formulation

I. Low-Grade Malignant Lymphoma
   A. Small lymphocytic
   B. Follicular, predominantly small cleaved cell
   C. Follicular mixed, small and large cell

II. Intermediate-Grade Malignant Lymphoma
   D. Follicular, predominantly large cell
   E. Diffuse small cleaved cell
   F. Diffuse mixed, small and large cell
   G. Diffuse large cell, cleaved/noncleaved

III. High-Grade Malignant Lymphoma
   H. Diffuse large cell immunoblastic
   I. Small noncleaved cell (Burkitt's/non-Burkitt's)
   J. Lymphoblastic (convoluted/nonconvoluted)

IV. Miscellaneous
   Composite
   Mycosis fungoides
   Other

American Joint Committee on Cancer—1992

PEDIATRIC CANCERS

Pediatric tumors are classified according to the recommendations of the Societe Internationale d'Oncologie Pediatrique (SIOP). The TNM classification used in this edition of the Manual for pediatric tumors is the same as that published in the 1988 edition. Tumors are staged clinically before definitive treatment and pathologically after examination of the resected specimen. The prognosis of childhood cancers has improved dramatically in the last 15 years. In clinical trials and cooperative group protocols, a different or modified staging classification may be used.

Malignant tumors of childhood include neuroblastomas, nephroblastomas or Wilms' tumor, and the soft tissue sarcomas, which include the rhabdomyosarcomas. Neuroblastomas are the most common tumor found at birth. Nephroblastomas have had over 75 synonyms, which will not be listed. Rhabdomyosarcoma is the most common soft tissue sarcoma of childhood.

These pediatric cancers may be present at birth or may develop during the first several years of life. Some pediatric cancers, especially Wilms' tumor, may be associated with congenital anomalies in other organs. Cancers in children are staged the same as in adults, except in one respect. For children, it is necessary to include a category for those cases in which a surgical exploration was carried out and a nonresectable tumor found. Such cases are designated with a "c" in the T category; for example, pT3c means that a nonresectable tumor was found on surgical exploration. The other two staging elements—that is, the N and M—are completed and the stage assigned according to all three categories.

49

Nephroblastoma (Wilms' Tumor)

C64.9 Kidney

Nephroblastoma, or Wilms' tumor, most commonly occurs in the kidney of young children, sometimes bilaterally. Histologically, these tumors are often mixed; that is, composed of stromal and epithelial derivatives in various stages of differentiation. Nephroblastomas are most commonly seen in children under age 8 years, with peak incidence occurring in the second year of life. Bilateral and familial nephroblastomas tend to occur at a younger age than nephroblastomas in general. The younger the child, the better the prognosis. Nephroblastomas typically present as an abdominal mass; plasma and urine erythropoietin levels are commonly elevated. Treatment for these cancers has improved dramatically in the past 15 years. These tumors are staged clinically and pathologically.

ANATOMY

Primary Site. Nephroblastomas arise from the kidneys. These tumors may be bilateral and multiple.

Regional Lymph Nodes. The regional lymph nodes are: the hilar nodes, the para-aortic nodes, and the paracaval nodes located between the diaphragm and the bifurcation of the aorta. All other lymph nodes involved are considered distant metastases and must be coded as M1.

Metastatic Sites. Distant metastases are most common in the lungs, liver, and regional lymph nodes. Tumor may also extend along the renal vein and the inferior vena cava. Involvement of the opposite kidney is classified as T4.

RULES FOR CLASSIFICATION

This classification applies only to nephroblastoma (Wilms' tumor).

Clinical Staging. Clinical classification is based on the surface area of the primary tumor as revealed by imaging, whether tumor occurs bilaterally or unilaterally, and whether or not the tumor has broken through and ruptured its capsule. Extension of the tumor through its capsule worsens the prognosis. Clinical classification is based on evidence acquired from clinical, radiologic, endoscopic, and other relevant studies prior to the decision about definitive treatment. When TNM is used without a prefix, it implies clinical classification (cTNM).

Pathologic Staging. Pathologic classification is based on regional extension beyond the confines of the kidney. This is determined by evidence acquired prior to the decision about definitive treatment and is supplemented or modified by the additional evidence acquired from definitive surgery and from the examination of the resected specimen.

DEFINITION OF TNM

Clinical Classification (cTNM)

Primary Tumor (cT)

TX   Primary tumor cannot be assessed
T0   No evidence of primary tumor
T1   Unilateral tumor 80 cm² or less in area (including the kidney)*
T2   Unilateral tumor more than 80 cm² in area (including the kidney)*
T3   Unilateral tumor rupture before treatment
T4   Bilateral tumors

Note: The area is calculated by multiplying the vertical and horizontal dimensions of the radiologic shadow of the tumor and kidney.

Regional Lymph Nodes (cN)

NX   Regional lymph nodes cannot be assessed
N0   No regional lymph node metastasis
N1   Regional lymph node metastasis

Distant Metastasis (cM)

MX   Presence of distant metastasis cannot be assessed
M0   No distant metastasis
M1   Distant metastasis

Pathologic Classification (pTNM)

Primary Tumor (pT)

pTX   Primary tumor cannot be assessed
pT0   No evidence of primary tumor
pT1   Intrarenal tumor completely encapsulated; excision complete and margins histologically free
pT2   Tumor invades beyond the capsule or renal parenchyma*; excision complete
pT3   Tumor invades beyond the capsule or renal parenchyma*; excision incomplete or preoperative or operative rupture
    pT3a   Microscopic residual tumor limited to the tumor bed

    pT3b   Macroscopic residual tumor or spillage or malignant ascites
    pT3c   Surgical exploration; tumor not resected
pT4   Bilateral tumors

Note: This includes breach of the renal capsule or tumor seen microscopically outside the capsule; tumor adhesions microscopically confirmed; infiltrations of or tumor thrombus within the renal vessels outside the kidney; and infiltration of the renal pelvis and/or ureter, peripelvic, and pericalyceal fat.

Regional Lymph Nodes (pN)

pNX   Regional lymph nodes cannot be assessed
pN0   No regional lymph node metastasis
pN1   Regional lymph node metastasis
pN1a   Regional lymph node metastasis completely resected
pN1b   Regional lymph node metastasis incompletely resected

Distant Metastasis (pM)

pMX   Presence of distant metastasis cannot be assessed
pM0   No distant metastasis
pM1   Distant metastasis

CLINICAL STAGE GROUPING (cTNM)

Stage I	T1	N0	M0
Stage II	T2	N0	M0
Stage III	T1	N1	M0
	T2	N1	M0
	T3	Any N	M0
Stage IVA	T1	Any N	M1
	T2	Any N	M1
	T3	Any N	M1
Stage IVB	T4	Any N	Any M

PATHOLOGIC STAGE GROUPING (pTNM)

Stage I	pT1	pN0	M0*
Stage II	pT1	pN1a	M0
	pT2	pN0	M0
	pT2	pN1a	M0
Stage IIIA	pT3a	pN0	M0
	pT3a	pN1a	M0
Stage IIIB	pT1	pN1b	M0
	pT2	pN1b	M0
	pT3a	pN1b	M0
	pT3b	Any pN	M0
	pT3c	Any pN	M0

(continued on next page)

Stage IVA	pT1	Any pN	M1
	pT2	Any pN	M1
	pT3a	Any pN	M1
	pT3b	Any pN	M1
	pT3c	Any pN	M1
Stage IVB	pT4	Any pN	Any M

Note: For pathologic stage grouping, a clinical M is acceptable.

HISTOPATHOLOGIC TYPE

These are a distinctive group of tumors that show various histologies, differentiation, and components. A number of synonyms include angiomyosarcoma, adenosarcoma, mesoblastic nephroma, and embryoma. The various synonyms, of which there are over 75, reflect the different tissue components that may be present.

NATIONAL WILMS' TUMOR STUDY GROUP (NWTSG)

Most children with Wilms' tumor treated in the United States are staged and treated on the basis of the NWTSG protocol. The pathologic stage grouping is identical to that of the AJCC, with the only exception being a separate category (Stage IV) for bilateral Wilms' tumor.

BIBLIOGRAPHY

1. Beckwith JB, Palmer NF: Histopathology and prognosis of Wilms' tumor: Results from the First National Wilms' Tumor Study. Cancer 41:1937–1948, 1978
2. Bennington JL, Beckwith JB: Tumors of the kidney, renal pelvis, and ureter. Atlas of Tumor Pathology, Second Series, Fascicle 12. Washington DC, Armed Forces Institute of Pathology, 1975.
3. Coppes MJ, Wilson PC, Weitzman S: Extrarenal Wilms' tumor: Staging, treatment, and prognosis. J Clin Oncol 9:167–174, 1991
4. D'Angio GJ, Breslow N, Beckwith JB, el al: Treatment of Wilms' tumor: Results of the third national Wilms' tumor study. Cancer 64:349–360, 1989
5. Grundy P, Breslow N, Green DM, et al: Prognostic factors for children with recurrent Wilms' tumor: Results from the second and third national Wilms' tumor studies. J Clin Oncol 7:638–647, 1989
6. Hrabovsky EE, Othersen HB Jr, deLorimier A, et al: Wilms' tumor in the neonate. J Pediatr Surg 21:385–387, 1986
7. Jereb B, Sanstedt B: Structure and size versus prognosis in nephroblastoma. Cancer 31:1473–1481, 1973
8. Klapproth HJ: Wilms' tumor: A report of 45 cases and an analysis of 1,351 cases reported in the world literature from 1940 to 1958. J Urol 81:633–648, 1959
9. Kumar APM, Huster O, Fleming ID, et al: Capsular and vascular invasion: Important prognostic factors in Wilms' tumor. J Pediatr Surg 10:301–309, 1975
10. Layfield LJ, Ritchie AW, Ehrlich R: The relationship of deoxyribonucleic acid content to conventional prognostic factors in Wilms' tumor. J Urol 142:1040–1043, 1989

Data Form for Cancer Staging

Patient identification
Name _____
Address _____
Hospital or clinic number _____
Age _____ Sex _____ Race _____

Institution identification
Hospital or clinic _____
Address _____

Oncology Record

Anatomic site of cancer _____
Histologic type _____
Grade (G) _____
Date of classification _____

Chronology of classification
[ ] Clinical (use all data prior to first treatment)
[ ] Pathologic (if definitively resected specimen available)

Clin	Path		
		DEFINITIONS	
		Primary Tumor (T)	
[ ]		TX	Primary tumor cannot be assessed
[ ]		T0	No evidence of primary tumor
[ ]		T1	Unilateral tumor 80 cm^2 or less in area (including kidney)*
[ ]		T2	Unilateral tumor more than 80 cm^2 in area (including kidney)*
[ ]		T3	Unilateral tumor rupture before treatment
[ ]		T4	Bilateral tumors

* *Note:* The area is calculated by multiplying the vertical and horizontal dimensions of the radiologic shadow of the tumor and kidney.

Lymph Node (N)

Clin	Path		
[ ]		NX	Regional lymph nodes cannot be assessed
[ ]		N0	No regional lymph node metastasis
[ ]		N1	Regional lymph node metastasis

Distant Metastasis (M)

Clin	Path		
[ ]		MX	Presence of distant metastasis cannot be assessed
[ ]		M0	No distant metastasis
[ ]		M1	Distant metastasis

Primary Tumor (pT)

Clin	Path		
	[ ]	pTX	Primary tumor cannot be assessed
	[ ]	pT0	No evidence of primary tumor
	[ ]	pT1	Intrarenal tumor completely encapsulated; excision complete and margins histologically free
	[ ]	pT2	Tumor invades beyond the capsule or renal parenchyma;* excision complete
	[ ]	pT3	Tumor invades beyond the capsule or renal parenchyma;* excision incomplete *or* preoperative or operative rupture
	[ ]	pT3a	Microscopic residual tumor limited to tumor bed
	[ ]	pT3b	Macroscopic residual tumor or spillage or malignant ascites
	[ ]	pT3c	Surgical exploration only, tumor not resected
	[ ]	pT4	Bilateral tumors

* *Note:* This includes breach of the renal capsule or tumor seen microscopically outside the capsule; tumor adhesions microscopically confirmed; infiltrations of or tumor thrombus within the renal vessels outside the kidney; and infiltration of the renal pelvis and/or ureter, peripelvic, and pericalyceal fat.

Lymph Node (pN)

Clin	Path		
	[ ]	pNX	Regional lymph nodes cannot be assessed
	[ ]	pN0	No regional lymph node metastasis
	[ ]	pN1	Regional lymph node metastasis
	[ ]	pN1a	Regional lymph node metastasis completely resected
	[ ]	pN1b	Regional lymph node metastasis incompletely resected

Distant Metastasis (pM)

Clin	Path		
	[ ]	pMX	Presence of distant metastasis cannot be assessed
	[ ]	pM0	No distant metastasis
	[ ]	pM1	Distant metastasis

(continued on next page)

Clin	Path				
		Clinical Stage Grouping (cTNM)			
[ ]	[ ]	I	T1	N0	M0
[ ]	[ ]	II	T2	N0	M0
[ ]	[ ]	III	T1	N1	M0
			T2	N1	M0
			T3	Any N	M0
[ ]	[ ]	IVA	T1	Any N	M1
			T2	Any N	M1
			T3	Any N	M1
[ ]	[ ]	IVB	T4	Any N	Any M
		Pathologic Stage Grouping (pTNM)			
[ ]	[ ]	I	pT1	pN0	M0
[ ]	[ ]	II	pT1	pN1a	M0
			pT2	pN0	M0
			pT2	pN1a	M0
[ ]	[ ]	IIIA	pT3a	pN0	M0
			pT3a	pN1a ·	M0
[ ]	[ ]	IIIB	pT1	pN1b	M0
			pT2	pN1b	M0
			pT3a	pN1b	M0
			pT3b	Any pN	M0
			pT3c	Any pN	M0
[ ]	[ ]	IVA	pT1	Any pN	M1
			pT2	Any pN	M1
			pT3a	Any pN	M1
			pT3b	Any pN	M1
			pT3c	Any pN	M1
[ ]	[ ]	IVB	pT4	Any pN	Any M

Staged by _____ M.D.

_____Registrar

Date _____

Histopathologic Type

These are a distinctive group of tumors that show various histologies, differentiation, and components. A number of synonyms include angiomyosarcoma, adenosarcoma, mesoblastic nephroma, and embryoma. The various synonyms, of which there are over 75, reflect the different tissue components that may be present.

50

Neuroblastoma

Neuroblastomas usually arise from the adrenal glands. These tumors are highly malignant, with a 5-year survival of approximately 30% when discovered in the first year of life. Spontaneous regression of neuroblastomas does occur, especially in very young infants. For this reason, these tumors are of great interest to oncologists and medical scientists. Neuroblastomas are almost always found in children under age 8 years. These tumors may elaborate epinephrine and norepinephrine. Neuroblastomas can cause widespread and rapid metastases. Clinical manifestations vary, depending on the tumor site and extent. In addition to staging, a number of prognostic factors have been identified for neuroblastoma. As a prognostic indicator, amplification of the *c-myc* oncogene is under extensive study. In the future, the extent of amplification may be incorporated formally into the staging system.

ANATOMY

Primary Site. Neuroblastomas usually originate in the adrenal medulla. However, they may be found at other sites; for example, in the posterior mediastinum or anywhere along the course of the sympathetic chain, from the cervical region to the pelvis. These tumors may be multicentric in origin.

Regional Lymph Nodes. The regional lymph nodes are defined as follows:

Cervical region: cervical and supraclavicular nodes
Thoracic region: intrathoracic and infraclavicular nodes
Abdominal and pelvic regions: subdiaphragmatic, intra-abdominal, and pelvic nodes, including the external iliac nodes
Other regions: the appropriate regional lymph nodes

Metastatic Sites. Metastases are usually found in the liver, orbit, and bones, although nearly every organ can be affected. When the tumor develops in utero, the placenta may also be involved.

RULES FOR CLASSIFICATION

Clinical Staging. Because it is often impossible to differentiate between the primary tumor and the adjacent lymph nodes, the T assessment relates to the total mass. When there is doubt about multicentricity and metastasis, the latter is presumed. Size is estimated clinically or radiologically; for classification, the larger measurement should be used. There should be histologic confirmation of the disease and/or confirmation by biochemical tests.

Pathologic Staging. All clinical data and that found on examination of the surgically resected specimen is to be used. Definitions of pTNM differ from cTNM.

DEFINITION OF TNM

Clinical Classification (cTNM)

Primary Tumor (T)

TX Primary tumor cannot be assessed
T0 No evidence of primary tumor
T1 Single tumor 5 cm or less in greatest dimension
T2 Single tumor more than 5 cm but not more than 10 cm in greatest dimension
T3 Single tumor more than 10 cm in greatest dimension
T4 Multicentric tumors occurring simultaneously

Regional Lymph Nodes (N)

NX Regional lymph nodes cannot be assessed
N0 No regional lymph node metastasis
N1 Regional lymph node metastasis

Distant Metastasis (M)

MX Presence of distant metastasis cannot be assessed
M0 No distant metastasis
M1 Distant metastasis

DEFINITION OF TNM

Pathologic Classification (pTNM)

Primary Tumor (pT)

pTX   Primary tumor cannot be assessed
pT0   No evidence of primary tumor
pT1   Excision of tumor complete and margins histo-
      logically free
pT2   The category does not apply to neuroblastoma
pT3   Residual tumor
    pT3a   Microscopic residual tumor
    pT3b   Macroscopic residual tumor or grossly
        incomplete excision
    pT3c   Surgical exploration tumor not resected
pT4   Multicentric tumors

Regional Lymph Nodes (pN)

pNX   Regional lymph nodes cannot be assessed
pN0   No regional lymph node metastasis
pN1   Regional lymph node metastasis
    pN1a   Regional lymph node metastases com-
        pletely resected
    pN1b   Regional lymph node metastases incom-
        pletely resected

Distant Metastasis (pM)

pMX   Presence of distant metastasis cannot be assessed
pM0   No distant metastasis
pM1   Distant metastasis

CLINICAL STAGE GROUPING (cTNM)

Stage	T	N	M
Stage I	T1	N0	M0
Stage II	T2	N0	M0
Stage III	T1	N1	M0
	T2	N1	M0
	T3	Any N	M0
Stage IVA	T1	Any N	M1
	T2	Any N	M1
	T3	Any N	M1
Stage IVB	T4	Any N	Any M

PATHOLOGIC STAGE GROUPING (pTNM)

Stage	pT	pN	pM
Stage I	pT1	pN0	M0*
Stage II	pT1	pN1a	M0
Stage IIIA	pT3a	pN0	M0
	pT3a	pN1a	M0
Stage IIIB	pT1	pN1b	M0
	pT3a	pN1b	M0
	pT3b	Any pN	M0
	pT3c	Any pN	M0
Stage IVA	pT1	Any pN	M1
	pT3a	Any pN	M1
	pT3b	Any pN	M1
	pT3c	Any pN	M1
Stage IVB	pT4	Any pN	Any M

*Note: For pathologic stage grouping, a clinical M is acceptable.

HISTOPATHOLOGIC TYPE

Depending on the extent of cellular differentiation, these tumors can be designated by several terms, including sympathicoblastomas, sympathicogoniomas, malignant ganglioneuromas, and gangliosympathicoblastomas. Ganglioneuroma, apparently a well-differentiated neuroblastoma, is also covered by this staging classification, even though it behaves in a benign manner.

BIBLIOGRAPHY

1. Bigotti G, Coli A: Histopathologic and immunohistochemical features of neuroblastoma: A tool for evaluating prognosis. Tumori 76:374–378, 1991
2. Cohen MD, Weitman RM, Provisor AJ, et al: Efficacy of magnetic resonance imaging in 139 children with tumors. Arch Surg 121:522–529, 1986
3. Combaret V, Wang Q, Favrot MC, et al: Clinical value of N-myc oncogene amplification in 52 patients with neuroblastoma included in recent therapeutic protocols. Eur J Cancer Clin Oncol 25:1607–1612, 1989
4. Evans AE, D'Angio GJ, Sather HN, et al: A comparison of four staging systems for localized and regional neuroblastoma: A report from the Children's Cancer Study Group. J Clin Oncol 8:678–688, 1990
5. Garvin J Jr, Bendit I, Nisen PD: N-myc oncogene expression and amplification in metastatic lesions of stage IV-S neuroblastoma. Cancer 65:2572–2575, 1990
6. Hata Y, Naito H, Sasaki F, et al: Fifteen years' experience of neuroblastoma: A prognostic evaluation according to the Evans and UICC staging systems. J Pediatr Surg 25:326–329, 1990
7. Hayashi Y, Kanda N, Inaba T, et al: Cytogenetic findings and prognosis in neuroblastoma with emphasis on marker chromosome 1. Cancer 63:126–132, 1989
8. Hsiao RJ, Seeger RC, Yu AL, et al: Chromogranin A in children with neuroblastoma: Serum concentration parallels disease stage and predicts survival. J Clin Invest 85:1555–1559, 1990
9. Hughes M, Marsden HB, Palmer MK: Histologic pat-

terns of neuroblastoma related to prognosis and clinical staging. Cancer 34:1706–1711, 1974

10. Jaffe N: Neuroblastoma: Review of the literature and an examination of factors contributing to its enigmatic character. Cancer Treat Rev 3:61–82, 1976
11. Massad M, Slim MS, Mansour A, et al: Neuroblastoma: Report on a 21-year experience. J Pediatr Surg 21:388–391, 1986
12. Phillips WS, Stafford PW, Duvol-Arnold B, et al: Neuroblastoma and the clinical significance of N-myc oncogene amplification. Surg Gynecol Obstet 172:73–80, 1991
13. Silber JH, Evans AE, Fridman M: Models to predict outcome from childhood neuroblastoma: The role of serum ferritin and tumor histology. Cancer Res 51:1426–1433, 1991
14. Squire R, Fowler CL, Brooks SP, et al: The relationship of class I MHC antigen expression to stage IV-S disease and survival in neuroblastoma. J Pediatr Surg 25:381–386, 1990

Data Form for Cancer Staging

Patient identification
Name _____
Address _____
Hospital or clinic number _____
Age _____ Sex _____ Race _____

Institution identification
Hospital or clinic _____
Address _____

Oncology Record

Anatomic site of cancer _____
Histologic type _____
Grade (G) _____
Date of classification _____

Chronology of classification
[ ]   Clinical (use all data prior to first treatment)
[ ]   Pathologic (if definitively resected specimen available)

Clin	Path	
		DEFINITIONS
		Primary Tumor (T)
[ ]		TX Primary tumor cannot be assessed
[ ]		T0 No evidence of primary tumor
[ ]		T1 Single tumor 5 cm or less in greatest dimension
[ ]		T2 Single tumor more than 5 cm but not more than 10 cm in greatest dimension
[ ]		T3 Single tumor more than 10 cm in greatest dimension
[ ]		T4 Multicentric tumors occurring simultaneously
		Lymph Node (N)
[ ]		NX Regional lymph nodes cannot be assessed
[ ]		N0 No regional lymph node metastasis
[ ]		N1 Regional lymph node metastasis
		Distant Metastasis (M)
		MX Presence of distant metastasis cannot be assessed
		M0 No distant metastasis
		M1 Distant metastasis
		Primary Tumor (pT)
	[ ]	pTX Primary tumor cannot be assessed
	[ ]	pT0 No evidence of primary tumor
	[ ]	pT1 Excision of tumor complete and margins histologically free
	[ ]	pT2 The category does not apply to neuroblastoma
	[ ]	pT3 Residual tumor
	[ ]	pT3a Microscopic residual tumor
	[ ]	pT3b Macroscopic residual tumor or grossly incomplete excision
	[ ]	pT3c Surgical exploration tumor not resected
	[ ]	pT4 Multicentric tumors
		Lymph Node (pN)
	[ ]	pNX Regional lymph nodes cannot be assessed
	[ ]	pN0 No regional lymph node metastasis
	[ ]	pN1 Regional lymph node metastasis
	[ ]	pN1a Regional lymph node metastases completely resected
	[ ]	pN1b Regional lymph node metastases incompletely resected
		Distant Metastasis (pM)
	[ ]	pMX Presence of distant metastasis cannot be assessed
	[ ]	pM0 No distant metastasis
	[ ]	pM1 Distant metastasis

(continued on next page)

Clin	Path				
		Clinical Stage Grouping (cTNM)			
[ ]	[ ]	I	T1	N0	M0
[ ]	[ ]	II	T2	N0	M0
[ ]	[ ]	III	T1	N1	M0
			T2	N1	M0
			T3	Any N	M0
[ ]	[ ]	IVA	T1	Any N	M1
			T2	Any N	M1
			T3	Any N	M1
[ ]	[ ]	IVB	T4	Any N	Any M
		Pathologic Stage Grouping (pTNM)			
[ ]	[ ]	I	pT1	pN0	M0
[ ]	[ ]	II	pT1	pN1a	M0
[ ]	[ ]	IIIA	pT3a	pN0	M0
			pT3a	pN1a	M0
[ ]	[ ]	IIIB	pT1	pN1b	M0
			pT3a	pN1b	M0
			pT3b	Any pN	M0
			pT3c	Any pN	M0
[ ]	[ ]	IVA	pT1	Any pN	M1
			pT2	Any pN	M1
			pT3a	Any pN	M1
			pT3b	Any pN	M1
			pT3c	Any pN	M1
[ ]	[ ]	IVB	pT4	Any pN	Any M

Staged by _____ M.D.

_____Registrar

Date _____

Histopathologic Type

These tumors can be designated by several terms, including sympathicoblastomas, sympathicogoniomas, malignant ganglioneuromas, and ganglisympathicoblastomas, depending on the extent of cellular differentiation. Ganglioneuroma, which apparently is a well differentiated neuroblastoma, is also covered by this staging classification, even though it behaves in a benign fashion.

51

Soft-Tissue Sarcoma—Pediatric

Malignant soft-tissue tumors can occur in infants and in children. Found in many sites, these tumors include various histologic types. The most important is the embryonic rhabdomyosarcoma, or sarcoma botryoides, which can arise in numerous organs. Some histologic types of sarcomas are found only in children. These tumors commonly have an embryonic appearance histologically, and usually are highly malignant. These tumors can be staged clinically and pathologically.

ANATOMY

Primary Site. Soft-tissue sarcomas can involve nearly all anatomic sites. In children, these tumors may even affect unusual sites, such as the vagina or extrahepatic bile ducts, which are rarely involved in adults.

The primary tumor site should be indicated according to the following notations:

ORB Orbit
HEA Head and neck
LIM Limbs
PEL Pelvis (including walls, genital tract, and viscera)
ABD Abdomen (including walls and viscera)
THO Thorax (including walls, diaphragm, and viscera)
OTH Other

Regional Lymph Nodes. The regional lymph nodes are those appropriate to the location of the primary tumor, as in the following:

Head and neck: cervical and supraclavicular lymph nodes
Abdominal and pelvic: subdiaphragmatic, intra-abdominal, and ilioinguinal lymph nodes
Upper limbs: ipsilateral epitrochlear and axillary lymph nodes
Lower limbs: ipsilateral popliteal and inguinal lymph nodes

In the case of unilateral tumors, all contralateral involved lymph nodes are considered distant metastases and should be coded as M1.

Metastatic Sites. Because these tumors are found in many sites, they can involve numerous organs either by direct extension or by distant spread, usually through the bloodstream.

RULES FOR CLASSIFICATION

Clinical Staging. There is a clinical and pathologic TNM classification for pediatric soft-tissue tumors. Clinical staging is based on clinical examination, including imaging and laboratory studies.

Pathologic Staging. Pathologic classification is based on information obtained from pretreatment clinical classification and from surgery and pathologic examination of the resected specimen.

The classification for soft-tissue sarcomas is designed to apply primarily to rhabdomyosarcomas in childhood, but it may also be used for other soft-tissue sarcomas. In rhabdomyosarcoma, bone marrow examination is recommended.

There should be histologic verification of the disease.

DEFINITION OF TNM

Clinical Classification (cTNM)

Primary Tumor (T)

TX Primary tumor cannot be assessed
T0 No evidence of primary tumor
T1 Tumor limited to the organ or tissue of origin
    T1a Tumor 5 cm or less in greatest dimension
    T1b Tumor more than 5 cm in greatest dimension
T2 Tumor invades contiguous organ(s) or tissue(s) and/or with adjacent malignant effusion
    T2a Tumor 5 cm or less in greatest dimension
    T2b Tumor more than 5 cm in greatest dimension

Note: The categories T3 and T4 do not apply. The existence of more than one tumor generally is considered as a primary tumor with distant metastases.

Regional Lymph Nodes (N)

NX Regional lymph nodes cannot be assessed
N0 No regional lymph node metastasis
N1 Regional lymph node metastasis

Distant Metastasis (M)

MX Presence of distant metastasis cannot be assessed
M0 No distant metastasis
M1 Distant metastasis

DEFINITION OF TNM

Pathologic Classification (pTNM)

Primary Tumor (pT)

pTX Primary tumor cannot be assessed
pT0 No evidence of primary tumor
pT1 Tumor limited to the organ or tissue of origin; excision complete and margins histologically free
pT2 Tumor invades beyond the organ or tissue of origin; excision complete and margins histologically free
pT3 Tumor invades beyond the organ or tissue of origin; excision incomplete
    pT3a Microscopic residual tumor
    pT3b Macroscopic residual tumor or adjacent malignant effusion
    pT3c Surgical exploration tumor not resected

Regional Lymph Nodes (pN)

pNX Regional lymph nodes cannot be assessed
pN0 No regional lymph node metastasis
pN1 Regional lymph node metastasis
    pN1a Regional lymph node metastasis completely resected
    pN1b Regional lymph node metastasis incompletely resected

Distant Metastasis (pM)

pMX Presence of distant metastasis cannot be assessed
pM0 No distant metastasis
pM1 Distant metastasis

CLINICAL STAGE GROUPING (cTNM)

It is recommended that the full TNM classification always be used.

Stage I	T1a	N0	M0
	T1b	N0	M0
Stage II	T2a	N0	M0
	T2b	N0	M0
Stage III	Any T	N1	M0
Stage IV	Any T	Any N	M1

When the regional lymph nodes cannot be assessed clinically or radiologically, NX should be considered N0 in Stages I and II. Further studies are required to determine the exact significance of N0, N1, and NX in such cases as pelvic tumors.

PATHOLOGIC STAGE GROUPING (pTNM)

Stage I	pT1	pN0	M0*
Stage II	pT1	pN1a	M0
	pT2	pN0	M0
	pT2	pN1a	M0
Stage IIIA	pT3a	pN0	M0
	pT3a	pN1a	M0
Stage IIIB	pT3b	Any pN	M0
	pT3c	Any pN	M0
	Any pT	pN1b	M0
Stage IV	Any pT	Any pN	M1

Note: For pathologic stage grouping, a clinical M is acceptable.

HISTOPATHOLOGIC TYPE

Histology can include the soft-tissue tumors found in adults. In general, soft-tissue sarcomas are relatively rare in children. Some sarcomas—for instance, osteogenic sarcomas found in children and young adolescents—are classified under the musculoskeletal system.

BIBLIOGRAPHY

1. Bell J, Averette H, Davis J, et al: Genital rhabdomyosarcoma: Current management and review of the literature. Obstet Gynecol Surv 41:257–263, 1986
2. Coffin CM, Dehner LP: Soft tissue tumors in first year of life: A report of 190 cases. Pediatr Pathol 10:509–526, 1990
3. Freedman AM, Reiman HM, Woods JE: Soft-tissue sarcomas of the head and neck. Am J Surg 158:367–372, 1989

4. Gehan EA, Glover FN, Mauer HM, et al: Prognostic factors in children with rhabdomyosarcoma. Natl Cancer Inst Monogr 56:83–92, 1981

5. Hays DM: The management of rhabdomyosarcoma in children and young adults. World J Surg 4:15–28, 1980

6. Horn RC, Enterline HT: Rhabdomyosarcoma: A clinicopathological study and classification of 39 cases. Cancer 11:181–199, 1959

7. Schmidt D, Reimann O, Treuner J, et al: Cellular differentiation and prognosis in embryonal rhabdomyosarcoma. Virchows Arch (A):409:183–194, 1986

Data Form for Cancer Staging

Patient identification
Name _____
Address _____
Hospital or clinic number _____
Age _____ Sex _____ Race _____

Institution identification
Hospital or clinic _____
Address _____

Oncology Record

Anatomic site of cancer _____
Histologic type _____
Grade (G) _____
Date of classification _____

Chronology of classification
[   ]   Clinical (use all data prior to first treatment)
[   ]   Pathologic (if definitively resected specimen available)

Clin	Path	DEFINITIONS
		Primary Tumor (T)
[ ]		TX Primary tumor cannot be assessed
[ ]		T0 No evidence of primary tumor
[ ]		T1 Tumor limited to the organ or tissue of origin
[ ]		T1a Tumor 5 cm or less in greatest dimension
[ ]		T1b Tumor more than 5 cm in greatest dimension
[ ]		T2 Tumor invades contiguous organs or tissue(s) and/or with adjacent malignant effusion
[ ]		T2a Tumor 5 cm or less in greatest dimension
[ ]		T2b Tumor more than 5 cm in greatest dimension
		Lymph Node (N)
[ ]		NX Regional lymph nodes cannot be assessed
[ ]		N0 No regional lymph node metastasis
[ ]		N1 Regional lymph node metastasis
		Distant Metastasis (M)
[ ]		MX Presence of distant metastasis cannot be assessed
[ ]		M0 No distant metastasis
[ ]		M1 Distant metastasis
		Primary Tumor (pT)
	[ ]	pTX Primary tumor cannot be assessed
	[ ]	pT0 No evidence of primary tumor
	[ ]	pT1 Tumor limited to organ or tissue of origin; excision complete and margins histologically free
	[ ]	pT2 Tumor invades beyond the organ or tissue of origin; excision complete and margins histologically free
	[ ]	pT3 Tumor invades beyond the organ or tissue of origin; excision incomplete
	[ ]	pT3a Microscopic residual tumor
	[ ]	pT3b Macroscopic residual tumor or adjacent malignant effusion
	[ ]	pT3c Surgical exploration tumor not resected
		Lymph Node (pN)
	[ ]	pNX Regional lymph nodes cannot be assessed
	[ ]	pN0 No regional lymph node metastasis
	[ ]	pN1 Regional lymph node metastasis
	[ ]	pN1a Regional lymph node metastasis completely resected
	[ ]	pN1b Regional lymph node metastasis incompletely resected
		Distant Metastasis (pM)
	[ ]	pMX Presence of distant metastasis cannot be assessed
	[ ]	pM0 No distant metastasis
	[ ]	pM1 Distant metastasis

(continued on next page)

Clin	Path				
		Clinical Stage Grouping (cTNM)			
[ ]	[ ]	I	T1a	N0	M0
			T1b	N0	M0
[ ]	[ ]	II	T2a	N0	M0
			T2b	N0	M0
[ ]	[ ]	III	Any T	N1	M0
[ ]	[ ]	IV	Any T	Any N	M1
		Pathologic Stage Grouping (pTNM)			
[ ]	[ ]	I	pT1	pN0	M0
[ ]	[ ]	II	pT1	pN1a	M0
			pT2	pN0	M0
			pT2	pN1a	M0
[ ]	[ ]	IIIA	pT3a	pN0	M0
			pT3a	pN1a	M0
[ ]	[ ]	IIIB	pT3b	Any pN	M0
			pT3c	Any pN	M0
			Any pT	pN1b	M0
[ ]	[ ]	IV	Any pT	Any pN	M1

Staged by _____ M.D.

_____Registrar

Date _____

Histopathologic Type

Histology can include the soft-tissue tumors that are found in adults. In general, soft-tissue sarcomas are relatively rare in children. Some sarcomas, for instance, osteogenic sarcomas that are found in children or young adolescents, are classified under the Musculoskeletal System.

PART III

Personnel of the American Joint Committee on Cancer

PERSONNEL OF THE AMERICAN JOINT COMMITTEE ON CANCER
FULL COMMITTEE MEMBERSHIP LISTING FOR THE FOURTH EDITION
(1959–1991)

W.A.D. Anderson, M.D.
Harvey W. Baker, M.D.
*Oliver H. Beahrs, M.D. (Ex-officio)
*Robert W. Beart, Jr., M.D.
*Harold E. Bowman, M.D.
David G. Bragg, M.D.
Weldon K. Bullock, M.D.
Paul R. Cannon, M.D.
Paul Carbone, M.D.
*David T. Carr, M.D. (Ex-officio)
William M. Christopherson, M.D.
Murray M. Copeland, M.D.
Michael P. Corder, M.D.
Anthony R. Curreri, M.D.
Sidney J. Cutler, Sc.D.
Herbert Derman, M.D.
Theodore P. Eberhard, M.D.
Jack Edeiken, M.D.
*Harmon J. Eyre, M.D.
*George M. Farrow, M.D.
*Irvin D. Fleming, M.D.
*Eugene P. Frenkel, M.D.
*Karen K. Fu, M.D.
Alfred Gellhorn, M.D.
*Eli Glatstein, M.D.
*Donald E. Henson, M.D.
Howard B. Hunt, M.D.
*Robert V.P. Hutter, M.D. (Ex-officio)
*B.J. Kennedy, M.D.
Alfred S. Ketcham, M.D.
Howard B. Latourette, M.D.
*Edward R. Laws, Jr., M.D.
Louis A. Leone, M.D.
*Seymour H. Levitt, M.D.
*Robert D. Lindberg, M.D.
Virgil Loeb, Jr., M.D.
Robert J. McKenna, M.D.
William A. Meissner, M.D.

William C. Moloney, M.D.
*Rodney R. Million, M.D.
William T. Moss, M.D.
Clifton F. Mountain, M.D.
Max H. Myers, Ph.D.
Gregory T. O'Conor, M.D.
John W. Pickren, M.D.
H. Marvin Pollard, M.D.
William E. Powers, M.D.
Antolin Raventos, M.D.
Guy F. Robbins, M.D.
William L. Ross, M.D.
Philip Rubin, M.D.
R. Wayne Rundles, M.D.
William O. Russell, M.D.
Edward F. Scanlon, M.D.
Robert L. Schmitz, M.D.
Milford D. Schultz, M.D.
Wendell G. Scott, M.D.
Robert J. Schweitzer, M.D.
*Robert E. Scully, M.D.
Paul Sherlock, M.D.
Danely Slaughter, M.D.
Charles R. Smart, M.D.
Robert R. Smith, M.D.
Edward H. Soule, M.D.
Samuel G. Taylor III, M.D.
Willis J. Taylor, M.D.
Louis B. Thomas, M.D.
Frank Vellios, M.D.
*David P. Winchester, M.D. (Ex-officio)
Morris J. Wizenberg, M.D.
David A. Wood, M.D.
John W. Yarbro, M.D.
John L. Young, Dr.P.H.
Robert C. Young, M.D.
John Ziegler, M.D.

*Current Members of the AJCC Full Committee (see also p. 282)